Preventing Childhood Obesity
Evidence Policy and Practice

Edited by

Elizabeth Waters MPH, DPhil
Jack Brockhoff Chair of Child Public Health,
McCaughey Centre
Melbourne School of Population Health
University of Melbourne
Melbourne, Australia

Jacob C. Seidell PhD
Professor of Nutrition and Health
Director, Institute of Health Sciences
EMGO Institute for Health and Care Research
VU University and VU University Medical Center
Amsterdam, The Netherlands

Boyd A. Swinburn MBChB, MD, FRACP
Professor of Population Health
School of Exercise and Nutrition Sciences
Director, WHO Collaborating Centre for Obesity
Prevention
Deakin University
Melbourne, Australia

Ricardo Uauy PhD MD
Professor, Nutrition and Public Health
London School of Hygiene & Tropical Medicine
London, UK and
Institute of Nutrition
INTA - University of Chile
Santiago, Chile

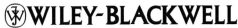
A John Wiley & Sons, Ltd., Publication

BMJ Books

BMJ Books is an imprint of BMJ Publishing Group Limited, used under licence by Blackwell Publishing which was acquired by John Wiley & Sons in February 2007. Blackwell's publishing programme has been merged with Wiley's global Scientific, Technical and Medical business to form Wiley-Blackwell.

Registered office: John Wiley & Sons Ltd, The Atrium, Southern Gate, Chichester, West Sussex, PO19 8SQ, UK

Editorial offices: 9600 Garsington Road, Oxford, OX4 2DQ, UK

111 River Street, Hoboken, NJ 07030-5774, USA

The Atrium, Southern Gate, Chichester, West Sussex, PO19 8SQ, UK

For details of our global editorial offices, for customer services and for information about how to apply for permission to reuse the copyright material in this book please see our website at www.wiley.com/wiley-blackwell

Library of Congress Cataloging-in-Publication Data

Preventing childhood obesity : evidence, policy, and practice / edited by
Elizabeth Waters ... [et al.].
   p. ; cm.
  Includes bibliographical references.
  ISBN 978-1-4051-5889-3
  1. Obesity in children–Prevention. I. Waters, Elizabeth, 1966–
  [DNLM: 1. Obesity–prevention & control.   2. Child Health Services.   3. Child Nutritional
Physiology Phenomena.   4. Child.   5. Evidence-Based Medicine–methods.   WD 210 P435 2010]
  RJ399.C6P74 2010
  618.92′398–dc22

                  2009038756

A catalogue record for this book is available from the British Library.

Set in 9.5/12pt Minion by Toppan Best-set Premedia Limited

1 2010

Contents

Evidence-Based Medicine Series

Updates and additional resources for the books in this series are available from:
www.evidencebasedseries.com

Contributors

Mulugeta Abebe BSocSc

Health Promotion Officer
Merri Community Health Services
Victoria, Australia

Rebecca Armstrong MPH, BN, BAppSci (Health Promotion) (Hon)

Senior Research Fellow
Cochrane Public Health Review Group
Jack Brockhoff Child Health and Wellbeing Program,
McCaughey Centre
Melbourne School of Population Health
University of Melbourne
Victoria, Australia

Louise A. Baur PhD, FRACP

Professor, Discipline of Paediatrics and Child Health
University of Sydney; Director, Weight Management
Services
The Children's Hospital at Westmead
Sydney, Australia

A. Colin Bell PhD

Co-joint Associate Professor
University of Newcastle
Wallsend, Australia

Jean-Michel Borys MD

EPODE's Director, Paris, France
Nutritionist, Centre Kennedy
Armentieres, France

Sue Bowker MSc

Head of Branch, Young and Older People
Health Improvement Division
Welsh Assembly Government
Cardiff, UK

Johannes Brug PhD

Director, EMGO Institute for Health and Care Research
Chair of Division VI; Head, Department of Epidemiology
and Biostatistics
VU University Medical Center Amsterdam
The Netherlands

Goof J. Buijs MSc

Manager Schools for Health in Europe Network
(SHE Network)
Netherlands Institute for Health Promotion NIGZ
Woerden, The Netherlands

Matthew Burke PhD

Research Fellow, Urban Research Program
Griffith University, Brisbane
Australia

Cate Burns PhD

Deakin University, WHO Collaborating Centre for Obesity
Prevention
Faculty of Health, Medicine, Nursing and Behavioural
Sciences
Melbourne, Australia

Georgina Cairns BSc, MBA

Research Fellow, Institute for Social Marketing
University of Stirling and the Open University
Stirling, UK

Rishi Caleyachetty MBBS, MSc

Doctoral Student
MRC Epidemiology Unit
Addenbrooke's Hospital
Cambridge
UK

Rob Carter PhD

Head, Health Economics Unit
Deakin University
Victoria
Australia

Mickey Chopra MD, PhD

Health Systems Research Unit
Medical Research Council
Western Cape, South Africa
Extraordinary Professor
School of Public Health
University of the Western Cape
Parow
South Africa

Deborah A. Cohen MD, MPH

Senior Natural Scientist
The RAND Corporation
Santa Monica
Parow
CA, USA

Camila Corvalán MPH, MD, PhD

Professor, School of Public Health
Faculty of Medicine
University of Chile
Santiago, Chile

Carey Curtis PhD, DipTP, CertTHE, MRPTI, MPIA

Australasian Centre for the Governance and
Management of Urban Transport and
Professor, WA Planning and Transport Research Centre
Curtin University of Technology
School of Built Environment
Bentley, Australia

Inez de Beaufort PhD

Professor of Healthcare Ethics
Erasmus Medical Center
Rotterdam, The Netherlands

Ilse De Bourdeaudhuij PhD

Full Professor, Department of Movement and Sport
Sciences
Ghent University
Gent, Belgium

Andrea de Silva-Sanigorski, MHN, PhD

Senior Research Fellow, WHO Collaborating Centre for
Obesity Prevention
Deakin University & Melbourne School of Population
Health
University of Melbourne
Victoria, Australia

William H. Dietz MD, PhD

Director, Division of Nutrition, Physical Activity, and
Obesity
National Center for Chronic Disease Prevention and
Health Promotion
Centers for Disease Control and Prevention
Atlanta, USA

Colleen Doak MA, PhD

Assistant Professor, Faculty of Earth and Life Sciences
Department of Health Sciences
VU University
Amsterdam, The Netherlands

Maureen Dobbins RN, PhD

Associate Professor, McMaster University School of
Nursing
and Department of Clinical Epidemiology and
Biostatistics
Faculty of Health Sciences and Career Scientist
Ontario Ministry of Health and Long-Term Care
Hamilton, ON, Canada

Mitch J. Duncan PhD

Senior Post-Doctoral Research Fellow
Institute for Health and Social Science Research
CQUniversity Australia
Rockhampton, Australia

Christina Economos PhD

New Balance Chair in Childhood Nutrition
Dorothy R. Friedman School of Nutrition Science and
Policy
Tufts University
Associate Director, John Hancock Center for Physical
Activity and Nutrition
Boston, USA

C. Raina Elley BA(Hons), MBCHB, FRNZCGP, PhD

Senior Lecturer, Department of General Practice and Primary Health Care
School of Population Health
University of Auckland
Auckland, New Zealand

Eva Elliott PhD

RCUK Academic Fellow, Cardiff Institute of Society and Health
School of Social Sciences
Cardiff University
Cardiff, UK

Edward A. Frongillo Jr. PhD

Professor and Chair, Department of Health Promotion, Education, and Behavior
University of South Carolina
Columbia, SC, USA

Lisa Gibbs PhD

Senior Research Fellow, Community Partnerships & Health Equity Research
Jack Brockhoff Child Health and Wellbeing Program, McCaughey Centre
Melbourne School of Population Health
University of Melbourne
Victoria, Australia

Gerard Hastings PhD, OBE

Director, Institute for Social Marketing
Stirling and the Open University
UK

Nadine Henley PhD

Professor of Social Marketing
Director of the Centre for Applied Social Marketing Research
Faculty of Business and Law
Edith Cowan University
Joondalup, Australia

Rebecca Hillier MBBS, BA (Hons)

Honorary Research Fellow & G.P. Registrar
Department Public Health Policy
London School of Hygiene & Tropical Medicine
London, UK

Karen Hoare MSc, AdvDip Health Sciences, NP, RN, FCNA (NZ), RGN, RSCN, RHV (UK)

Lecturer, Goodfellow Unit and School of Nursing
University of Auckland
Auckland, New Zealand

Søren Holm BA, MA, MD, PhD, DrMedSci

Professor of Bioethics
Centre for Social Ethics and Policy
School of Law
University of Manchester
Manchester, UK

Laura M. Irizarry MS

Center for Research in Nutrition and Health
National Institute of Public Health
Cuernavaca
Morelos, Mexico

Rachel Jackson-Leach MSc Nutrition

Senior Policy Officer
International Association for the Study of Obesity (IASO)
London, UK

W. Philip T. James MD, FRCP

President, International Association for the Study of Obesity
London School of Hygiene and Tropical Medicine
London, UK

Sonya Jones PhD

Center for Research in Nutrition and Health Disparities
University of South Carolina
Columbia, SC, USA

Juliana Kain MPH

Institute of Nutrition and Food Technology (INTA)
University of Chile
Santiago, Chile

Stef Kremers PhD, MPH

Department of Health Promotion
NUTRIM School for Nutrition, Toxicology and Metabolism
Maastricht University Medical Centre
Maastricht
The Netherlands

Shiriki Kumanyika PhD, MPH

Professor of Epidemiology
Department of Biostatistics and Epidemiology
and Department of Pediatrics (Gastroenterology;
Nutrition Section)
University of Pennsylvania School of Medicine
Philadelphia, PA, USA

Mark Lawrence BSc (Hons), Grad Dip Nutr and Diet, Grad Dip Epidem and Biostats, MSc, PhD

Director Food Policy Unit
WHO Collaborating Centre for Obesity Prevention
Deakin University
Melbourne, Australia

Tim Lobstein PhD

Director of Policy and Programmes
International Association for the Study of Obesity
London, UK
Research Fellow, SPRU—Science and Technology Policy
Research
University of Sussex
Brighton, UK

Karen Lock BMBCh, PhD

Clinical Senior Lecturer in Public Health
London School of Hygiene and Tropical Medicine
London, UK

Jane Martin BA (Hons), MPH

Senior Policy Adviser
Obesity Policy Coalition
Carlton, Australia

Helen Mavoa PhD (Anthropology)

WHO Collaborating Centre for Obesity Prevention
Melbourne, Australia
[formerly School of Psychology, Deakin University]

Marj Moodie DrPH

Senior Research Fellow, Deakin Health Economics
Deakin University
Melbourne, Australia

Laurence Moore PhD, FFPH, FRSS

Director, Cardiff Institute of Society and Health
School of Social Sciences
Cardiff University
Cardiff, UK

Luis A Moreno MD, PhD

Professor E.U. Ciencias de la Salud
Universidad de Zaragoza
Zaragoza, Spain

Ladda Mo-suwan MD

Associate Professor, Department of Pediatrics
Prince of Songkla University
Hat Yai, Songkhla
Thailand

Simon Murphy PhD, CPsychol

Senior Research Fellow
Cardiff Institute of Society and Health
School of Social Sciences
Cardiff University
Cardiff, UK

Naomi Priest PhD

Jack Brockhoff Child Health and Wellbeing Program,
McCaughey Centre
Melbourne School of Population Health
University of Melbourne
Victoria, Australia

Lauren Prosser BAppSci, PhD

Research Fellow, The McCaughey Centre
VicHealth Centre for the Promotion of Mental Health and
Community Wellbeing
Melbourne School of Population Health
University of Melbourne
Victoria, Australia

Sandrine Raffin MMAA

Co-founder of EPODE
Paris, France

André M.N. Renzaho PhD, MPH, MPHAA

Senior Research Fellow, WHO Collaborating Centre for
Obesity Prevention
Public Health Research Evaluation and Policy Cluster
Faculty of Health, Medicine, Nursing and Behavioural
Sciences
Deakin University
Burwood, Australia

Neville Rigby

European Policy Adviser to the Obesity Forum
Neville Rigby & Associates
London, UK

**Elisha Riggs BAppSc(Health Promotion)
(Hons)**

Research Fellow, The McCaughey Centre
Melbourne School of Population Health
Faculty of Medicine, Dentistry and Health Sciences
University of Melbourne
Carlton, Australia

Juan A. Rivera PhD

Center for Research in Nutrition and Health
National Institute of Public Health
Cuernavaca, Morelos, Mexico

Vivian Romero PhD

MURP Research Associate, GAMUT
University of Melbourne
Windsor, Australia

Andrea M. Sanigorski MHN, PhD

Senior Research Fellow, WHO Collaborating Centre for
Obesity Prevention
Deakin University & Melbourne School of Population
Health
University of Melbourne
Victoria, Australia

Anne Simmons MND

Research Fellow, Deakin University School of Exercise and
Nutrition Sciences
Geelong, Australia

Saskia te Velde PhD

Post-doctoral Researcher
Department for Epidemiology & Biostatistics
EMGO Institute for Health and Care Research and
VU University Medical Center
Amsterdam, The Netherlands

Marieke ten Have MA

Researcher at the Department of Medical Ethics and
Department of Public Health at the Erasmus University
Rotterdam
Rotterdam, The Netherlands

Paul Tranter PhD

Associate Professor in Geography
School of Physical, Environmental and Mathematical
Sciences
University of New South Wales
Australian Defence Force Academy
Canberra, Australia

Tommy L.S. Visscher PhD

Research Coordinator, Research Centre for Overweight
Prevention
EMGO Institute for Health and Care
VU University
Amsterdam, The Netherlands

Carolyn Whitzman PhD

Certified Practicing Planner
Planning Institute of Australia
Senior Lecturer in Urban Planning
Faculty of Architecture, Building and Planning
University of Melbourne
Parkville, Australia

Yang Gao PhD, MPH, Bmed

Instructor, School of Public Health and Primary Care
The Chinese University of Hong Kong
Hong Kong, SAR China

Foreword

Obesity became a major health threat for higher income countries in the last decades of the 20th Century and now early in the 21st Century, most of the world must consider this challenge to our ongoing quest for better health and longer healthy life for all our citizens. A particular concern, both for the long term impact of its sequelae and because it may be more amenable to prevention, is childhood obesity. Preventing childhood obesity must be one of the top priorities of public health and clinical medicine and indeed, public policy.

Preventing Childhood Obesity, with multiple chapters by global experts from diverse fields, offers a breadth of material and thought on this health challenge that can serve as a thorough introduction for those new to the field and a useful text for those already engaged in it. While, many books, monographs and papers have been written with a particular national focus, this book offers a truly global perspective. After setting the nature and extent of the problem ("The context"), it then examines the evidence for prevention in multiple settings and how that evidence can be applied to interventions, policies and practice.

Included in the discussions on childhood obesity are important perspectives on: economics, programme evaluation, monitoring, advocacy, social determinants, politics and stigmatization.

Countries well beyond Europe, North America, Australia and New Zealand are now recognizing childhood obesity as national health threats , for example Brazil, Chile, South Africa, India and China. *Preventing Childhood Obesity* offers us all a concise clear examination of the elements, challenge, setting and complexity of obesity prevention and control while providing the basis for taking steps to address the challenges. It has taken several decades for our environment and lifestyle to include multiple elements that promote excess caloric intake and diminished caloric expenditure. It will likely take decades for us to reverse such trends but we all need to make this effort.

Jeffrey P. Koplan, MD, MPH
Director, Emory Global Health Institute
Emory University
Atlanta, Georgia, USA
February 2010

Preface

If we had all the evidence, practice experience and policy insight, what would be the best investments to improve the health and well-being of children, reduce the likelihood and impact of increased weight gain, improve health outcomes and minimize the potential increased morbidity associated with being less advantaged?

In September 2006, the first international meeting on Community-based Interventions for Child Obesity Prevention was held in Geelong, Australia, to accompany the 10th International Congress on Obesity. This was an outstanding event that attracted a remarkable collection of those working in this area internationally. It was accompanied by site visits to two major community-based interventions in Victoria: *Fun'n' Healthy in Moreland!*—a five-year school community intervention in an inner urban metropolitan area of Melbourne, and *Be Active Eat Well*, in the rural town of Colac, which provided attendees with opportunities to engage with community partners involved with innovating and implementing programs designed to increase healthy eating sustainably, increase physical activity and enjoyment, address social determinants such as parental employment and social participation, and address neighborhood renewal and local government policies.

The two-day meeting that followed was the first time that evidence, policy, practice and passion provided the foundation for discussions between researchers, policy-makers, practitioners and community. What was eminently clear was the vast array of issues that impact on decisions and programs required to address the seemingly unstemmable tide of childhood obesity and the commonality of challenges that the international community faces.

However, while childhood obesity presents us with a particular set of risks for children and the population as a whole, we are still working with children, adolescents, families and communities on an issue that is core to health and well-being—healthy eating, physical activity, and feeling happy and connected. There is a vast history of successful and unsuccessful initiatives to improve population health outcomes, and understanding what has worked for whom and why is pivotal to solutions. If this particular health issue is conceptualized in isolation from other issues for children, families, communities, politics and policy, then it is unlikely that we will see improvements in health and well-being for children and reductions in health concerns associated with obesity. We clearly need to be working together to find efficient ways of understanding the evidence base, using comparable high quality methods for understanding what is, and is not, working, and developing effective solution-oriented partnerships between researchers, policy-makers and practitioners.

It is easy to be overwhelmed by the complexity of the factors that have contributed to the problem, the scale at which changes may need to occur, and the sectors that need to be talking together. This book aims to help. The full range of chapters has been brought together to highlight cutting-edge research, and to provide a review of current practice. The closely connected interface between the research and policy agenda has catalysed new ideas and perspectives based on research findings. The book is written by leading researchers in the field internationally. It has been designed to be relevant to both developing and developed countries, those with resources and those with less, those with strong effective policy frameworks and those without.

The book is separated into four sections: the context, evidence synthesis, evidence generation and policy and practice. We aimed to have those writing about the evidence base making recommendations for policy and practice, and vice versa. The content area is one in which a vast amount of research is currently underway, and one that is challenging governments and industry, in terms of solutions.

PART 1

The context

This section of five chapters paints the big picture for childhood obesity prevention. The problem needs to be well articulated before the solutions, which are the focus for most of the book, can be defined. The rise in obesity has many societal and environmental drivers so the options for solutions to reduce childhood obesity must be multi-dimensional and sustained. The solutions are at once simple, from a behavioral action point of view (eating less and moving more), and highly complex, from a societal, economic and cultural point of view. The solutions must also give primacy to what should be a prevailing societal responsibility to provide safe and healthy environments for children. The human rights approach to childhood obesity, therefore, provides an important frame of reference for solutions to be developed and communicated.

The epidemiology of the childhood obesity epidemic gives us many clues about its determinants and Chapter 1, led by Tim Lobstein from the International Obesity Taskforce, plots the global trends in prevalence rates. The rise has been rapid but varied, and much of the variation in prevalence is likely to be explained by environmental and socio-cultural factors—
—a neglected area of obesity research. The increasing demands on pediatric health services and the tracking of obesity into adulthood, and thus the future demand on adult health services, are two enormous challenges we face. We need to look widely for the answers to the obesity epidemic and there are many valuable lessons to be learned from the successful control of other epidemics. This important evidence, which is explored in Chapter 2 by Mickey Chopra, is known to many epidemiologists and public health researchers who work across different health issues, but the lessons need to be applied systematically to obesity. The central role of policy is one crucial lesson that has yet to be well applied in obesity prevention.

Terms "life-course", "multi-sector", multi-strategy", "whole-of-society" are often used to describe the approaches to obesity prevention and these are discussed in Chapter 3 by Ricardo Uauy and colleagues. What becomes an inescapable conclusion is that we cannot hope to reduce childhood obesity in the face of the continuing barrage of commercial marketing of "junk" food to children. Something must be done to reduce this overwhelming driver of obesogenic environments as a central plank of childhood obesity prevention. Taking an ethics-based, child rights approach is vital to give gravity to society's response. It also ensures that the ethical dilemmas intrinsic to obesity prevention, such as the potential for risk and the balance between paternalism and individualism, are assessed and managed in the best interests of child health. Chapter 4, led by Marieke ten Have, and Chapter 5, led by Naomi Priest, enter this important territory and, again, food marketing to children arises as a fundamental problem.

CHAPTER 1

The childhood obesity epidemic

Tim Lobstein,[1,2] *Louise A Baur*[3] and *Rachel Jackson-Leach*[1]
[1] International Association for the Study of Obesity, London, UK
[2] SPRU—Science and Technology Policy Research, University of Sussex, Brighton, UK
[3] Discipline of Paediatrics and Child Health, University of Sydney, Sydney, Australia

Summary

- Childhood obesity can be measured in various ways, but applying a single method across all available data shows a rapid rise in the numbers of children affected.
- Very few countries have shown a reversal of this trend, but prevalence levels vary across populations, and according to social demographics.
- The rise in child obesity will almost certainly lead to a rise in adult obesity rates.
- Child obesity is a health concern itself and will increase the demand for pediatric treatment.

Introduction

In many developed economies child obesity levels have doubled in the last two decades.[1] The impending disease burden in these countries has been described by medical professionals as "a public health disaster waiting to happen",[2] "a massive tsunami",[3] and "a health time-bomb".[4] In emerging and in less developed economies, child obesity prevalence levels are also rising,[5] especially among populations in urban areas where there may be less necessity for physical activity, greater opportunities for sedentary behavior and greater access to energy-dense foods and beverages.

This chapter looks at the figures and predictions, and considers the implications in terms of children's

Preventing Childhood Obesity. Edited by
E. Waters, B.A. Swinburn, J.C. Seidell and R. Uauy.
© 2010 Blackwell Publishing.

obesity-related health problems and the need for policy development for both pediatric treatment services and public health preventive action.

Measuring the prevalence of obesity

Policy-makers will need to evaluate the trends in child obesity and the success of any interventions, but they face an initial problem in agreeing a clear definition of what constitutes excess body weight in a child. Among adults, obesity is generally defined as a BMI greater than $30\,kg/m^2$, and overweight as a BMI between 25 and $30\,kg/m^2$, but for children there are difficulties in defining a single standard as normally-growing children show significant fluctuations in the relationship between weight and height. Charts showing weight, height and BMI for children by age and gender are commonly used, but with different cut-off points for overweight and obesity, such as 110% or 120% of ideal weight for height, or weight-for-height greater than 1 or 2 standard deviations above a predefined mean, or a BMI-for-age at the 85th, 90th, 95th or 97th percentiles, based on various reference populations.[1]

For young children, it has been common practice to use "weight-for-height" rather than BMI. This stems from existing definitions used in the assessment of underweight and stunting, where "weight-for-age", "height-for-age" and "weight-for-height" are used to assess infant growth. The measures are still occasionally used for assessing overweight in young children, usually by taking a value of two standard deviations (Z >+2.0) above a reference population mean as the criteria for excess weight for a given age and gender.

In recent years, BMI has been increasingly accepted as a valid indirect measure of adiposity in older children and adolescents for survey purposes,[1,6] leading to various approaches to selecting appropriate BMI cut-off values to take account of age and gender differences during normal growth.[7–12] A number of different BMI-for-age reference charts have been developed, such as those from the US National Centre for Health Statistics,[9] the United Kingdom[10] and France.[11]

An expert panel convened by the International Obesity TaskForce (IOTF) proposed a set of BMI cut-offs based on pooled data collected from Brazil, Britain, Hong Kong, Singapore, the Netherlands and the USA. The IOTF definitions of overweight and obesity are based on BMI centile curves that passed through the adult cut-off points of BMI 25 and 30. The resulting set of age- and gender-specific BMI cut-off points for children was published in 2000.[12]

The World Health Organization (WHO) has for many years recommended using a set of cut-offs based on a reference population derived from the USA, but more recently the WHO has been reviewing their recommendations. There had been concern that the USA data included large numbers of formula-fed infants with growth patterns that differed from breast-fed infants, and which underestimated the true extent of overweight in younger children. WHO has now published a new "standard" set of growth charts for children aged 0–5 years, based on data from healthy breast-fed babies.[13] It is unclear at this stage what BMI cut-off values should be used from this healthy population to define overweight and obesity, with both centile and Z-score options available in published tables. Further reference charts are available for children aged 5–19 years, based on a revision of US data collected in 1977 adapted to match the standards for 0–5-year-olds.

Care should be taken when looking at published prevalence figures for overweight and obesity. Some authors use "overweight" to define all members of a population above a specified cut-off, while others mean "overweight" to mean those above one cut-off but not above a higher cut-off that defines obesity. Thus, in some reports the prevalence value for "over-weight" children includes obese children and in other reports it does not. In this section "overweight" includes obese, so the term should properly be understood to mean "overweight including obese". Readers should also note that prevalence levels using reference curves from the USA sometimes refer to "at risk of overweight" and "overweight" for the top two tiers of adiposity, and sometimes to "overweight" and "obese".

It should also be noted that the definitions are very helpful for making comparisons between different population groups, or monitoring a population over time. However, for the clinical assessment of children, serial plotting of BMI on nationally recommended BMI-for-age charts should be coupled with more careful examination of the child in order to be sure that, for example, a high BMI is not due to extra muscle mass or to stunted linear growth.

In this chapter the prevalence levels will be based on the IOTF international classification scheme, as most survey evidence is available using this approach, and the results tend to be more conservative than some other approaches.[1]

Prevalence levels

Policy-makers face a second hurdle in understanding the circumstances surrounding obesity in children and adolescents, namely, a lack of representative data on what is happening in the population that is of interest. Only in a few countries are children monitored routinely and data on their nutritional status gathered, analysed and reported consistently.

Even where data are available, they need to be examined carefully. Firstly, data may be collected using proper measurement procedures, or may be self-reported, but self-reported measures tend to underestimate BMI, especially among more overweight respondents. Data may come from nationally representative surveys or from smaller surveys—for example, in the more accessible urban areas—which do not represent national populations. And, when comparing two surveys across a period of time, surveys need to be properly comparable in terms of the children's ages, and their ethnic and socio-demographic mix.

The figures presented here are based on the latest and most reliable available, some of which were previ-

Table 1.1 Estimated prevalence of excess bodyweight in school-age children in 2010.

Region[a]	Obese	Overweight (including obese)
Americas	15%	46%
Mid East & N Africa	12%	42%
Europe & former USSR	10%	38%
West Pacific	7%	27%
South East Asia	5%	23%
Africa	>1%	>5%

[a] Countries in each region are according to the World Health Organization.
Source: Wang and Lobstein[5].

ously published in 2006 by Wang and Lobstein.[5] Unless otherwise stated, the IOTF definitions of overweight and obesity in childhood are used.

Global figures

Taking an estimate for the world as a whole, in 2004 some 10% of school-age children (aged 5–17) were defined as overweight, including some 2–3% who were obese. This global average reflects a wide range of prevalence levels in different regions and countries, with the prevalence of overweight in Africa and Asia averaging well below 5% and in the Americas and Europe above 20%. Projections to the year 2010 are shown in Table 1.1.

Region: Americas

The most comprehensive and comparable national representative data on trends in the prevalence of obesity are from the USA, where nationally representative surveys undertaken in the 1960s were followed by the series of National Health and Nutrition Examination Surveys (NHANES) from 1971 onwards. The most recent publications (for surveys conducted in 2003–2004) show that 36% of children aged 6–17 were overweight, including 13% obese. These figures are based on the international (IOTF) criteria for overweight and obesity,[12] and compare with 36% and 18% respectively using US-defined cut-offs.[14]

In Canada 26% of younger children and 29% of older children were found to be overweight in a 2004 survey, almost exactly double the prevalence levels found among children 25 years earlier.[15] In Brazil, the prevalence of overweight among school-aged children

was 14% in 1997, compared with 4% in 1974. In Chile, in 2000 the prevalence of overweight among school children was 26%.

There are few data available for schoolchildren in most other South and Central American countries, but some data have been collected for pre-school children. In Bolivia, the prevalence of overweight (defined as one standard deviation above a reference mean) was 23% in 1997, and in the Dominican Republic it was 15% in 1996. In a few countries in the region, obesity prevalence has fallen: in Columbia it fell from 5% to 3% between 1986 and 1995.

Region: Europe

A number of studies have examined childhood overweight and obesity prevalence in European countries. The highest prevalence levels are observed in southern European countries. A survey in 2001 found that 36% of 9-year-olds in central Italy were overweight, including 12% who were obese. In 1991, 21% of school-age children in Greece were overweight or obese, whereas a decade later, in 2000, 26% of boys and 19% of girls in Northern Greece were overweight or obese, while data from Crete in 2002 show 44% of boys aged 15 years to be overweight or obese. In Spain, 35% of boys and 32% of girls aged 13–14 years were overweight in a survey in 2000.

Northern European countries tend to have lower prevalence values. In Sweden in 2000–2001, the prevalence was 18% for children aged 10 years. In the Netherlands the figures are particularly low, with only 10% of children aged 5–17 overweight, including only 2% obese, in a 1997 survey. In France, the figures are a bit higher, at 15% overweight and 3% obese in a northern French survey in 2000, and these figures appear to have remained stable, according to recent preliminary results of surveys in 2007.[16] In England, prevalence rates have climbed to 29% overweight, including 10% obese, in a 2004 survey.

The reasons for a north–south gradient are not clear. Genetic factors are unlikely to be the explanation, as the gradient can be shown even within a single country, such as Italy and virtually all countries have shown a marked increase in prevalence in recent decades. A range of factors influencing regional barriers or promoters of population levels of physical activity may be important. The child's household or family income may be another relevant variable, possibly mediated through income-related dietary factors such as maternal nutrition during pregnancy, or breast- or bottle-feeding in infancy, as well as the quality of the diet during childhood.

Regions: North Africa, Eastern Mediterranean and Middle East

Several countries in this region appear to be showing high levels of childhood obesity. In Egypt, for example, the prevalence of overweight (based on local reference charts and a z score >1) was over 25% in pre-school children and 14% in adolescents. Similar figures are found in other parts of the region. A fifth of adolescents aged 15–16 years in Saudi Arabia were defined as overweight (based on BMI >120% reference median value). In Bahrain in 2002, 30% of boys and 42% of girls aged 12–17 were overweight, including over 15% obese in both groups (defined by IOTF cut-offs).

Regions: Asia and Pacific

The prevalence of obesity among pre-school children is around 1% or less in many countries in the region, for example Bangladesh (1.1%), the Philippines (0.8%), Vietnam (0.7%) and Nepal (0.3%), but it should be noted that no data are available for some countries in the region (e.g., the Pacific islands) where adult obesity prevalence rates are known to be high.

In more economically developed countries, the prevalence figures for pre-school and school-age children are considerably higher. Among Australian children and adolescents aged 7–15 years, the prevalence of overweight (including obesity) doubled from 11% to 21% between 1985 and 1995, and was found to be 27% in a regional survey of 4–12-year-olds in 2003–4.[17]

In mainland China, whose population accounts for one-fifth of the global population, the prevalence of obesity has been rising in both adults and children during the past two decades. A survey in 1992 showed the prevalence of overweight, including obesity, among schoolchildren to be 4% – this rose to 7% in 2002. In urban areas the prevalence was 10%, and in the largest cities nearly 20% (see Table 1.3).

While the epidemic of obesity has affected a wide range of countries in this region, under-nutrition is still a major problem. In China, the prevalence of underweight (<5th percentile BMI of the US reference) was 9% among children aged 6–9 years, and 15% among children aged 10–18, in 1997. In Indonesia, over 25%, and in Bangladesh and India over 45% of children under 5 years old are underweight. Thus, several of the most populous countries in this region are facing a double burden of continued under-nutrition and rising over-nutrition.

Region: Sub-Saharan Africa

The burden of under-nutrition remains very high in this region, with continuing poverty, war, famine and disease, especially HIV/Aids, and very high rates of child mortality. There are very few surveys from African countries that can provide prevalence figures for childhood obesity, as most public health nutrition programs have been focused on under-nutrition and food safety problems. In general, the prevalence of childhood obesity remains very low in this region, except for countries such as South Africa where obesity has become prevalent in adults, particularly among women, and where childhood obesity is also rising. Data from South Africa show the prevalence of overweight (including obesity) among young people aged 13–19 years to be over 17%, with boys generally less at risk (7%) than girls (25%). Prevalence was highest (over 20% for both boys and girls) in white and Indian population groups.

Trends over time

The prevalence of excess weight among children is increasing in both developed and developing countries, but at different rates and in different patterns. North America and some European countries have the highest prevalence levels, and in recent years have shown high year-on-year increases in prevalence. Data from Brazil and Chile show that rates of increasing overweight among children in some developing countries is comparable to that in the USA or Europe.

Other countries are showing only modest increases. China has shown a small rise in the prevalence of overweight among rural children, but a more marked increase among urban children.[18] The rapid rise in the prevalence of overweight is shown in most developed economies, but an interesting exception is Russia, where the economic downturn in the early 1990s may explain the decline in the prevalence of overweight children during the period (Table 1.2).

Demographics of child adiposity

If policies to prevent child obesity are to be successful they need to consider the distribution of the problem among different demographic groups within the child population. Some population groups are more easily accessed than others but they may not be those most in need of attention. Treatment may be accessed more easily by some groups, but not necessarily by those that need it most.

Examination of differences in the distribution of overweight and obesity among children coming from different social classes (defined by family income levels or educational levels of the main income earner) shows a complex pattern. In more economically developed, industrialized countries, children in lower socio-economic groups tend to show higher prevalence levels of overweight and obesity. Moreover, programmes to tackle obesity may be assisting better-off families while obesity levels continue to rise among poorer families.

In contrast, in countries that are not economically developed, or are undergoing economic development, overweight and obesity levels tend to be highest among families with the highest incomes or educational attainment. In Brazil, in 1997, 20% of children in higher-income families were overweight or obese, compared with 13% of children in middle-income families and only 6% of children in lower-income families. In China, there is a clear positive association between child overweight and both income level and educational level, and by urban–rural differences (Table 1.3).

These figures need to be considered in developing policies targeting obesity prevention. Economic development in urban and rural areas is likely to be closely related to the development of environments that reduce physical activity, encourage sedentary behavior and encourage the consumption of energy-dense foods and beverages. Physical activity is likely to be highest in rural areas in less developed economies, where there is likely to be only limited access to pre-processed, long-shelf-life, mass-produced products—soft drinks, fatty snack foods, confectionery and fast food outlets—compared with urban areas and among

Table 1.2 Examples of the rise in the prevalence of overweight children in developed and developing economies.

	Date of survey	Prevalence of overweight
USA	1971–74	14%
	1988–94	25%
	2003–4	36%
Canada	1978–79	14%
	2004	29%
Australia	1985	11%
	1995	21%
New Zealand	1989	13%
	2000	30%
Japan	1976–80	10%
	1992–2000	19%
England	1984	7%
	1994	12%
	2004	29%
Greece (boys)	1991	21%
Greece North (boys)	2000	26%
Greece Crete (boys)	2002	44%
Iceland	1978	12%
	1998	24%
Netherlands	1980	5%
	1996–97	11%
Spain	1980	13%
	1995	19%
	2000–2	34%
Brazil	1974	4%
	1997	14%
Chile	1987	13%
	2000	27%
China rural	1992	4%
	2002	5%
China urban	1992	7%
	2002	10%
Russia	1992	15%
	1998	9%
	2005	12%[a]

[a] Based on self-reported height and weight.

wealthier families. In contrast, in highly-developed economies, the large majority of the population is likely to have less need of physical activity and to have extensive access to processed, energy-dense foods and beverages.

For children, economic development sees a move from agricultural labor and domestic labor to TV watching, while active transport (walking, cycling) is replaced with motorized transport, even for short

Table 1.3 Prevalence of overweight and obesity (combined) among children aged 7–12 years in rural and urban populations and various income and education levels defined by parental status, China, 2002.

	Boys	Girls
Urban/rural		
Large city	24%	15%
Small city	10%	7%
Village	5%	3%
Family income (yuan/year/person)		
>10,000	22%	13%
5000–10,000	15%	10%
2000–5000	10%	7%
<2000	7%	3%
Education level of father		
College and higher	20%	12%
Senior high school	15%	9%
Junior high school	7%	5%
Primary or less	4%	2%

Source: Li.[18]

Table 1.4 Proportion of children who had a BMI >27.5 kg/m^2 as young adults (before age 30 years) according to obesity status in childhood.

Age	BMI normal range for age	BMI >85th centile for age	BMI >95th centile for age
1–2 years	15%	19%	26%
3–5 years	12%	36%	52%
6–9 years	11%	55%	69%
10–14 years	10%	75%	83%
15–17 years	9%	67%	77%

Source: Whitaker et al.[21]

journeys such as getting from home to school or to shops. Traditional staple foods give way to highly marketed and promoted branded food and beverage products.

When economic development suffers a reversal, as was witnessed in some Eastern European economies and in the Russian Federation during the late 1980s and early 1990s, child overweight levels may actually show decreasing prevalence, as the data for Russia indicate here. A study of children's body height and mass in Poland from 1930 until 1994 indicated that the lowest values for both traits were found immediately post-war (1948–49), increasing to the end of the 1970s, and falling again during the recession of the 1980s.[19] When the economy recovers, the prevalence of overweight and obesity may increase sharply, as has been shown in data for East Germany (school-age children) and Croatia (pre-school children) in the years following unification and national independence, respectively.

Child obesity and tracking to adulthood

One of the most pressing considerations to emerge from the dramatic rise in child obesity is the likely impact that this will have on adult disease rates in the next few years. The persistence, or tracking, of obesity from childhood and adolescence to adulthood has been well documented.[20] In the USA, Whitaker et al[21] demonstrated that if a child was obese during childhood, the chance of being obese in young adulthood ranged from 8% for 1- or 2 year-olds without obese parents to 79% for 10–14-year-olds with at least one obese parent. Evidence from a longitudinal study of children, the Bogalusa Heart Study, suggests that children who have overweight onset before the age of 8 are at significantly increased risk of obesity in adulthood.[22] Comparing racial groups, tracking of adiposity was stronger for black compared with white youths, especially for females (Table 1.4).[23]

In a review of evidence on child adiposity undertaken by the US Preventive Task Force, persistence of overweight was consistently seen in 19 longitudinal studies of children of both genders and all ages, with the greatest likelihood of overweight persistence seen for older children and those most severely overweight, for both genders.[24] Parental overweight also substantially increases the risk of child obesity and subsequent adult obesity.

Co-morbidities of child obesity

Besides being a risk factor for adult obesity and chronic disease, excess adiposity in childhood raises the risk of a number of adverse physical and psychosocial health outcomes in childhood itself[1,25] summarized in Table 1.5.

Table 1.5 Health problems concurrent with child and adolescent obesity.

Endocrine
    Insulin resistance/impaired glucose tolerance
    Type 2 diabetes
    Menstrual abnormalities
    Polycystic ovary syndrome
    Hypercorticolism

Cardiovascular
    Hypertension
    Dyslipidaemia
    Fatty streaks
    Left ventricular hypertrophy

Gastroenterological
    Cholelithiasis
    Liver steatosis / non-alcoholic fatty liver
    Gastro-oesophageal reflux

Pulmonary
    Sleep apnea
    Asthma
    Pickwickian syndrome

Orthopedic
    Slipped capital epiphyses
    Blount's disease (tibia vara)
    Tibial torsion
    Flat feet
    Ankle sprains
    Increased risk of fractures

Neurological
    Idiopathic intracranial hypertension (e.g., pseudotumour cerebri)

Other physical
    Systemic inflammation/raised C-reactive protein

Psycho-social
    Anxiety
    Depression
    Low self-esteem
    Social discrimination

Table 1.6 Estimated prevalence of disease indicators among obese children.

	Mean	95% CI
Raised blood triglycerides	25.7%	21.5%–30.5%
Raised total blood cholesterol	26.7%	22.1%–31.8%
High LDL cholesterol	22.3%	18.9%–26.3%
Low HDL cholesterol	22.6%	18.7%–27.0%
Hypertension	25.8%	21.8%–30.2%
Impaired glucose tolerance	11.9%	8.4%–17.0%
Hyperinsulinaemia	39.8%	33.9%–45.9%
Type 2 diabetes	1.5%	0.5%–4.5%
Metabolic syndrome, 3 factors	29.2%	23.9%–35.3%
Metabolic syndrome, 4 factors	7.6%	4.6%–12.2%
Hepatic steatosis	33.7%	27.9%–41.8%
Raised serum aminotransferase	16.9%	12.8%–22.0%

Note: Definitions of obesity and of the indicators differ between source surveys. Mean and confidence intervals based on weighted averages of survey findings.
Source: Lobstein and Jackson-Leach.[26]

The lack of adequate information can be a significant problem in the planning of pediatric services to respond to the rising levels of child obesity. One estimate, based on clinical surveys in a number of countries, suggests that a substantial proportion of obese children are likely to be affected by one or more concurrent disease indicator, as shown in Table 1.6.

Type 2 diabetes

Obesity in childhood is a major risk factor for the development of Type 2 diabetes – a disease that until recently was considered to occur only later in adulthood. The American Diabetes Association's (ADA) consensus report indicated that up to 85% of children diagnosed with Type 2 diabetes are overweight or obese at diagnosis.[27] Small sample surveys in the USA suggest that up to 3% of clinically obese children may be affected, the majority of them without awareness.[26] These patients may present with glycosuria without ketonuria, and absent or mild polyuria and polydipsia.

Figures for the numbers of children affected by co-morbidities are remarkable hard to obtain. BMI or obesity status may not be recorded when diagnoses of ill-health are made in pediatric clinics, while in the population at large the early stages of chronic disease may not be diagnosed among overweight and obese children.

Impaired glucose tolerance and insulin resistance

Before Type 2 diabetes develops, there is a period of altered glucose metabolism. Oral glucose tolerance testing (OGTT) appears to be more sensitive than fasting blood glucose to detect the pre-diabetic condition of impaired glucose tolerance (IGT). Children with IGT have elevated insulin levels in the fasting state and in response to OGTT. Around 10% of clinically obese children may be affected.[27] Central adiposity represents an additional independent risk factor.

Metabolic syndrome and cardiovascular disorders

The metabolic syndrome or insulin-resistance syndrome, is a well-known obesity-associated condition found in at least 20% of all adults in the USA[28] and is increasingly observed among obese children and adolescents. The syndrome has a range of definitions, but is usually diagnosed based on the presence of several of the following conditions: abdominal obesity, elevated triglycerides, low high-density lipoprotein (HDL) cholesterol, hypertension and elevated fasting glucose. The overall prevalence among adolescents in the USA in 1999–2000 was estimated to be over 6%,[29] and it increased from less than 1% among normal weight adolescents to 10% among those who were overweight, and to more than 30% among those who were obese.

Approximately 4% of normal-weight US adolescents have high blood pressure, while the prevalence rises to over 25% among obese adolescents. Low levels of circulating HDL cholesterol are found among 18% and 39% or normal weight and obese adolescents, respectively, and high levels of blood triglycerides are found among 17% and 46%, respectively. Results from a study conducted in Hungary suggests that the number of metabolic syndrome components increases with the duration of the obesity.[30]

Evidence from the Bogalusa Heart Study indicates that atherosclerotic changes are present in blood vessels of even very young children.[31] The extent and severity of asymptomatic coronary and aortic disease in young people increases with age, and is strongly correlated with BMI, blood pressure, cholesterol and triglyceride levels.[31] Additionally, very overweight children show signs of severe cardiovascular deconditioning in tests of physical fitness, and some already have left ventricular hypertrophy.[32] These findings suggest that cardiovascular risk factors present in childhood may not only impact long-term risk, but may also have more immediate consequences, further highlighting the importance of addressing cardiovascular risk factors well before adulthood.[31,32]

Hyperandrogenism/polycystic ovary syndrome

Polycystic ovary syndrome (PCOS) is a condition where there is chronic anovulation and evidence of excess androgen, for which there is no other explanation. Although the prevalence of PCOS among adolescents is difficult to determine, girls who are oligomenorrheic and are overweight or obese appear to be at greatest risk for developing PCOS.[33] Insulin resistance may be an important underlying factor.

Cholelithiasis

The increase of total body synthesis of cholesterol that occurs in obesity leads to a higher ratio of cholesterol to solubilizing lipids in bile, and predisposes the individual to gallstone formation.[34] Although cholelithiasis and cholecystitis are relatively uncommon in children, pediatric hospital discharges for gall bladder disease in the USA have tripled in the period 1980 to 1999.[35] Obese children with gall bladder disease may present with non-specific abdominal pain with or without vomiting. Asymptomatic presentations are not uncommon, with gallstones being detected by abdominal ultrasound.

Non-alcoholic fatty liver disease

A further complication of pediatric obesity is non-alcoholic fatty liver disease or liver steatosis. Liver function tests are often abnormal, with greater elevations in aminotransferase (ALT) relative to aspartate aminotransferase (AST). Up to 77% of obese Chinese children referred for medical assessment had radiological evidence of fatty liver disease.[36] In a multi-center review of liver biopsies in Boston area hospitals, all 14 children with varying degrees of hepatosteatosis and steatohepatitis were obese.[37] In a similar study conducted in Australia, 16 of 17 children with steatohepatitis were 125–218% of ideal body weight.[38] Liver biopsies in these children generally show inflammation and fibrosis, but there have been occasional reports of cirrhosis.[38,39] As in adults, improvements in liver function tests have been reported among children who lost weight, and both ALT and BMI have been shown to be strong independent predictors of fatty liver disease.[36]

Apnea and Asthma

Obstructive sleep apnea, one part of a spectrum of sleep-disordered breathing, is another potentially dangerous consequence of childhood obesity. Two independent studies of obese US children referred for assessment of sleep-associated breathing disorders reported that 37%[40] to 94%[41] had abnormal polysomnographic findings. All were reported to be snorers and up to 50% had episodes of apnea.

Among US children with asthma, severe obesity is more than twice as prevalent as it is among children without asthma,[42] and asthma is about twice as common in obese children compared with non-obese children in studies conducted in Israel, Germany and the USA.[43–45] Despite this evidence supporting a cross-sectional association between obesity and asthma in children and adolescents, a recent survey in Canada failed to detect a statistically significant association between obesity and asthma in a large population of 4–11-year-olds.[46] Studies differ in their definitions of obesity and/or asthma, and it is plausible that the direction of causation is reversed, with the presence of asthma leading to physical inactivity, which results in weight gain.

Orthopedic/musculoskeletal effects

Excessive body weight in childhood adds mechanical stress to unfused growth plates and bones that are undergoing ossification, making overweight and obese children susceptible to orthopedic abnormalities, namely Blount disease and slipped capital femoral epiphysis. Obese children may also be predisposed to excess fractures, as well as bone and joint pain. Calculations of plantar force and pressure during standing and walking indicate that obese children may be at increased risk of developing foot pain or pathologies.

Psychological effects

Much of the work that has been done in this area is cross-sectional, so that the directionality of the associations is uncertain. However, the stigmatization, bullying and teasing experienced by overweight children may be internalized in feelings of low self-worth, depressive symptoms or suicidal thinking. Whereas one longitudinal study in the USA showed no effect of BMI on self-esteem in adolescents and young adults,[47] a second study identified important racial/ethnic differences in the relationship between changes in self-esteem and overweight in girls.[48] In Hispanic and white girls, but not among black girls, those who were overweight experienced significant decreases in self-esteem compared with their non-obese counterparts.[48] The lack of a similar association for black girls is consistent with an earlier cross-sectional study reporting normal self-esteem among obese inner-city black children, suggesting that, at least in this subgroup, obese children may not be motivated to lose weight by the promise of improved self-esteem.[49]

Psychosocial effects

Possibly the most pervasive consequences of obesity in many Western societies are psychosocial.[50] Cross-sectional associations between obesity risk and bullying, social marginalization and poor academic performance have been documented in studies conducted in Canada, the USA and Sweden.[25] Awareness of the stigma associated with obesity can lead to concerns about weight and fear of obesity even in children as young as 5 or 6.[50]

Adolescent obesity appears to affect socio-economic outcomes: data from the US National Longitudinal Survey of Youth demonstrated that overweight in adolescence and young adulthood may be a significant socio-economic handicap, especially for females.[47] Adolescent and young adult women who were overweight at baseline completed fewer years of school, were 20% less likely to be married, had lower household income and had higher rates of household poverty than non-overweight women when surveyed seven years later. Overweight men were 11% less likely to be married than were non-overweight men in the cohort. A British cohort study also identified poorer economic outcomes in young women (but not men) independent of parental socio-economic status and academic ability.[51]

Treatment implications

The impact of child obesity on children's health raises several questions for pediatric services. Are the services prepared, and adequately resourced, to act as a screening service to prevent later disease? Should screening be offered to children who are overweight as well as those who are obese? If screening leads to the detection of early indications of disease, are there sufficient resources for treatment—and are the treatments used for adults suitable for adolescents, and for even younger children?

Certainly, some disease risk factors are likely to improve if the child loses weight, or at least "grows into" their weight, if they are still showing growth in height. However, experience gained so far suggests that weight control interventions organized by pediatric services require a multi-disciplinary team of staff working with both the child and the child's family over an extended period of time, if there is to be a good chance of success.

This leads to two conclusions. The first is that obesity treatment may need to be conducted in a broader context than that currently being discussed. Successful treatment is likely to involve more than just the family and the pediatric services, and will almost certainly require support in the school and the wider community. It may be futile to ask the child to restrain his behavior in the context of what is increasingly accepted to be an "obesogenic" environment, with frequent opportunities for the consumption of food (along with its widespread marketing and promotion) and frequent opportunities for sedentary behavior. This type of environment is a challenge for children and their parents, potentially leading to difficult family dynamics and a sense of personal failure.

The second point is that child obesity is becoming a public health issue rather than a health services issue, with the emphasis moving from treatment of individuals to prevention in the population at large. Prevention of weight gain among normal weight children will require much the same set of policies to tackle obesogenic environments as are needed to support weight control among overweight and obese children. Measures such as those proposed by the World Health Organization[52] and by other expert groups[53–55] include those that are taken "downstream" in the school, home and neighborhood environment, and "upstream" in terms of policies for food supplies, commercial marketing and the encouragement of healthier lifestyles through the creation of health-promoting environments.

References

1 Lobstein T, Baur L, Uauy R: IASO International Obesity TaskForce. Obesity in children and young people: a crisis in public health. *Obes Rev* 2004; **5**(Supp. 1):4–104.
2 Olshansky SJ: University of Illinois. Cited by J Ritter in "Obesity may cut US lifespans", Chicago Sun-Times, 17 March 2005. www.highbeam.com/doc/1P2-1567779.html (accessed 11 June 2008).
3 Ludwig D: Children's Hospital, Boston. Cited by D DeNoon in "Will obesity shorten the American lifespan?" *Medcsape Today*, 16 March 2005. www.medscape.com/viewarticle/527397 (accessed 11 June 2008).
4 Chief Medical Officer, UK Department of Health. Annual: Report of the Chief Medical Officer 2002. London: Department of Health, 2003.
5 Wang Y, Lobstein T: Worldwide trends in childhood overweight and obesity. *Int J Pediatr Obes* 2006; **1**:11–25.
6 Dietz WH, Robinson TN: Use of the body mass index (BMI) as a measure of overweight in children and adolescents. *J Pediatr* 1998; **132**:191–193.
7 Kuczmarski RJ, Ogden CL, Grummer-Strawn LM et al: CDC growth charts: United States. *Adv Data* 2000; **314**:1–27.
8 World Health Organization: Physical status: the use and interpretation of anthropometry. WHO Technical Report Series No. 854. Geneva: WHO, 1995:161–311.
9 Must A, Dallal GE, Dietz WH: Reference data for obesity: 85th and 95th percentiles of body mass index (wt/ht2) and triceps skinfold thickness. *Am J Clin Nutr* 1991; **53**:839–846. Erratum in *Am J Clin Nutr* 1991; 54:773.
10 Cole TJ, Freeman JV, Preece MA: Body mass index reference curves for the UK, 1990. *Arch Dis Child* 1995; **73**:25–29.
11 Rolland-Cachera MF, Cole TJ, Sempe M, Tichet J, Rossignol C, Charraud A: Body Mass Index variations: centiles from birth to 87 years. *Eur J Clin Nutr* 1991; **45**:13–21.
12 Cole TJ, Bellizzi MC, Flegal KM, Dietz WH: Establishing a standard definition for child overweight and obesity worldwide: international survey. *BMJ* 2000; **320**:1240–1243.
13 World Health Organization: Growth Reference Data for 5-19 Years. Internet publication. Geneva: WHO, 2007. www.who.int/growthref/ (accessed 4 April 2008).
14 Lobstein T, Jackson-Leach R: Child overweight and obesity in the USA: prevalence rates according to IOTF definitions. *Int J Pediatr Obes* 2007; **2**:62–64.

15 Shields M: Overweight and obesity among children and youth. *Statistics Canada Health Report* 2006; **17**:27–42.

16 European Congress on Obesity. Child obesity "levelling off" in France. Media release, 15 May 2008. See abstracts nos: T5: PS.66 and T5: PS.113 at www.nature.com/ijo/journal/v32/n1s/pdf/ijo200847a.pdf (accessed 11 June 2008).

17 Sanigorski AM, Bell AC, Kremer PJ, Swinburn BA: High childhood obesity in an Australian population. *Obesity (Silver Spring)* 2007; **15**:1908–1912.

18 Li Y, Schouten EG, Hu X, Cui Z, Luan D, Ma G: Obesity prevalence and time trend among youngsters in China, 1982–2002. Wageningen: Wageningen University, 2007. *Asia Pac J Clin Nutr* 2008; **17**:131–137.

19 Stolarczyk H, Malinowski A: Secular changes of body height and mass in children and adolescents of Lodz. *Z Morphol Anthropol* 1996; **81**:167–177.

20 Power C, Lake JK, Cole TJ: Body mass index and height from childhood to adulthood in the 1959 British birth cohort. *Am J Clin Nutr* 1997; **66**:1094–1101.

21 Whitaker R, Wright J, Pepe M, Seidel K, Dietz W: Predicting obesity in young adulthood from childhood and parental obesity. *N Engl J Med* 1997; **337**:869–873.

22 Freedman DS, Khan LK, Serdula MK, Dietz WH, Srinivasan SR, Berenson GS: The relation of childhood BMI to adult adiposity: the Bogalusa Heart Study. *Pediatrics* 2005; **115**:22–27.

23 Freedman DS, Khan LK, Serdula MK, Dietz WH, Srinivasan SR, Berenson GS: Racial differences in the tracking of childhood BMI to adulthood. *Obes Res* 2005; **13**:928–935.

24 Whitlock EP, Williams SB, Gold R, Smith PR, Shipman SA: Screening and interventions for childhood overweight: a summary of evidence for the US preventive services task force. *Pediatrics* 2005; **116**:E125–E144.

25 Must A, Hollander SA, Economos CD: Childhood obesity: a growing public health concern. *Expert Rev Endocrinol Metab*, 2006; **1**:233–254.

26 Lobstein T, Jackson-Leach R: Estimated burden of paediatric obesity and co-morbidities in Europe. Part 2. Numbers of children with indicators of obesity-related disease. *Int J Pediatr Obes* 2006; **1**:33–41.

27 American Diabetes Association: Type 2 diabetes in children and adolescents. *Am Diabetes Assoc Diabetes Care* 2000; **23**:381–389.

28 Ford ES, Giles WH, Dietz WH: Prevalence of the metabolic syndrome among US adults. *JAMA* 2002; **287**:356–359.

29 Duncan GE, Li SM, Zhou XH: Prevalence and trends of a metabolic syndrome phenotype among U.S. adolescents, 1999–2000. *Diabetes Care* 2004; **27**:2438–2443.

30 Csabi G, Torok K, Jeges S, Molnar D: Presence of metabolic cardiovascular syndrome in obese children. *Eur. J Pediatr* 2000; **159**:91–94.

31 Berenson GS, Srinivasan SR, Bao W, Newman WP, Tracy RE, Wattigney WA: Association between multiple cardiovascular risk factors and atherosclerosis in children and young adults. *N Engl J Med* 1998; **338**:1650–1656.

32 Gidding SS, Nehgme R, Heise C, Muscar C, Linton A, Hassink S: Severe obesity associated with cardiovascular deconditioning, high prevalence of cardiovascular risk factors, diabetes mellitus/hyperinsulinemia, and respiratory compromise. *J Pediatr* 2004; **144**:766–769.

33 Guttmann-Bauman I: Approach to adolescent polycystic ovary syndrome (PCOS) in the pediatric endocrine community in the USA. *J Pediatr Endocrinol Metab* 2005; **18**:499–506.

34 Grundy SM: Cholesterol gallstones: a fellow traveler with metabolic syndrome? *Am J Clin Nutr* 2004; **80**:1–2.

35 Wang G, Dietz W: Economic burden of obesity in youths aged 6 to 17 years: 1979–1999. *Pediatrics* 2002; **109**:E81.

36 Chan DF, Li AM, Chu WC et al: Hepatic steatosis in obese Chinese children. *Int J Obes* 2004; **28**:1257–1263.

37 Baldridge AD, Perez-Atayde AR, Graeme-Cook F, Higgins L, Lavine JE: Idiopathic steatohepatitis in childhood: a multicenter retrospective study. *J Pediatr* 1995; **127**: 700–704.

38 Manton ND, Lipsett J, Moore DJ, Davidson GP, Bourne AJ, Couper RT: Non-alcoholic steatohepatitis in children and adolescents. *Med J Aust* 2000; **173**:476–479.

39 Rashid M, Roberts EA: Nonalcoholic steatohepatitis in children. *J Pediatr Gastroenterol Nutr* 2000; **30**:48–53.

40 Mallory GB, Fiser DH, Jackson R: Sleep-associated breathing disorders in morbidly obese children and adolescents. *J Pediatr* 1989; **115**:892–897.

41 Silvestri JM, Weese-Mayer DE, Bass MT, Kenny AS, Hauptmann SA, Pearsall SM: Polysomnography in obese children with a history of sleep-associated breathing disorders. *Pediatr Pulmonol* 1993; **16**:124–129.

42 Gennuso J, Epstein LH, Paluch RA, Cerny F: The relationship between asthma and obesity in urban minority children and adolescents. *Arch Pediatr Adolesc Med*, 1998; **152**:1197–1200.

43 Bibi H, Shoseyov D, Feigenbaum D et al: The relationship between asthma and obesity in children: is it real or a case of over diagnosis? *J Asthma* 2004; **41**:403–410.

44 von Kries R, Hermann M, Grunert V, von Mutius E: Is obesity a risk factor for childhood asthma? *Allergy* 2001; **56**:318–322.

45 von Mutius E, Schwartz J, Neas LM, Dockery D, Weiss ST: Relation of body mass index to asthma and atopy in children: the National Health and Nutrition Examination Study III. *Thorax* 2001; **56**:835–838.

46 To T, Vydykhan TN, Dell S, Tassoudji M, Harris JK: Is obesity associated with asthma in young children? *J Pediatr* 2004; **144**:162–168.

47 Gortmaker SL, Must A, Perrin JM, Sobol AM, Dietz WH: Social and economic consequences of overweight in adolescence and young adulthood. *N Engl J Med* 1993; **329**: 1008–1012.

48 Strauss RS: Childhood obesity and self-esteem. *Pediatrics* 2000; **105**:E15.

49 Kaplan KM, Wadden TA: Childhood obesity and self-esteem. *Pediatrics* 1986; **109**:367–370.

50 Dietz W: Health consequences of obesity in youth: childhood predictors of adult diseases. *Pediatrics* 1998; **101**: 518–525.

51 Sargent JD, Blanchflower DG: Obesity and stature in adolescence and earnings in young adulthood: analysis of a British birth cohort. *Arch Pediatr Adolesc Med*, 1994; **148**: 681–687.

52 World Health Organization. Global Strategy on Diet, Physical Activity and Health. Adopted by the World Health Assembly, May 2004. Geneva: WHO, 2004.

53 Lobstein T, Baur LA: Policies to prevent childhood obesity in the European Union. *Eur J Public Health* 2005; **15**: 576–579.

54 Stockley L: Toward public health nutrition strategies in the European Union to implement food based dietary guidelines and to enhance healthier lifestyles. *Public Health Nutr* 2001; **4**:307–324.

55 Swinburn B, Gill T, Kumanyika S: Obesity prevention: a proposed framework for translating evidence into action. *Obes Rev* 2005; **6**:23–33.

CHAPTER 2

Lessons from the control of other epidemics

Mickey Chopra
School of Public Health and Systems Research Unit, Medical Research Council, University of Western Cape, Parow, South Africa

Summary

The causes of childhood obesity, both at an individual and at the population level, are now mostly well understood. Fundamentally overweight and obesity result from an imbalance between calorie intake and expenditure. However, changing diets and lifestyles, as other authors in this book have pointed out, is a complex undertaking that requires a multi-pronged approach. Other chapters in this book and review articles outline the evidence for an effective and comprehensive approach towards the prevention and management of childhood obesity. Some of the components being promoted include: a recognition of the need for more than individual level educational and behavioral interventions; taking a settings approach in schools, public institutions, workplace, and so on; the responsibility of governments in "making healthy choices the easy choice".

Introduction

For these strategies to have an impact, there is a need for a broader evidence base of their efficacy in different settings (especially in low-resource settings) and for them to be implemented at scale so that they reach those who require it the most. However, experience of converting evidence into policy and practice is not well documented for childhood obesity. There is good reason to believe that conversion of evidence to policy will be particularly difficult for combating changes in childhood diet and physical activity. Critical drivers of

the childhood obesity epidemic, such as the marketing of high-fat foods, poor provision of facilities for physical activities and the increasing popularity of sedentary activities are intimately bound with modern development and globalization.[1] In this sense it shares many of the challenges of other non-communicable diseases that are also increasing rapidly in both developed and developing countries.

This chapter aims to learn from the experience of attempting to scale up the response to non-communicable diseases especially in resource poor settings. What are the strategic lessons to be learnt from the experience of responding to other non-communicable diseases?

Despite a continual struggle to move from non-communicable diseases being regarded as the problems of the rich, and having to confront the interests of some powerful private industries, there have been significant policy developments even in low- and middle-income countries. China and India have started to pull together the various initiatives around smoking, cardiovascular disease, diabetes and so on, into coherent national plans that go beyond individual level education or warnings on cigarette packets. Pakistan launched a National Action Plan on Non-communicable Diseases in 2003, which is now being scaled up as a major public health programme; and Vietnam, using the WHO recommended approach, has invested in the stepwise approach to the surveillance, prevention, and control of non-communicable diseases. The lifelong treatment of HIV/Aids is now being scaled up across a number of resources-poor settings and is giving rise to a number of innovations with respect to the way long-term care is to be delivered.

A comprehensive approach to childhood obesity shares many of the challenges that have been faced by

Preventing Childhood Obesity. Edited by
E. Waters, B.A. Swinburn, J.C. Seidell and R. Uauy.
© 2010 Blackwell Publishing.

other non-communicable disease epidemics, such as tobacco control, cancer control, diabetes and HIV/Aids. This chapter does not aim to re-state the control strategies being employed or go into details of specific interventions. Rather, it seeks to identify essential principles that have been critical for scaling up approaches to the various non-communicable disease epidemics in order to suggest some priority actions for addressing the childhood obesity epidemic.

In no particular order they are as follows:

Shifting from an individual to public health approach

Traditional responses to the control of non-communicable disease arose from the results of large longitudinal studies of men in places such as Framingham in the United States.[2] These studies followed up thousands of middle-aged men in order to isolate a number of important risk factors for heart disease and other non-communicable diseases. The control strategies that arose from such an approach focused on isolating individuals with risky lifestyles or risk factors and prescribed relevant behavior changes through health education to the population and, possibly, treatment for those at "high risk". However, this approach has been very expensive and in itself had limited impact. In particular, it has been the realization that a large number of people at a small risk may give rise to more cases of disease than the small number who are at high risk,[3] that shifted attention to interventions that could make a difference at a population level as exemplified by this insight into controlling blood pressure: "… a 2% reduction in of mean blood pressure … has the potential to prevent 1.2 million deaths from stroke (about 15% of all deaths from stroke) and 0.6 million from coronary heart disease every year by 2020 in the Asia Pacific region alone … and could be readily achieved in many populations by reducing the salt content of manufactured food".[4]

Analysis of large-scale examples of significant reversals in the prevalence of risk factors or reductions in mortality from non-communicable diseases from places such as Norway, Poland and Mauritius[5–7] has identified important structural interventions. Such interventions include a combination of selective agricultural subsidies, price manipulation, retail regula-

tions, and clear labeling. For example, in the case of Norway this was based on a wide range of measures that included:[5]

- public and professional education and information;
- setting of consumer and producer price and income subsidies jointly in nutritionally justifiable ways;
- the adjustment of absolute and relative consumer food price subsidies, ensuring low prices for food grain, skimmed and low-fat milk, vegetables and potatoes;
- the avoidance of low prices for sugar, butter and margarine;
- the marking of regulations to promote provision of healthy foods by retail stores, street vendors and institutions; and
- the regulation of food processing and labeling.

Shifting from an international to a global public health approach

Traditionally, international public health approaches have viewed national governments as the primary agents and locus of control for public health. Global threats are primarily conceived of as problems of border control and dealt primarily through cross-border cooperation between governments. The legal instruments are confined to national legislation and regulations. The scope of activities is also mostly focused on targeting risk factors in prevention programmes based in the Ministry of Health.[8]

However, experiences from global efforts to control tobacco consumption or restrict the marketing of breast-milk substitutes suggest that such an approach is not sufficient.[9] In both cases attempts to influence the production, marketing and distribution of these products through general education, national campaigns or appeals to industry have been found to be necessary but not sufficient to have a real impact.[10] The accelerating pace of globalization has resulted in many health determinants being constituted beyond national or even regional boundaries.[8]

Quite clearly, the de-linking of many health determinants from national space, requires a much broader response than that traditionally associated with the international approach. A wider range of actors and stakeholders, both governmental and non-governmental, need to be involved. It also suggests that a wider range of tools and approaches are required. One approach has been the development and adoption of codes of conduct that specify the control of marketing and trade of goods felt to damage public health.[11] Perhaps the most famous example is that of the International Code of Conduct on Breastfeeding Substitutes. This is a non-binding recommendation adopted by the World Health Assembly in 1981, with the purpose of promoting breastfeeding and regulating the marketing of breast-milk substitutes. However, this example also illustrates the limitation of voluntary codes with numerous documented transgressions of the Code by the breast-milk substitute industry.[12] This has led to the recognition of the need to develop more binding instruments.

In terms of binding instruments, the International Health Regulations were adopted by the Assembly in 1948 in order to control the international spread of communicable diseases. Most recently, the Framework Convention on Tobacco Control (FCTC), is a binding international convention, which aims to circumscribe the global spread of tobacco use and tobacco products (Box 2.1).

Legally binding instruments have the distinct advantage that State Parties tend to comply, and the disadvantage of a drawn-out process and the need for global political support for a single solution. Approaches which endorse binding international instruments on food-related health issues have been limited to food safety and security and, more recently, discussions of rights-based approaches to undernutrition. The non-binding intergovernmental resolution has the advantage of flexibility. Potential international standards and instruments in this area might address issues such as marketing restrictions for unhealthy food products, restrictions on the advertising and availability of unhealthy products in schools, standard packaging and labeling of food products, and potential price or tax measures to reduce the demand for unhealthy products. There is also the advantage of the public attention surrounding the drafting of such an instrument and the fact that it may set general standards for corporate conduct without actually being passed through legislation.

More recently, the importance of international trade has put the relationship between trade agreements and public health more in the spotlight. The World Trade Organization (WTO) has become the

Box 2.1 WHO Framework Convention on Tobacco Control (FCTC)

The WHO FCTC is the first global health treaty to be negotiated under the auspices of the WHO. It was developed in response to the globalization of the tobacco epidemic and asserts the importance of a broad range of strategies for demand reduction. These include: price and tax measures; protection from exposure to environmental tobacco smoke; regulation and disclosure of the contents of tobacco products; packaging and labeling; education, communication, training and public awareness; comprehensive ban and restriction on tobacco advertising, promotion and sponsorship; and tobacco dependence and cessation measures. There are also a number of measures relating to a reduction in the supply of tobacco including: elimination of the illicit trade of tobacco products; restriction of sales to and by minors and support for economically viable alternatives for growers.

The treaty came into force on 27 February 2005, and with almost 150 parties it is one of the most widely embraced treaties in UN history. Notably absent from the list of signatory countries are Russia and Indonesia; the USA has signed but not ratified the treaty. The challenge of implementation of the WHO FCTC involves putting in place the required technical foundation, translating the treaty into national laws, creating strong mechanisms for enforcement, and then monitoring their implementation. With about 25% of adults smoking, there is a long way to go before achieving full implementation of the treaty and a reduction in the prevalence of smoking. The early signs are encouraging with governments in low- and middle-income countries such as South Africa moving rapidly to legislate most of the provisions in the Convention. National surveys show that the adoption of this suite of broad legal and voluntary measures has reduced smoking among the poorest sections of the population by at least 30%.

arbiter of conflicts around the desire to reduce trade barriers, on the one hand, and the need to protect populations from harmful practices and goods, on the other. For example, a government's ability to establish and maintain legitimate, non-discriminatory food safety and food-related consumer information labeling policies has been challenged as a barrier to free trade. There are provisions that allow public health concerns to "override" the desire for more free trade in the WTO but the drawbacks of relying upon WTO exemptions include economic disincentives associated with violation of WTO rules that may prevent States from giving priority to public health when conflicts arise, and may also impede the negotiation, ratification and implementation of international public health instruments.

Optimize effectiveness (in terms of quality and coverage) of existing efficacious interventions especially in health sector

There are a number of efficacious and effective interventions that can prevent or reduce the morbidity and mortality associated with non-communicable diseases. However, too often, the inverse care law applies in terms of the coverage of these interventions: those who need the interventions the most are the least likely to receive them. Within countries, there are differences in coverage between the rich and poor and between urban and rural areas. There are also large differences in access to care between countries.

Unfortunately, the evidence for what works in terms of scaling up interventions for non-communicable diseases is limited. Reviews of relatively successful non-communicable disease programmes have highlighted some common features including: routine patient monitoring; shared decision making between health professionals and patients; self-management support that allow patients to successfully manage their symptoms, treatments and preventive health behaviors on a day-to-day basis; and community linkages that allow interventions such as population-based health promotion and disease prevention, integration of people with NCDs into community life, and provision of complementary and home-based health services.[13] However, nearly all these lessons are based on non-communicable care models in the USA or UK with very little evidence of what works at scale in resource-poor settings. The approach of WHO with regards to the non-communicable care and treatment of people living with HIV/Aids is interesting in that it focuses on a slightly different set of principles (Box 2.2).

Box 2.2 Scaling up HIV treatment

The huge burden of unmet care and treatment for HIV has led to a plethora of treatment options for those infected, especially in Southern Africa where the epidemic is at its worst. Difficulty in accessing efficacious drug treatments has led many HIV patients to spend significant amounts of resources in accessing substandard care and treatment. Governments and agencies are now responding by scaling up the introduction of long-term treatment of HIV with the provision of anti-retroviral treatment (ART). The challenges of providing non-communicable care in the context of weak health systems have led WHO to adopt what they termed a "public-health approach to ART treatment". A number of innovations marked a shift from previous attempts to provide ART:
1) standardization of first-line and second-line treatment along with a prescriptive approach, facilitating the development of fixed-dose first line combinations, and driving down the price of these drugs;
2) simplification of clinical decision making with an attempt to manage without necessarily having any immunological monitoring;
3) decentralization of treatment to the district level through the development and training in adapted integrated management of adult illness (IMAI) guidelines;
4) task shifting of essential activities such as initiation and monitoring of treatment from physicians to nurses;
5) procurement and supply management strengthening, with a focus on reducing the number of commodities and drugs and being more specific of exact requirements. Such an approach has allowed a significant scaling up of the provision of ART and early results suggest that while early mortality is high the medium-term outcomes for those on the programmes is good.[14]

Decentralized care focused at the primary health care level

The example of the scale-up of treatment for HIV/Aids emphasizes the shift in the care of patients from specialists and hospitals to nurse-led care at a primary health care center. There is now good evidence from well resourced settings that primary-care-led patient models can lead to similar and often better outcomes than specialist, tertiary level care. There is also some evidence that such an approach is also effective in low income settings.

Essential to the success of a primary health care approach is the identification of core competencies required by the primary health care team and then building the capacity of such a team. WHO has highlighted five basic competencies, which apply to all members of the workforce caring for patients with non-communicable diseases: patient-centered-care; partnering; quality improvement; information and communication technology; and public health perspective.

Achieving these results across a wide range of settings has also required some innovation in order to overcome the increasing shortages of highly specialized and skilled health workers, especially in more disadvantaged areas. Examples of such innovation include task shifting where different cadres of workers take on tasks traditionally assigned to a more specialized level. For example, a number of rigorous studies have shown that capable nurses can manage clinical challenges at primary level just as competently as general practitioners.[15] In the United States a large number of non-physician clinicians and nurse practitioners have been developed and been shown to be just as competent as physicians.[16] However, the success of such approaches does require a multi-disciplinary teamwork approach so that carers can be provided with support and there are good referral mechanisms for more complex cases.

Increasing attention is also being paid to the potential of non-professionals, including community members and "expert patients" in the prevention and management of many non-communicable diseases. Interventions to increase the capacity of either individual or groups of individuals in the self-management of the disease has led to improvements in outcomes such as pain control, reductions in disability and depression as well as self-efficacy (confidence about managing their own condition).

More sophisticated advocacy responses

Moving from policy to implementation remains a challenge. Analysis of attempts to address global and regional determinants of poor social outcomes has highlighted three major deficits that need to be over-come. These are: first, "democracy" deficits as power is concentrated in the hands of a few governments (e.g., G8) often heavily influenced by big industrial interests in these matters; second, "coherence" deficits between different Ministries within governments and sometimes between different international agencies work to inhibit the necessary intersectoral action; third, the shortcomings of democratic participation, accountability and coherence contribute to "compli-ance" deficits as international institutions and national governments fail to implement decisions they make.

Regardless of the exact deficiency, it is clear from the experience of other non-communicable diseases that strong political will and leadership is required to achieve the necessary coordination of the planning and implementation of priority policies and prgrammes. Unlike other communicable epidemics in the past, there are now far more stakeholders including the private sector, non-governmental organizations and civil society, operating at many different levels and settings, who need to be brought together. In particular, most of these epidemics are occurring in the context of urbanized settings where achieving changes to physical and environmental structures requires high levels of policy and advocacy skills (along with plenty of patience). Building coalitions, especially with non-governmental organizations and other parts of civil society, has been important in the fight against tobacco and HIV/Aids.

Developing appropriate monitoring systems

The lack of timely, reliable and comparable data on prevalence, risk factors and trends has traditionally hampered attempts to raise awareness of the problem of non-communicable disease. Proper planning and implementation of prevention and control strategies depend on the availability of reliable and comparable information for monitoring the burden of non-communicable diseases and their risk factors; information needs are greatest in the poorest countries. The generation of simple but valid data concerning the contribution of non-communicable diseases to premature mortality and disability, together with the high health care costs – and ensuing high economic costs – have been important in raising awareness of the problem for even poor and middle income countries.

The usefulness of data for monitoring and evaluation can be seen from the experience of the establishment of Chinese cancer registries. This began in 1963 in Shanghai, and data from registries has been used extensively to raise the profile of cancer control efforts and influence policy-making. One example is the careful charting of the impact of cervical cancer screening programme, which saw a dramatic decline in mortality from cervical cancer in the Jing'an county of Jiangxi province, decreasing to 9·6 per 100,000 in 1985, from 42·0 per 100,000 in 1974. Documented success such as this has encouraged the Chinese national authorities to develop and implement a national Program of Cancer Prevention and Control in China (2004–2010), which contains a national programme for rapid diagnosis and screening for cervical cancer.

Realizing that establishing large-scale national surveillance systems can be expensive, WHO has suggested a simple stepwise approach to risk factor surveillance, leading to policy actions. It starts with a focus on measuring the prevalence of eight key risk factors: tobacco use, harmful alcohol consumption, unhealthy diet (low fruit and vegetable consumption), physical inactivity, raised blood pressure, overweight and obesity, raised blood sugar and abnormal blood lipids/cholesterol. Depending on the available resources, it suggests starting with the standardized collection of core data from household surveys before expanding into collection of blood samples. The distribution of risk factors among the population is the key information required for planning.

Developing an evidence base for action and focusing on key research questions

The history of tobacco control illustrates the critical importance of using research to build a solid evidence base to support advocacy and policy actions. Starting with the meticulously conducted observational studies by Richard Doll and colleagues, it was the accumulation of a large body of evidence that finally persuaded policy-makers to implement wide ranging anti-tobacco measures. In terms of research priorities, the challenge of moving from having a good understanding of risk factors and interventions to pre-

venting and treating many non-communicable disease to actually reducing the burden of disease is proving the big challenge. This stresses that the need for support from funding agencies is crucial for implementation research—that is, for research that explores the most practical and efficient methods of applying existing knowledge for the available interventions.

References

1 Hawkes C: Uneven Dietary Development: Linking the Policies and Processes of Globalization with the Nutrition Transition, Obesity and Diet-Related Chronic Diseases. Globalization and Health, 2006.
2 Chopra M: A new epidemiology and public health for a new South Africa. S Afr Med J 2000; 90(9):875–876.
3 Rose G: The Practice of Prevention. London UK: Tavistock, 1992.
4 Beaglehole R: Global cardiovascular disease prevention: time to get serious. Lancet 2001; 358:661–663.
5 Norum KR: Some aspects of Norwegian nutrition and food policy. In: Shetty P, McPherson K, eds. Diet, Nutrition and Chronic Disease: Lessons From Contrasting Worlds. London: John Wiley & Sons, Ltd, 1997:72–86.
6 Zatonski WA, McMichael AJ, Powles JW: Ecological study of reasons for sharp decline in mortality from ischaemic heart disease in Poland since 1991. BMJ 1998; 316(7137):1047–1051.
7 Dowse GK, Gareeboo H, Alberti KG et al: Changes in population cholesterol concentrations and other cardiovascular risk factor levels after five years of the non-communicable disease intervention programme in Mauritius. Br Med J 1995; 311:1255–1259.
8 Lee K: Global health promotion: how can we strengthen governance and build effective strategies? Health Promot Int 2006; 21(Suppl. 1):42–50.
9 Chopra M, Darnton-Hill I: Tobacco and obesity epidemics: not so different after all? BMJ 2004; 328(7455):1558–1560.
10 James WPT: The policy challenge of coexisting undernutrition and nutrition-related chronic diseases. Matern Child Nutr 2005; 1(3):197–203.
11 Chopra M, Galbraith S, Darnton-Hill I: A global response to a global problem: the epidemic of overnutrition. Bull World Health Organ 2002; 80(12):952–958.
12 Aguayo VM, Ross JS, Kanon S, Ouedraogo AN: Monitoring compliance with the International Code of Marketing of Breastmilk Substitutes in west Africa: multisite cross sectional survey in Togo and Burkina Faso. BMJ 2003; 326(7381):127.
13 Tsai AC, Morton SC, Mangione CM, Keeler EB: A meta-analysis of interventions to improve care for chronic illnesses. Am J Manag Care 2005; 11(8):478–488.

14 Gilks CF, Crowley S, Ekpini R et al: The WHO public-health approach to antiretroviral treatment against HIV in resource-limited settings. *Lancet* 2006; **368**(9534):505–510.

15 Laurant M, Reeves D, Hermens R, Braspenning J, Grol R, Sibbald B: Substitution of doctors by nurses in primary care. *Cochrane Database Syst Rev* 2005; 2 (Art. No.: CD001271).

16 McPherson K, Kersten P, George S et al: A systematic review of evidence about extended roles for allied health professionals. *J Health Serv Res Policy* 2006; **11**(4):240–247.

CHAPTER 3

Childhood obesity prevention overview

Ricardo Uauy,[1,2] *Rishi Caleyachetty*[3] and *Boyd Swinburn*[4]
[1] Nutrition and Public Health Intervention Research Unit, London School of Hygiene and Tropical Medicine, London, UK
[2] Institute of Nutrition and Food Technology, University of Chile, Santiago, Chile
[3] MRC Epidemiology Unit, Institute of Metabolic Science, Cambridge, UK
[4] WHO Collaborating Centre for Obesity Prevention, Deakin University, Melbourne, Australia

Summary

- The childhood obesity epidemic demands a concerted prevention effort from governments, international organizations, the private sector and civil society.
- A life-course approach to preventing childhood obesity provides multiple opportunities for intervention and many childhood settings offer opportunities for access to children and parents.
- Government policies are needed to provide the backbone for health promotion activities.
- International agencies and multinational food companies have critical supporting roles to play.
- Marketing of unhealthy foods to children is a multi-billion dollar commercial enterprise and these practices severely undermine the efforts of parents, governments and health and education professionals to provide a healthy environment for children.

Introduction

The rising prevalence of childhood obesity in most populations around the world is a matter of grave concern because the physical, psychological and social consequences of obesity in childhood are substantial.[1] The increase in the prevalence of obesity has been accompanied by a more rapid increase in the severity of obesity with more children becoming severely obese, indicating that obesity-related medical conditions will rise at least as rapidly as the overall obesity prevalence rate. Furthermore, as these children carry that risk of excess weight into adulthood, the impact of obesity on the management of chronic disease and disability will continue to grow as the epidemic gains momentum.[2] The consequences of the obesity burden and related diseases include not only the known health consequences but also lost educational opportunity and lost economic contribution from the lost days of employment by an older adolescent, or by a parent or carer in the family if the child requires medical attention. Furthermore, there are many intangible costs such as the psycho-social consequences of obesity.[1]

Since the early 1990s, the prevalence of overweight and obesity in children has increased in virtually every country of the world: in some it has doubled and in others it has tripled.[3] It is now recognized that there are many societal and environmental drivers of unhealthy weight gain[4,5] and yet most of the research efforts are directed at the individual level, particularly the genetic level, and most of the current prevention efforts center on education and social marketing approaches rather than underlying determinants. This is shown schematically in Figure 3.1. This chapter provides an overview of some of the approaches to reducing the rapidly increasing epidemic of childhood obesity and calls for multiple interventions across the life course backed by a much greater focus on reversing some of the underlying drivers of the epidemic. We also examine one of the critical drivers of childhood obesity: food marketing that targets children.

Preventing Childhood Obesity. Edited by
E. Waters, B.A. Swinburn, J.C. Seidell and R. Uauy.
© 2010 Blackwell Publishing.

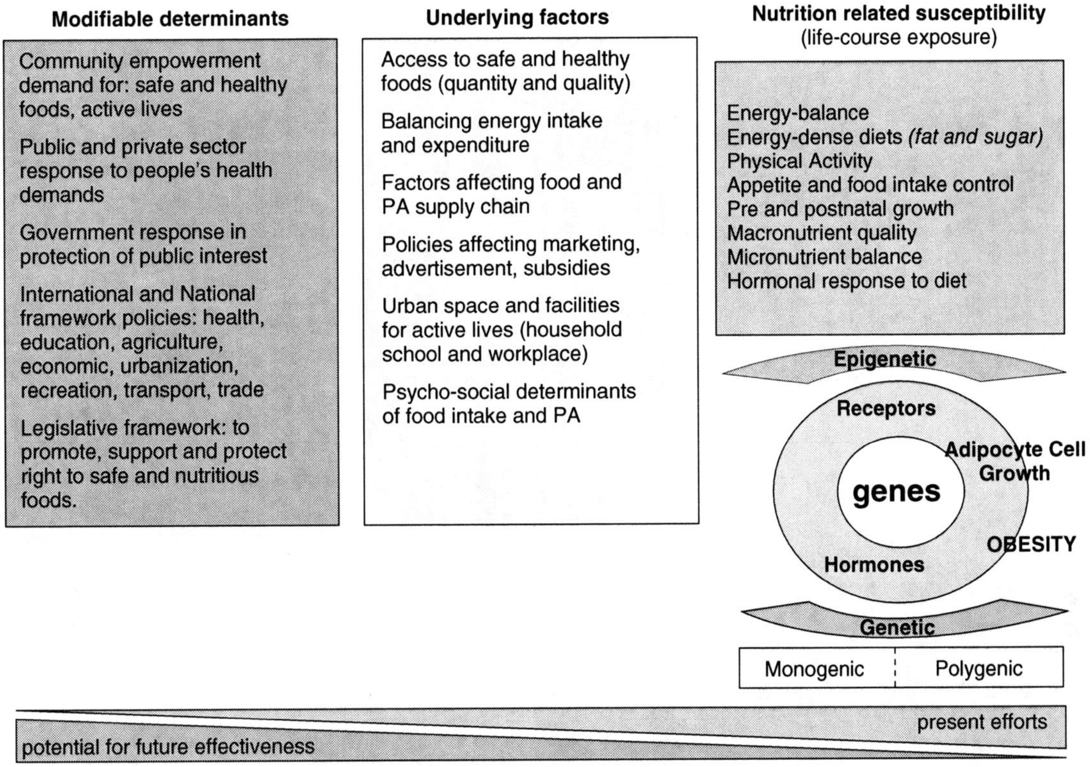

Modifiable determinants

Community empowerment demand for: safe and healthy foods, active lives

Public and private sector response to people's health demands

Government response in protection of public interest

International and National framework policies: health, education, agriculture, economic, urbanization, recreation, transport, trade

Legislative framework: to promote, support and protect right to safe and nutritious foods.

Underlying factors

Access to safe and healthy foods (quantity and quality)

Balancing energy intake and expenditure

Factors affecting food and PA supply chain

Policies affecting marketing, advertisement, subsidies

Urban space and facilities for active lives (household school and workplace)

Psycho-social determinants of food intake and PA

Nutrition related susceptibility
(life-course exposure)

Energy-balance
Energy-dense diets *(fat and sugar)*
Physical Activity
Appetite and food intake control
Pre and postnatal growth
Macronutrient quality
Micronutrient balance
Hormonal response to diet

Epigenetic

Receptors

genes

Adipocyte Cell Growth

OBESITY

Hormones

Genetic

| Monogenic | Polygenic |

present efforts

potential for future effectiveness

Figure 3.1 The hierarchy of determinants of childhood obesity from basic societal determinants (which have the greatest potential for prevention efforts) to individual and genetic predisposition (which is where the greatest efforts are currently based).

A life-course approach to obesity prevention

The concept that obesity should be prevented using a life-course approach is relatively new. The old concept that children would outgrow overweight and obesity has been abandoned based on the currently available data which show that as obesity prevalence rises the tracking of increased adiposity into adulthood becomes stronger and more clearly defined.[6] The evidence indicates that the time to consider obesity and chronic disease prevention is from early life and continues throughout every stage of the life course, Figure 3.2 offers a graphic depiction of this concept.

Preconception This is an important time to ensure, if possible, that maternal body mass index (BMI) is normal (i.e., between 18.5 and 25 kg/m^2) and that micronutrient status is normal (i.e., any anemia is corrected and folate intake is adequate through ade-

quate diet, fortified foods or supplements). Monitoring maternal weight gain is important to reduce the risk of low birth weight (<2.5 kg) as well as macrosomia (birth weight >4.0 kg). The relationship between birth weight and obesity is that of an open J-shaped curved: that is, both low birth weight and high birth weight are associated with a higher risk of later obesity. While the mechanisms by which intrauterine undernutrition or overnutrition predisposes to later unhealthy weight gain are beginning to be elucidated,[7] the key message is that we should change what is considered good nutrition during infancy, from a focus on weight gain to one where linear growth and the proportionality of weight relative to length are truly important.

Infants and young children The main preventive strategies for these groups are to: promote and support the practice of exclusive breastfeeding for the first six months of life as the preferred mode of feeding; avoiding the use of added sugars and starches when feeding

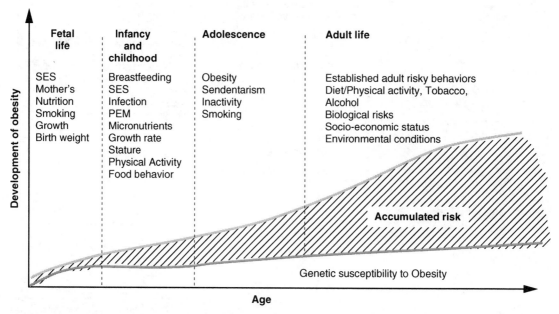

Figure 3.2 The life-course approach to obesity prevention considers age specific actions at each stage of the life course, the objective of these actions is to ameliorate the burden of obesity that is preventable by diet and physical activity interventions.

artificial formula, considering that flow of milk from the bottle is faster than from the breast, so it is easier to provide excess energy; instructing mothers to accept their child's ability to regulate energy intake rather than feeding until the plate is empty; and assuring the appropriate micronutrient intake needed to promote optimal linear growth.

Older children and adolescents The main preventive strategies in these age groups are to: promote an active lifestyle, limit television viewing, promote the intake of fruits and vegetables; restrict the intake of energy-dense, micronutrient-poor foods (e.g., packaged snacks); restrict the intake of sugar-sweetened soft drinks. Additional measures to support these behavioral approaches include: modifying the environment to enhance physical activity in schools and communities; creating more opportunities for family interaction (e.g., eating family meals); limiting the exposure to aggressive marketing practices of energy-dense, micronutrient-poor foods; and providing the necessary information and skills to make better food choices. In lower income countries, special attention

should be given to avoidance of overfeeding stunted population groups. Nutrition programmes designed to control or prevent undernutrition need to assess stature in combination with weight to prevent providing excess energy to children of low weight-for-age but normal weight-for-height.[8,9] In countries undergoing rapid growth and demographic transition, and as populations become more sedentary and able to access energy-dense foods, there is a need to maintain the healthy components of traditional diets (e.g., high intake of vegetables, fruits and non-starch polysaccharides).[10]

Education provided to parents from disadvantaged communities that are food insecure should stress that overweight and obesity do not represent good health. Low-income groups globally and populations in countries in economic transition often replace traditional micronutrient-rich foods by heavily marketed, sugar-sweetened beverages (such as soft drinks) and energy-dense fatty, salty and sugary foods.[10]

These trends, coupled with reduced physical activity, are associated with the rising prevalence of obesity.

Strategies are needed to improve the quality of diets by increasing the consumption of fruits and vegetables, in addition to increasing physical activity, to stem the epidemic of obesity and associated diseases.

Linking community, national and global approaches

The opportunities for action can be viewed not only by life stages but also by the settings and sectors where specific action can take place. While these are explored in detail in the other chapters in this book, this section provides an overview of the major options in relation to specific childhood settings and the government policies and sector changes which are essential to support healthy eating and physical activity. Food marketing to children is dealt with separately because it is such an important policy strategy to support parents and to provide a healthier environment for children.

Communities and settings

Homes and families
The home and family environment has by far the most powerful influence on children and many aspects of parenting and home life have been shown to be associated with unhealthy weight gain in children and adolescents.[11,12] However, when it comes to health promotion, access to parents is relatively limited with the main options being through social marketing directly and through childhood and health-care settings.

Preschool settings
Health promotion efforts in preschool settings (nurseries, child-care kindergarten etc.) provide essential access to young families, especially first-time parents who are in a rapid learning period about caring for children's food and activity needs. Preventive services should ensure that the needs of nutritionally-at-risk infants and children were met, paying special attention to linear growth of pre-term and/or low birth weight infants, and that interventions are monitored to avoid excess weight relative to length gain increases the risk of obesity in later life. Parents should be encouraged to actively play and interact with their children,

starting from infancy, to promote active living and motor development.

Nurseries and kindergartens should ensure that they do not restrict physical activity and promote sedentary habits during the growing years. Children in nurseries should be involved in active play for at least one hour a day, so appropriate staffing and physical facilities for active and safe play should be a requirement for nurseries caring for young children.

Schools
Schools represent a unique opportunity for obesity prevention. They can serve to exemplify the preferred approaches to good nutrition and active living, and their practices should set an example not only for the students but also for their families. A coherent, comprehensive "whole school" approach (children, parents and all staff including food services) to health promotion (active living and healthy diets) is needed because it is more likely to be sustainable, and there are broader benefits for the child (e.g., improved educational, social and self-esteem outcomes) and the community at large. Funding of schools including sports and athletic facilities needs to be independent of commercial sources to prevent pressures that counter the ethos of obesity prevention. Raising funds for school programmes by sponsorships from unhealthy snacks and sugary drinks manufacturers sends the wrong message to both pupils and the larger school community. Teachers may need additional training in health promotion, including personal advice in terms of healthy weight and active living, since they are role models for the pupils they teach. Further training of staff may be needed to ensure obese children are not stigmatized or bullied by others in the school. Consistent policies are needed to ensure the nutritional value of foods made available in schools. Physical education is also a vital part of the curriculum in all grades. Chapters 10, 11 and 30 on the evidence for school-based interventions and working in schools provide much more detail on this crucial setting for childhood obesity prevention.

Health care services
Health care facilities need to provide a range of preventive services and health promoting activities, and

should liaise with schools and community services to ensure that their messages are given prominence. Health care staff also have a role in monitoring children's growth to recognize early signs of "mis-nourishment", including stunting and overweight, and to provide appropriate responses. The contacts between parents and the maternal/child health nurses are especially important "learning moments" and should be utilised to encourage breastfeeding and teach parents about appropriate growth trajectories and feeding practices for their children. The evidence on effective primary care management is very limited (as outlined in Chapter 12) and many of the existing structures in primary care, especially the funding structures that dictate the short consultation periods, conspire against this setting being used to its full potential (see Chapter 31).

Community-wide approaches

Enabling environments must encompass all communities and must also operate within a given community, affecting transport policies, urban design policies and access to healthy diets. Community-wide approaches play an important role in providing the broader approach, and these are covered in more detail in Chapters 7, 26, 27. However, it is worth emphasizing the need to ensure adequate access to healthy foods for low-income families. This may require programs and policies to ensure that healthy food is more readily available, affordable and better promoted than the unhealthy alternatives.

National policies

While there are several key players in obesity prevention (governments, international organizations, the private sector and civil society/non-governmental organizations), governments need to take the lead and to drive the policy changes. Each country should select a mix of promising policies and actions that are in accord with national capabilities, laws and economic realities.[13] Ministries of health have a crucial convening role in bringing together other ministries that are needed for effective policy design and implementation. However, it is important to realize that while health usually takes a large slice of national budget, ministers of health are not usually the most powerful members of cabinet. Governments need to work together with the private sector, health professional bodies, consumer groups, academics, the research community and other non-governmental bodies if sustained progress is to occur.

National policies and programs should explicitly address equality and diminish disparities by focusing on the needs of the more disadvantaged communities and population groups. Furthermore, since women generally make decisions about household nutrition, strategies need to be gender sensitive. Continued support for the full implementation of the WHO-UNICEF Code of Marketing of Breast Milk Substitutes is vital in all countries. Recommendations for local and central governments are delineated in the WHO Global Strategy on Diet, Physical Activity and Health (DPAS)[14] and, in addition to the specific measures to address childhood obesity, they also have a fundamental role in providing the support strategies for effective obesity prevention, as shown in the box below.

> ## Support functions for governments in addition to specific obesity prevention interventions
>
> - Monitoring programs on outcomes (obesity), and determinants (e.g., behaviors and environments) should report to a parliamentary scrutiny committee or an "obesity observatory".
> - Coordination to ensure cross-departmental, cross-sectoral polices can be implemented and these should managed centrally by government but monitored by a separate agency.
> - Capacity should be built at national and at local levels, through training programs and other support structures and funding.
> - State support for commerce (e.g. food enterprises, agricultural enterprises) should include health criteria.
> - Political donations from food companies should be restricted.
> - Access to and affordability of fruits and vegetables should be improved, especially for low-income and disadvantaged population groups.
> - National governments should support WHO moves to ensure that all UN agencies have policies that are consistent with the Global Strategy.

Global approaches

While governments have jurisdiction over many aspects of promoting optimal diets and healthy living, there are some limits to what individual countries can do alone. The environments which influence physical activity are largely under national control, but the food supply is already very global. Strategies need to draw substantially on existing international standards that provide a reference in international trade. WHO and other UN and international organizations such as the World Bank, the International Monetary Fund and the World Trade Organization play a very important role in food security and a healthy food supply. The Food and Agriculture Organization (FAO) has a special role to play since it deals with issues relating to the production, trade, marketing of food and agricultural commodities and provides guidelines ensuring the safety and nutritional adequacy of food and food products.

Large, multinational food companies such as Nestle, Unilever and Kraft are highly influential in determining the composition, price, availability and promotion of many of the foods eaten today and therefore must be an important part of the global solutions to obesity.

International non-governmental organizations such as the global peak bodies for obesity, diabetes, heart disease, nutrition, cancer and pediatrics have a major role to play in international advocacy for change. Their voices, especially if they are all promoting the same messages to decision makers, can be powerful catalysts for change. The International Obesity Taskforce developed a set of principles (the Sydney Principles) to guide substantial reductions in marketing to children, which underwent a global consultation process and is now calling for an international code to embody the principles for national governments to incorporate into regulations.[15]

Food marketing to children

Given the importance of protecting children and the present priority given to addressing the need to limit the food marketing to children, we discuss these issues in greater detail in this chapter. Additional practical approaches and policies to achieve this are provided in Chapters 15 and 28.

Today's children live in a media-saturated environment where media, celebrity, shopping brand names and aggressive marketing practices are ubiquitous and are creating the "commercialization of childhood". Central to this development is children's role in defining family purchases and their direct access to income.[16] Children have become a valuable target for advertisers as they represent a fast-growing market-segment. However, this is not new; the advertising industry has a long-standing history of targeting children as food consumers. In 1916, the advertising traders' journal *Printers Ink* ran an advertisement by a children's magazine, *St Nicholas*, criticizing a nameless food company for not joining the efforts of other companies already targeting 9–17-year-olds.[17] By the 1920s, the Cream of Wheat campaign was making functional claims, warning that, "Children are often slow to learn and intellectually simple because they have not eaten the right kind of breakfast." By the early 1930s, advertisements were promising good nutrition and suggesting that food was effective for peaceful parenting.[17] More recently, the WHO expert consultation on diet, nutrition and prevention of chronic disease (TRS 916) categorized aggressive food marketing to children as a probable determinant of childhood overweight and obesity.[16] The impact of marketing and television viewing, in light of the childhood obesity epidemic affecting children globally and specially lower-income and under-served minorities, was also recognized.

Children's exposure to marketing

In the USA, children between the ages of 4 and 12 spent a reported $6.1 billion in purchases from their own money in 1989, $23.4 billion in 1997, and $30 billion in 2002.[18] A third of children's total expenditures is on sweets, snacks and beverages, making up the largest product category for spending.[16] The food industry is a major player in the field of advertising. For every $1 spent by the World Health Organization (WHO) on trying to improve the nutrition of the world's population, $500 is spent by the food industry on promoting processed food.[19] Total UK advertising spending per annum in the categories of food, soft drinks and chain restaurants is £743 million, with £522 million spent on television advertising and £32 million spent in children's airtime.[20] In the United States, the food and beverage industries spend more than $10 billion per year on marketing to children. American children receive an average 65 messages from television advertising every day (about half are for food) with numerous additional marketing messages from websites, schools and in retail stores.[21] For now, television remains one of the most influential sources of communication despite the introduction of other technological advances such as the Internet and the mobile phone, presently also used for marketing purposes.[22] Television is both the main electronic medium with which children engage,[23] and the primary source of advertising used by the food industry.

A 1996 a cross-cultural study of children's television in 13 industrialized countries found that food advertising accounted for almost half of all advertising broadcast and represented by far the largest category of advertisements shown during children's TV viewing times.[24] The study demonstrated that over half of all food advertisements were dominated by confectionary, pre-sweetened breakfast cereals and fast food restaurants. Savoury snacks, high-sugar dairy products, ready prepared foods, soft drinks, cakes, biscuits and desserts were also often advertised in most countries.[19] In America, where most children who are at risk of becoming obese are African American children[25] from low-income families,[26] African American prime-time television shows contain 60% more food commercials (fast food, candy and snacks) compared with general prime-time market shows.[27]

The impact of food marketing to children

Central to the discussion around the impact of limiting food advertising to young children is the nature of children's comprehension of advertising.[28] Food advertising to young children draws considerable public concern. Numerous studies have documented that young children whose advertising literacy is lower are more susceptible to media effects.[29,30] Prior to age 7 or 8 years, children tend to view advertising as fun and do not tend to differentiate advertising from programs, regarding advertising as entertaining, unbiased information.[29,31]

The majority of studies on the effect of television food advertising on children's food choices were North American, and took place during in the 1970s and 1980s. Goldberg's study[32] in Quebec demonstrated that the more television advertisements a child sees for sugared cereals, the more likely the product will be present in the household. Taras et al[32,33] found that for children aged 4 to 8, weekly television viewing time was significantly correlated with requests for specified advertised products as well as overall energy intake. Borzekowski and Thomas's experiment[34] demonstrated with 2- to 6-year-old low-income children that even a brief exposure to food advertisements led children to choose advertised products more often. Recently, Hastings et al[35] systematically reviewed the effects of advertising on food consumption in children, concluding that food promotion has an effect on their preferences, purchase behavior and consumption.

In contrast, Livingstone and Helsper suggest that the effects of television advertising on young children's (2–6-year-olds) food choice are weak, concluding that young children are no more affected by advertising than teenagers. They asserted that if children of all ages, at different stages of advertising literacy are similarly influenced by advertising, then this must mask some underlying differences in persuasion.[31] Livingstone and Helsper applied the Elaboration Likelihood Model of Persuasion,[36] which holds that the process responsible for advertisement effectiveness is one of two routes to persuasion. The first, known as the "central route", involves effortful cognitive activity, whereby the person focuses their attention on message relevant information and draws on prior experience and knowledge to assess and elaborate on the presented information. The other mode of persuasion is known as the "peripheral route", whereby a person does not think much about message content but they may be still persuaded by non-content elements (peripheral cues).[37] They suggest that younger children are more likely to be persuaded by the peripheral route and teenagers are more likely to be persuaded by the central route. Young children, as less media-literate viewers, are more interested in such peripheral cues such as celebrity sources, jingles and colorful and entertaining images.[31] As Fischer et al[38] demonstrated, 2–6-year-olds can recognize well-known brand names and associate them with products particularly when brands use visual cues such as bright color, pictures and cartoon characters.[39]

References

1 Lobstein T, Bauer L, Uauy R: Counting the costs: the physical, psychosocial and economic consequences of childhood obesity. *Obes Rev* 2004; **5**:4–32.

2 Lobstein T, Baur L, Uauy R: Obesity in children and young people: a crisis in public health. *Obes Rev* 2004; **5** (Suppl. 1):4–104.

3 Wang Y, Lobstein T: Worldwide trends in childhood overweight and obesity. *Int J Pediatr Obes* 2006; **1**(1):11–25.

4 Jones A, Bentham G, Foster C, Hillsdon M, Panter J: Obesogenic Environments Evidence Review: Office of Science and Innovation, Foresight Tackling Obesities: Future Choices project.

5 Moodie R, Swinburn B, Richardson J, Somaini B: Childhood obesity—a sign of commercial success but market failure. *Int J Pediatr Obes* 2006; **1**(3):133–138.

6 Magarey AM, Daniels LA, Boulton TJ, Cockington RA: Predicting obesity in early adulthood from childhood and parental obesity. *Int J Obes Relat Metab Disord* 2003; **27**(4):505–513.

7 Power C, Li L, Manor O, Davey Smith G: Combination of low birth weight and high adult body mass index: at what age is it established and what are its determinants? *J Epidemiol Community Health* 2003; **57**:969–973.

8 Corvalan C, Dangour AD, Uauy R: Need to address all forms of childhood malnutrition with a common agenda. *Arch Dis Child* 2008; **93**:361–362.

9 Uauy R, Kain J: The epidemiological transition: need to incorporate obesity prevention into nutrition programmes. *Public Health Nutr* 2002; **5**(1a):223–229.

10 Albala C, Vio F, Kain J, Uauy R: Nutrition transition in Chile: determinants and consequences. *Public Health Nutr* 2002; **5**(1A):123–128.

11 Campbell K, Crawford D: Family food environments as determinants of preschool-aged children's eating behaviours: implications for obesity prevention policy: a review. *Aust J Nutr Diet* 2001; **58**(1):19–25.

12 Campbell KJ, Crawford DA, Salmon J, Carver A, Garnett SP, Baur LA: Associations between the home food environment and obesity-promoting eating behaviors in adolescence. *Obesity* (Silver Spring, Md) 2007; **15**(3):719–730.

13 Swinburn B, Gill T, Kumanyika S: Obesity prevention: a proposed framework for translating evidence into action. *Obes Rev* 2005; **6**(1):23–33.

14 World Health Organization: Prevention and control of noncommunicable diseases: implementation of the global strategy. Report by the Secretariat. 2008. www.who.int/gb/ebwha/pdf_files/A61/A61_8-en.pdf (accessed 15 December 2008).

15 Swinburn B, Sacks G, Lobstein T et al: The 'Syndey Principles' for reducing the commercial promotion of foods and beverages to children. *Public Health Nutr* 2008; 881–886.

16 Kelly B, Chapman K: Food references and marketing to children in Australian magazines: a content analysis. *Health Promot Int* 2007; **22**(4):284–291.

17 Lovett L: The popeye principle: selling child health in the first nutrition crisis. *J Health Polit Policy Law* 2005; **30**(5):803–838.

18 Schor J, Ford M: From tastes great to cool: children's food marketing and the rise of the symbolic. *J Law Med Ethics* 2007; **35**(1):10–21.

19 Dalmeny K, Hanna E, Lobstein T: Broadcasting Bad Health: Why Food Marketing to Children Needs to be Controlled. The International Association of Consumer Food Organizations, 2003.

20 Office of communications (Ofcom). Childhood Obesity—Food Advertising in Context: Children's Food Chioices, Parents' Understanding and Influence, and the Role of Food Promotions. United Kingdom: Office for communications, 2004.

21 Batada A, Wootan M: Nickelodeon markets nutrition-poor foods to children. *Am J Prev Med* 2007; **33**(1):48–50.

22 Kunkel D, Gantz W: Children's television advertising in the multichannel environment. *J Commun* 1992; **42**(3): 134–152.

23 Linn S: Food marketing to children in the context of a marketing maelstrom. *J Public Health Policy* 2004; **25**(3–4): 367–378.

24 Dibb S: A spoonful of sugar: television food advertising aimed at children: An international comparative survey. UK: Consumers International, 1996.

25 Strauss R, Pollack H: Epidemic increase in childhood overweight, 1986–1998. *JAMA* 2001; **286**:2845–2848.

26 Sherry B, Mei Z, Scanlon K, Mokdad A, Grummer-Strawn L: Trends in state-specific prevalence of overweight and underweight in 2-through 4-year-old children from low-income families from 1989 through 2000. *Arch Pediatr Adolesc Med* 2004; **158**(12):1116–1124.

27 Henderson V, Kelly B: Food advertising in the age of obesity: content analysis of food advertising on general market and African American television. *J Nutr Educ Behav* 2005; **37**(4):191–196.

28 Story M, French S. Food advertising and marketing directed at children and adolescents in the US. *Int J Behav Nutr Phys Act* 2004; **1**(1):3.

29 John D: Consumer socialization of children: a retrospective look at twenty-five years of research. *J Consum Res* 1999; **26**(3):183–213.

30 Strasburger V: Children and TV advertising: nowhere to run, nowhere to hide. *J Dev Behav Pediatr* 2001; **22**(3): 185–187.

31 Livingstone S, Helsper E. Does advertising literacy mediate the effects of advertising on children? A critical examination of two linked research literatures in relation to obesity and food choice. *J Commun* 2006; **56**(3):560–584.

32 Goldberg M: A quasi-experimental assessing the effectiveness of TV advertising directed to children. *J Mark Res* 1990; **27**(4):445–454.

33 Taras H, Sallis J, Patterson T, Nader P, Nelson J: Television's influence on children's diet and physical activity. *J Dev Behav Pediatr* 1989; **10**(4):176–180.

34 Borzekowski D, Robinson T: The 30-second effect an experiment revealing the impact of television commercials on food preferences of preschoolers. *J Am Diet Assoc* 2001; **101**(1):42–46.

35 Hastings G, Stead M, McDermott L et al: Review of Research on the Effects of Food Promotion to Children. Glasgow: University of Strathclyde, 2003.

36 Petty R, Cacioppo J: Communication and Persuasion: Central and Peripheral Routes to Attitude Change. New York: Springer, 1986.

37 Lien N: Elaboration likelihood model in consumer resesarch: a review. *Proc Natl Sci Counc ROC (C)* **11**(4):301–310.

38 Fischer P, Schwartz M, Richards J, Goldstein A, Rojas T: Brand logo recognition by children aged 3 to 6 years. Mickey Mouse and Old Joe the Camel. *JAMA* 1991; **266**(22):3145–3148.

39 Macklin M: Preschoolers learning of brand names from visual cues. *J Consum Res* 1996; **23**(3):251–261.

CHAPTER 4

No country for fat children? Ethical questions concerning community-based programs to prevent obesity

Marieke ten Have,[1] *Inez de Beaufort*[1] and *Søren Holm*[2,3]
[1] Department of Healthcare Ethics, Erasmus Medical Center, Rotterdam, The Netherlands
[2] Centre for Social Ethics and Policy, The University of Manchester, Manchester, UK
[3] Section for Medical Ethics, University of Oslo, Oslo, Norway

Summary

Make the healthy choice the ethical choice: introduction

A personal letter from the Department of Health warning parents of overweight children,[1] compulsory membership of a soccer club,[2] banning soft drinks vending machines in schools,[3] supervision for the parents of obese children:[2] What are the ethical issues when it comes to interventions and programs aimed at preventing or combating obesity in children? What questions should be asked and answered before embarking on the implementation of different measures? That is the subject of this chapter.

Convictions on balancing the responsibilities of parents, state and companies differ. We set out here to provide those who develop and implement certain measures with "tools" to take into account the ethical dimension of their work, not because they are immune, ignorant or unsympathetic to that dimension, but in order to structure the debate. While doing so, however, we do not pretend that evaluating ethical issues always leads to clear-cut and shared answers for practice.

Introduction

In order to illustrate our analysis, we use examples of different measures, selected from a wide range, varying from very general information to the public, to increasing the possibilities to adopt a more healthy lifestyle, to interference with family eating habits. Across this range, the ethical issues and balancing will be different. Some measures may not give rise to grave, or even any, ethical worries (e.g., increasing traffic safety in order to enable children to walk or cycle to school) whereas others are more difficult. We focus on the complex ones. Think of putting children on a weighing scale in front of their classmates during physical education lessons, health promotion campaigns with a negative and stigmatizing message about overweight, banning *all* unhealthy snacks that pupils bring from home (even sugared muesli bars),[4] forcing overweight children to participate in classes or even summer camps for weight loss,[5] and advising stomach surgery and weight-loss pills for obese children.[6]

We suggest six ethical issues that should be discussed before a program is launched. The aim of our endeavor is to stimulate and structure the debate on the ethical implications. We do not think that "prefab" ethical answers that everyone will agree with exist.

In the background are three general ethical themes: the effects of moral panics; responsibility; and children's right to protection from unhealthy commercial influences. Before discussing the six issues, we offer some remarks on these background themes. The first two background themes are discussed briefly. The third issue will be elaborated more extensively, since this is a central topic in the current debate.

Preventing Childhood Obesity. Edited by
E. Waters, B.A. Swinburn, J.C. Seidell and R. Uauy.
© 2010 Blackwell Publishing.

The bad effects of moral panics

A factor that complicates the ethical debate, but also lies at the heart of it, is the sense of urgency that sometimes borders on panic. Children are growing fatter – many children all over the world – and they will suffer the consequences. The spectre has been raised that whole generations will die younger and be outlived by their parents. This has led policy makers to identify childhood obesity as an important and urgent policy priority. In one sense, this identification is correct. Doing something about the problem is urgent; doing nothing would be forsaking our duty to protect the affected and at-risk children. But overstating the urgency, on the other hand, might also incline us to become less critical about evidence and about respecting important moral constraints when it comes to interference with lifestyles. The view that, "We have to do something now. Doing nothing is not an option" may blind us to the fact that doing something where we have very little evidence that it works is, apart from in a political sense, unlikely to be much better than doing nothing. And we also have to remember that doing something without sufficient evidence may later be proved to be a bad idea. A balance is necessary, but certainly difficult.

Responsibility and the complex causal network

Underlying many ethical issues in the obesity debate (such as stigmatization, justice and interference) is a fundamental debate concerning responsibility. Whose fault is it anyway? Who is to blame – the individual or his obesogenic environment (with lazy or opportunistic governments, industries who only want to sell their fattening products to gullible people etc.)?

But framing the question this way exposes it as a false dichotomy. The responsibility question is very hard and it cannot be answered by positing just two sets of actors with possible responsibility and then demanding a choice between them. The causal network leading to obesity in the individual child is almost always complex, and the more general causal network creating the observed increase in childhood obesity is even more complex and spans many sectors of society, including the family, the education system, the food industry, the media, the transport sector,

designers of the built environment, the government and others. There is no good reason to apportion primary responsibility for the childhood obesity problem to only one of these sectors.[7] All are to some degree responsible and all have to be ready to implement some changes. It may well be the case that parental behavior and habits are the main causal factors in most individual cases of childhood obesity, but that does not imply that parental behavior is the only or even most legitimate target for intervention. The cumulative effect of small causal contributions to many individual cases of obesity can justify targeting interventions at, for instance, soft drinks companies.

This complex causal network has led to busy washing of dirty hands, to the competition of measuring blame ("I'm to blame but he is more to blame" etc.) and to games of responsibility ping pong: "It is not me. No, it is you". For instance, the American campaign "Parents step up" focuses exclusively on parental responsibility. To quote from its television spot: "How could you let your kid be so overweight? … He could get diabetes or cancer or heart disease. And don't blame it on videogames or fast food, you're letting him down as a parent."[8]

Sometimes those who are blamed but feel they are unjustly blamed or exclusively blamed whereas others are as blameworthy, translate this into responsibility for the future. ("If I'm only 5% to blame, then I only have to contribute 5% to the solution.") This obviously does not contribute to any solution. It distracts. The debate would profit from focusing on *responsibility for contributions to solving the problem* rather arguing about *responsibility for causing the problem* and blame and retribution.

Children's right to protection from unhealthy commercial influences

Children have a right to be protected against unhealthy influences. The precise scope of this right is difficult to determine because of the wide spectrum of types of such influences.

However, if childhood obesity is a public health problem of such a magnitude that it justifies intervention in family life, it probably also justifies measures affecting companies. In modern societies, the freedom of action of commercial actors is circumscribed in many ways and the relevant question is, therefore, not whether such circumscription is ever warranted, but under what circumstances and for what purposes it can be justified.

Community-based interventions in relation to childhood obesity may target commercial actors like food producers, food retailers or the media. This may include measures such as differential sales taxes on high energy foods, planning requirements restricting the site of certain kinds of food outlets in relation to schools or sports fields, or specific labeling requirements. The more intrusive those measures are, the stronger the requirement that they are evidence-based.

Research suggests that up to 80% of today's children have diets that are considered "poor" or "in need of improvement".[9] According to the Global Prevention Alliance, it is widely acknowledged that marketing plays a significant role in determining children's dietary behavior and preferences, thereby undermining the objectives of the WHO Global Strategy on Diet, Physical Activity and Health.[10] Parents are misinformed by confusing information about the health value of food products. And children (who influence household purchase decisions at an estimated value of $500 billion annually) are tempted through commercial messages from children's icons and brightly colored packages that often include toys.[11] The strong negative influence on children's diets, suggests that marketing aimed at children should be circumscribed.

Some people argue that the problem is not so much about misleading information, but about people's lack of equipment to distinguish facts about nutrition from fiction. Therefore, one should empower children and parents to cope with the temptations that will always be present in a commercial society, among other things, by providing correct information about nutritional value.

Others, however, stress that it is an illusion to think that information provided by governments and consumer organizations can ever counter the effect of information provided by the food industry, as the budget of the latter is extremely small compared to that of the former.

To what extent can we restrict the promotion of unhealthy behavior by corporations? The level of marketing restrictions that is accepted by the public and is morally justifiable is different for different types of unhealthy behavior. With regard to smoking tobacco, current health policy is probably most restrictive. In many countries, commercials are completely banned. Marketing strategies to promote alcoholic beverages are generally not as strict: commercial messages are permitted, provided that they contain a warning message about health risks. However, with regard to foods and beverages that are high in saturated fat, sugar and salt, but of poor nutritional quality, there is hardly any boundary to the freedom of corporations. Most countries seem to accept misleading messages about the health value of products ("consuming this light drink is equivalent to going to the gym") and allow the promotion of chocolates, potato chips, soft drinks and large fast food meals. It is quite unthinkable that a ban on eating hamburgers or oversized ice creams in public spaces would be accepted at the present time. Why are some marketing strategies that promote unhealthy behavior granted more freedom than others?

The willingness to accept restrictions is influenced by the awareness of health risks. Twenty years ago, even non-smokers opposed paternalistic anti-tobacco measures. But now that the health risks of smoking are common knowledge, the current strict non-smoking policy evokes less criticism. The idea that food products rich in saturated fats and sugars pose a threat to our health is relatively new. It will take time for society to become fully aware of the urgency of the problem. The growing public awareness will surely influence the arguments about (unjustified) paternalistic meddling in commercial freedom.

Restrictive policy is also more easily accepted if an unhealthy behavior comes to be understood as non-essential or even unnecessary behavior. Whereas cigarettes and alcoholic beverages are "luxury products", eating is a primary need in life. It would be absurd to stop corporations from marketing and selling food products altogether. Admittedly, having breakfast with a bottle of cola and a king-size bag of chips cannot be considered necessary at all. But with regard to many food products, it is difficult to draw the line between necessary products with nutritional value and luxury products, which are bad for health. Is butter healthy or unhealthy? What about strawberry yoghurt, for example? Should we only allow commercials for sugar-free cereals and mineral water? The necessity of eating and the difficulty in drawing a clear line between healthy and unhealthy food may be a reason why food policy is not as restrictive as anti-smoking policy.

A third reason for restricting the promotion of some behavior more than others involves harm to other people. Smokers and drunken persons pose a threat to their environment. Consuming junk food and soft drinks is *not* dangerous for others. I do not get diabetes if my neighbor is a junk food addict. But, so one could argue: there are other costs involved, such as increased costs of the health care system. We will not go into that argument here,[12,13] but do want to mention that such harms are of a very different nature, compared to direct threats to the health and the safety of third parties.

The promotion of unhealthy products poses a specific threat to children. Children are vulnerable to influences from their environment. It is often more difficult for them to separate fact from fiction in commercial messages. They are not capable of making autonomous choices about their lifestyle. They are, to a great extent, dependent on their parents, who are also misled by commercial information. The vulnerable position of children provides a good reason for restricting the marketing of products that are high in saturated fat, sugar and salt, either directly targeted at children or via their parents. This was recognized in December 2007 when eleven major European food and beverage companies announced a common commitment to change the way they advertise to children. They declared that they would neither advertise food and beverage products in primary schools, nor to children under the age of 12 (except for products that fulfil specific nutrition criteria).[14]

So far we have covered the background themes. In the following sections we explore some ethical issues that should be raised, analysed and thoroughly discussed before implementing interventions to prevent childhood obesity.

Evidence

The first issue concerns evidence and good reasons:

Do we have enough evidence or good reasons to support the proposed program?

No conclusive evidence is available on the effectiveness of most measures to promote healthy behavior, but recent reports from (among others) WHO have

stated that the urgency of the problem makes waiting for such evidence undesirable.[15] Although this strategy is based on sound reasons, we should ensure that in the process of implementing interventions we are not over pressured by government, or panic, or by some other pressure because something has to be done now.

The less clear the benefits of a campaign are, the stronger the moral burdens weigh. This raises important questions regarding effectiveness. Is a campaign only effective if it creates weight loss? Or when it creates awareness? Or should it make people feel happier about their weight? How sure must we be about the effectiveness of a measure before implementing it? These are important issues to think about. It is important to realize that an intervention always creates costs, in financial terms but also in moral terms, by intervening in lifestyle. The benefits have to outweigh the burdens.

But in many cases we are not sure about the effectiveness and this does not automatically mean that a campaign should be stopped. In June 2007 government funding for a Dutch clinic for obese children was stopped because politicians claimed it was too costly to proceed without evidence. But others argued that as long as scientific evidence for long-term effects was lacking, we should rely on experiences, which suggested effectiveness. Accordingly, the project had to continue precisely to *gather* scientific evidence.[16] More generally, there is an obligation to rigorously evaluate the effectiveness of interventions for which there is currently little evidence, so that the evidence base can be improved over time.

Stigmatization

The second issue is stigmatization:

Does the program or intervention target obesity as a state of being or the underlying behavior? What are the consequences in terms of possible stigmatization?

Targeting obesity and the creation of stigma

Overweight and obese children face stigmatization every single day of their lives. They are bullied, laughed at, called names and associated with bad moral character traits (being lazy, stupid etc.). In thinking about interventions for treatment and prevention of obesity it is important to note that they must necessarily differ from interventions aimed at reducing tobacco use or excessive consumption of alcohol. Obesity is a state, not a behavior, and whereas the action of smoking can be targeted directly (e.g., it can be prohibited in public places) targeting obesity would target the obese person, not the behaviors leading to obesity. Focusing on obesity directly, instead of on behaviors that are healthy whether or not a person is obese (e.g., physical activity, eating a balanced diet) may increase the social stigma already attached to obesity.

Those measures that aim to promote a healthy life-style in general, without focusing on overweight or emphasizing obesity, are often more acceptable, not only from the point of view of stigmatization but also from the perspective of fairness, as all participants may benefit from such measures. Healthy lifestyles are, after all, also healthy for slim children. We are aware that this can be used as a sham argument: pre-tending that "of course it is not focusing on over-weight", although actually it is.

Targeting vulnerable groups is also sensitive from the stigmatization angle. ("You get breakfast at school because your parents don't care for you and they are poor.") Special attention to the justification and pos-sible effects is necessary. Targeting, however, may sometimes be necessary, even ethically required, in order to reach persons and groups that will not be reached by general measures or programs. For American Indian and Alaska Native children, The American National Centre for Chronic Disease Prevention and Health Promotion designed "The Eagle's Books" program. To quote from the program: "The eagle represents balance, courage, healing, strength and wisdom, and is seen as a messenger or a teacher. In the Eagle Book series, the wise bird teaches children how to use these values to prevent diabetes and grow safe and strong. ... Mr. Eagle reminds the young boy of the healthy ways of his ancestors."[17]

Will children across the whole BMI range profit from the measure (even if they do not lose weight) because the proposed measure increases their possibilities/options for a healthier lifestyle? Or will they just hear that they are too heavy?

Measures to do something about obesity might reinforce stigmatization as, whatever measures are proposed, the underlying idea is that children should *not* be overweight and certainly not fat. What does this mean for those who already are fat, for example, chil-dren that are born in families where everyone has been obese for generations and did very well, thank you? What price will such children pay if the strongly pro-moted image is that one should not be overweight? Take, for example, the Singaporean "Trim and fit" campaign, which mentions on its website that over-weight children "tend to be clumsy". Parents are informed that "trim and fit children" are not only healthier and feel better, but also look better.[18]

Programs like "Epode", the French cities that aim to be a motivating environment for a healthy life-style,[19] are interesting examples of programs that would provide positive answers to the above ques-tions. Another positive example is the "Kids in balance" campaign from the Netherlands, which offers workshops to promote an active lifestyle for children. It stresses emotional health, instead of focus-ing on overweight. To quote from the program: "Feeling good about yourself, being emotionally fit, is just as important as eating brown bread and doing sports!" Those who do not lose weight but do develop a healthier lifestyle are not stigmatized as the "losers", "the ones for whom the program did not work".[20]

Several experts argue that negative, stigmatizing and scary campaigns are not only ethically problem-atic but also ineffective. Instead, people need positive tools and motivation to work on behavior change.

Parental involvement

The third cluster of questions has to do with parents.

In some cases, individual parental involvement is not an issue as the measure is on a very general level, for example, restricting commercials for sweets on television at certain hours. Parents are involved in a general way as citizens, of course, but not in a more personal, individual way. Other interventions, however, do involve the individual parents. After all, programs directed at informing children about a healthy diet and the importance of physical exercise are unlikely to be sufficient as long as the parents are not involved. What is the use of knowing that vegeta-bles contain vitamins when all that is ever offered at home are French fries?

Is it possible to inform and/or involve parents without undermining their parental autonomy? Can they be involved in a respectful way? Can they be convinced instead of overruled or bypassed?

Interventions that involve the individual parents vary from cooking classes in the local supermarket to supervision from social workers in families, or even putting obese children into care.[21] The balance between parental autonomy and the interests of the child, in particular with regard to health, is an important area of the ethical debate. It is an issue that is debated in many different fields: from child abuse, refusal of vaccination, school and leisure, to choices of diet. Parents need (and have the right) to raise their children in their own way, according to their views on what is proper or good for children. Interference against their will is controlled and limited to serious cases where the interests of a child leave no other option. What can be done if parents do not provide breakfast, give the child some money to buy a hamburger for breakfast and the kitchen is stocked with soft drinks and junk food, whereas apples are considered to be something exotic that led to dire consequences in paradise, anyway?

Programs can also involve parents in a harmless way, such as the Australian "Walking school bus" campaign, where parents take turns to accompany their children to school.[22] There are programs where schools provide what the parents do not provide, compensating for what is absent at home: for example, breakfast in the classroom, tasting classes, cooking classes, subsidized fruit and vegetables during school breaks.

And programs are often directed at informing the parents. Take, for example, the "Hello World!" campaign that provides information for future parents, such as health quizzes by email that can be stopped if they are unwelcome.[23] This kind of campaign enables parents, or is aimed at enabling them, with the possibilities to provide themselves what is good for their child. They may already know, but might simply not manage.

Are parents' arguments and reasons for having a particular lifestyle analysed and taken seriously?

Many, probably most, parents do want the best for their children and are not a priori against information and options to do the best for their children.

What if parents just do not change their lifestyle? Think of parents who during lunchtime brought their children hamburgers because they thought the lunches provided by Jamie Oliver, the well-known television cook who is campaigning for healthy food for young people in the UK, were not good, not enough, not good enough for their children. Is their right to respect for parental autonomy undermined by what seems to be a lack of responsibility? An answer to this question will, at least partly, depend on why the parents behaved in this way. Had they been involved in discussions about the changes to the school meals, had their views been taken into account, had the children been involved, and so forth? The fact that parents or children react against imposed policies is only a sign of irresponsibility if they have at least been engaged in discussion about the policies and their rationale. To involve parents in a serious way is probably not only ethically right but also helpful from a strategic point of view.

Durable skills, habits, virtues

The fourth issue has to do with the durability of proposed skills, virtues and habits:

Will the children develop skills/virtues/habits that will also serve them later in life?

In every society, in every individual life, there will be temptation. To be equipped to deal with temptation is a good thing. (And by the way does not necessarily mean that one always has to say no and never yield to temptation … to choose to yield is very different from impulsive surrender.)

In the prevention of obesity there are also virtues at stake. Self-control and carefulness and the ability to say "no" are probably the most important – skills that are also relevant in relation to use of alcohol, safe sex, internet addiction, gambling, and so on. Teaching these skills means that children can learn something they can profit from and let others profit from for the rest of their lives.

But don't parents have the right to spoil their children and turn them into little manipulating spoiled brats (obese or not obese) if they want to? Why is self-control an important skill? It is important because people without self-control, or who are out of control, often end up in difficult and unpleasant social and emotional situations. One needs self-control in order to survive in a society, and in order for societies to survive. Self control is, to some extent, something one has to learn, from one's parents, among others. Parents do not mind saying "no" (or rather yelling "no") when a child is going to touch a hot stove, and the direct prevention of harm is at stake. But many parents find it more difficult when it comes to restricting or denying pleasures. However, this is something the child will have to accept in his or her life. If it is not "no" to the sweets, it will be "no" to something else. One will have to live with requests being refused from time to time.

This means that one has to illustrate the advantages of self-control: the enjoyment of tasting instead of the "mindless stuffing", the idea that you are not the victim of habit, feeling or an urge stronger than you, but that you are the master of yourself. That is a reward in itself. Also, control is more effective if embraced rather than imposed. Self-control actually increases freedom. And it also has to be compared to the alternatives: bariatric surgery at the age of 14 is not an attractive proposition.

This does not mean that one can rely on self-control and that it is, therefore, not necessary, for example, to remove soft drinks vending machines in schools. But removing the vending machines without changing the *idea* that one needs gallons of soft drinks every day is not helpful either.

However, we also want to stress that the importance of engendering self-control and carefulness in relation to eating should not be conceived in an overly moralistic frame. Many obese adults and children do exhibit self-control and carefulness even in their eating. Although they eat too much for their caloric needs they do so in a controlled way. They do not stuff themselves but have become habituated to eating large portions. So what is needed in many cases is to re-set the perception of what is a normal meal.

Proportionality

The fifth question concerns proportionality:

Is there a balance between the goals, the chosen methods and the possible ethical impact?

Can a certain goal be reached with less intrusive measures? For example, to take all children with a BMI above 28 out of parental care and raise them in foster families or clinics is clearly disproportional (apart from being quite unrealistic).

How can one evaluate proportionality? The Nuffield Council has designed a framework to evaluate public health measures that can be used in the debate. It is a ladder that indicates different levels of intrusiveness,

from "do nothing" up to "eliminate choice". The higher up the ladder, the more intrusive a program is and the stronger its justification needs to be.[24]

We want to emphasize the distinction of enabling versus enforcing.

Enabling versus enforcing

Enabling means that the opportunities are provided for children and parents to choose the healthy habit or lifestyle, whereas enforcing means they have no choice. There are important arguments to prefer enabling to enforcing. The chances that a certain healthy lifestyle or certain eating habits will be integrated, incorporated or embraced is greater if people themselves learn to appreciate them and feel better, enjoy the advantages, rather than when they feel they are submitting to dictates put upon them by others as the internal motivation may then be lacking.

Slippery slope

The sixth question regards the slippery slope:

Are the measures sensitive to the argument of the slippery slope?

The slippery slope concept is that if one measure or intervention is permitted then this will result in further, more intrusive measures being taken in the future which would then significantly infringe upon an important right or ethical principle, such as adults choosing whether to exercise or not. Fears of "1984", total health control, or moral imperialism are enlisted in this argument along with the notion that we will all die sooner or later and that there is no point in living a frugal life with no pleasures. These slippery slope fears are often accentuated when proposed interventions are either novel or vague in their definitions and boundaries.

In many areas of public health, especially for injury prevention, tobacco control, and to some extent infectious disease control, regulations are enacted which place restrictions on individual behaviours in addition to changing the environment. Influencing personal choices regarding behaviour is also used in the prevention of overweight. This varies from the subtle pushing message "Please take the stairs" that one may encounter as health promotion notices at the base of the stairs[25], to employers forcing their employees to walk by locating the cafeteria far away from the office building[26], to imposing a 'fat tax' on fattening foods[27], imposing higher insurance premiums for obese people[28] or banning cars from city centres and around schools[29].

With programs requiring physical exercise for obese adolescents in Singapore[30] and university diplomas being withheld from obese students in Pennsylvania[31], it is understandable that people are concerned about a slippery slope in directive programs for the prevention of obesity.

Although fear of a slippery slope does not imply that there is an actual risk of a slippery slope, it is important to discuss whether enough safeguards against heading down slippery slopes have been incorporated, and whether the limits of the intervention are clearly communicated to the public.

Conclusion

These six issues are aimed at inspiring and structuring debate on the ethical presuppositions and goals of measures. They are not a simple set of criteria to be passed in order to have ethical "approval".

Within the process of developing and testing interventions to prevent overweight among children, it is crucial to pay attention to their normative aspects. Ethical analysis will help to develop measures in line with values that are deeply important to many of us. That analysis is worthwhile in its own right, and may also contribute to effectiveness.

References

1 Elliot F: Parents of fat children to be given a warning. *The Times*, 2007 (22 October). www.timesonline.co.uk (accessed 9 July 2008).

2 Simpson J: Lose weight or we'll take all six of your children away: outrage over social workers' "draconian ultimatum" to parents. *The Daily Mail*, 2008 (24 March). www.dailymail.co.uk (accessed 9 July 2008).

3 Johnson A: Setting the standard for school food. Department for Children, Schools and Families. 2006 (19 May). www.dfes.gov.uk/pns/DisplayPN.cgi?pn_id=2006_0074 (accessed 9 July 2008).

4 CBBC Newsround. School bans all unhealthy snacks (updated 31 August 2005). http://news.bbc.co.uk/cbbcnews/ (accessed 9 July 2008).

5 Walsh B: Singapore shapes up: the lion city's aggressive government programs show the benefits of a concerted, nationwide war on fat. *Time Asia Magazine*. 2004 (1 November). www.time.com/time/asia/covers/501041108/obesity_singapore.html (accessed 9 July 2008).

6 Hall S: Stomach surgery and drugs for children to tackle obesity epidemic. *The Guardian*. 2006 (13 December). www.guardian.co.uk (accessed 9 July 2008).

7 Holm S: Parental responsibility and obesity in children. *Public Health Ethics* 2008; **1**:21–29.

8 Parents step up. Parents Step Up/Familias en Marcha, an innovative, bilingual, childhood obesity public information campaign in South Florida. 2005. www.parentsstepup.com/ad.html (accessed 9 July 2008).

9 Nestle, M: What to Eat: An Aisle-By-Aisle Guide to Savvy Food Choices and Good Eating. New York: North Point Press 2006.

10 United Nations system of organizations. Global Prevention Alliance: Call to action on the marketing to foods and beverages to children. 2006. www.unsystem.org/scn/Publications/AnnualMeeting/SCN34/global_prevention_alliance.doc (accessed 9 July 2008).

11 Mikkelsen L, Merlo C, Lee, V, Chao C: Where's the fruit? Fruit content of the most highly advertised children's food and beverages. Prevention Institute. 2008 Jan. www.preventioninstitute.org/sa/fruit/wheresthefruit.pdf (accessed 9 July 2008).

12 De Beaufort ID: Individual responsibility for health. In: Bennett R, Erin CA eds. HIV and AIDS, Testing, Screening and Confidentiality. New York: Oxford University Press, 1999:107–24.

13 ten Have M, de Beaufort ID: Hogere premies, goedkope worteltjes en bemoeizuchtige collega's: eigen verantwoordelijkheid in de aanpak van overgewicht [Personal responsibility in the prevention of overweight]. Hartbulletin, 2007 Aug; 38 (4).

14 Private Sector EU Pledge: Food and drink companies pledge to change advertising to children (Press Release) 2007 (11 December). www.fachverbandwerbung.at/mmdb/1/2/602.pdf (accessed 9 July 2008).

15 World Health Organization: Global strategy on diet, physical activity and health. 2004 May. www.who.int/dietphysicalactivity/strategy/eb11344/strategy_english_web.pdf (accessed 9 July 2008).

16 Berkeljon S, Vos C. Klink stopt financiering kliniek voor obesitas (Klink stops funding for obesity clinic). *De Volkskrant*. 2007 (8 June). www.volkskrant.nl (accessed 9 July 2008).

17 National Center for Chronic Disease Prevention and Health Promotion: The eagles nest campaign. 2007. www.cdc.gov/diabetes/eagle/index.html (accessed 9 July 2008).

18 Keep your child trim and fit. Program to prevent childhood obesity. www.hpb.gov.sg/health_articles/trim_and_fit/ (accessed 9 July 2008).

19 Ensemble, Prévenons l'Obésité des Enfants: Prevention progam in French cities. www.epode.fr (accessed 9 July 2008).

20 Balance Matters: Kids in balance campaign. www.balance-matters.org/index.php?option=com_content&task=view&id=12&Itemid=26 (accessed 9 July 2008).

21 Templeton, S-K. Fat boy may be put in care. *The Times*. 2007 Feb 25. www.timesonline.co.uk (accessed 9 July 2008).

22 Walking School Bus: Starting a walking school bus. www.walkingschoolbus.org (accessed 9 July 2008).

23 Hallo Wereld (Hello World): Education program via email. www.hallowereld.nl (accessed 9 July 2008).

24 Nuffield Council on Bioethics. Public health: ethical issues. 2007. www.nuffieldbioethics.org/go/ourwork/publichealth/introduction.html (accessed 9 July 2008).

25 'Promoting stair climbing: intervention effects generalize to a subsequent stair ascent.' Webb O.J., Eves F.F., *Am J Health Promot*. 2007 Nov–Dec; **22**(2):114–119.

26 Fight against fat shifting to the workplace. *New York Times* 2003 (12 October). http://www.nytimes.com/2003/10/12/us/fight-against-fat-shifting-to-the-workplace.html (accessed 27 November 2009).

27 http://en.wikipedia.org/wiki/Fat_tax. (accessed 24 May 2009).

28 Insurers pile pounds on the overweight. *The Guardian* 2006 (1 January). http://www.guardian.co.uk/money/2006/jan/01/observercashsection.healthinsurance, (accessed 27 November 2009). Extra weight, higher costs. *The New York Times*, 2006 (2 December). http://www.nytimes.com/2006/12/02/business/02money.html?_r=1&pagewanted=print (accessed 27 November 2009).

29 Pupils get the measure of the walk to school. Gateshead Council 2008, (5 November). http://www.gateshead.gov.uk/Council%20and%20Democracy/news/News%20Articles/Pupils%20Get%20the%20Measure%20of%20the%20Walk%20to%20School.aspx (accessed 27 November 2009).

30 http://en.wikipedia.org/wiki/Trim_and_Fit, accessed at may 24, 2009, School link to eating disorders possible, Sandra Davie, *The Straits Times*, 2005 (16 May). http://www.moe.gov.sg/media/forum/2005/forum_letters/20050520.pdf (accessed 31 January 2010).

31 Rebecca R. Ruiz. A University Takes Aim at Obesity. *The New York Times* (27 November 2009), http://thechoice.blogs.nytimes.com/2009/11/27/a-university-takes-aim-at-obesity/?scp=1&sq=lincoln%20university%20overweight%20diploma&st=cse (accessed 3 December 2009).

CHAPTER 5

A human rights approach to childhood obesity prevention

Naomi Priest,[1] *Boyd Swinburn*[2] *and Elizabeth Waters*[1]
[1] Jack Brockoff Child Health and Wellbeing Program, McCaughey Centre, Melbourne School of Population Health, University of Melbourne, Melbourne, Australia
[2] WHO Collaborating Centre for Obesity Prevention, Deakin University, Melbourne, Australia

Summary

- Three sets of human rights are relevant to childhood obesity: UN Convention on the Rights of the Child (UNCROC), the right to adequate food, and the right to health.
- Within UNCROC, the "developmental rights" (right to develop to the fullest and the right to protection from harmful influences, abuse and exploitation) are to protect children from circumstances injurious to their well-being.
- The marketing of unhealthy food and beverages to children is an example of commercial exploitation of children.
- The right to adequate food was originally aimed at preventing undernutrition and food insecurity, but has now been broadened to include overnutrition in vulnerable populations.
- It is the right of everyone to enjoy the highest attainable standard of physical and mental health, and for children this may include freedom from obesity.
- The use of a human rights approach to preventing childhood obesity helps to ensure that the debates and actions centre on what is best for children and the Sydney Principles to guide substantial reductions in food marketing of unhealthy foods that targets children is one example of such an application.

Preventing Childhood Obesity. Edited by
E. Waters, B.A. Swinburn, J.C. Seidell and R. Uauy.
© 2010 Blackwell Publishing.

Introduction

The relationship between human rights and health is one that is now increasingly discussed throughout the world and rights-based approaches to public health issues are being promoted as having much to contribute to addressing health inequalities and achieving sustainable gains in population health.[1-4] To date, this relatively recent consideration of the relationship between human rights and health has largely concentrated on the right of individuals to health care and treatment and on the protection of individuals from physical harm.[5] For example, rights-based approaches have been used to advocate for strengthened health care systems, to target maternal mortality and reproductive health, mental health care, and neglected diseases, and to raise the profile of underlying determinants such as the right to water and sanitation.[6-10] The work of the UN Special Rapporteur on the right to health, a position established in 2002, has done much to promote greater global attention to health and human rights.[11] However, the health sector has also recently been critiqued for its relative silence on human rights, with the suggestion that there is a general lack of awareness within the field regarding human rights and what they mean in practice.[1]

Human rights are essentially freedoms and entitlements that are concerned with protecting the inherent dignity and quality of all human beings, and encompass civil, political, economic, social and cultural rights.[12,13] While human rights are inspired by, and grounded upon, moral values such as dignity, equality and access to justice they are also guaranteed legally and reinforced by international and national legal obligations.[2] The Universal Declaration of Human Rights (UDHR) ratified in 1948 is the foundation of international human rights law, and was the first global statement to recognize the inherent dignity and equality of all human beings.[14] Subsequently, however, in the context of Cold War tensions, human rights became polarized into two separate categories as States prepared to turn the provisions of the Declaration into binding law.[2] The West claimed civil and political rights were primary with economic and social rights mere aspirations; the Eastern bloc argued that civil and political rights were secondary to the essential rights to food, health and education.[2] As a result, in 1966 two separate treaties were formed—the International Covenant on Economic, Social and Cultural Rights (IESCR)[15] and the International Covenant on Civil and Political Rights (ICCPR).[16] Since then, human rights have been reiterated by numerous international treaties, declarations and resolutions that protect human rights to varying degrees.[13]

International human rights treaties, commonly referred to as covenants or conventions, are legally binding on States that ratify them while conversely, human rights declarations are non-binding, although many encompass principles that are consistent with binding customary international law.[2,13] Traditionally, human rights have focused on the relationship between the State and individuals, with those States that have ratified international human rights treaties assuming obligations that are binding under international law to effect the human rights outlined within them. Additionally, some States have national laws protecting some human rights; and some explicitly protect human rights within their constitutions.[2,13]

It is in this global context that the application of a human rights approach to childhood obesity prevention is gaining attention and is advocated as a particular lens through which childhood obesity prevention can be viewed.[5,17,18] Such an approach is increasingly considered as having an important contribution to make, although it is also acknowledged that a rights approach is likely to be most effective when utilized in combination with other paradigms.[17]

Human rights declarations applicable to childhood obesity

Within the array of human rights declarations, conventions and resolutions three are of particular relevance to the issue of childhood obesity: the UN Convention on the Rights of the Child,[19] the right to adequate food,[15] and the right to health.[20]

UN Convention on the Rights of the Child

The Convention on the Rights of the Child[19] was adopted and ratified by the United Nations in 1989 and is the first international instrument to incorporate the full range of human rights—civil, cultural, economic, political and social rights specifically in relation to children.[21] It was developed in recognition of a need for children to have a convention explicitly acknowledging that they often need special care and attention that adults do not, and was motivated by a desire to increase international awareness that children have human rights as well as adults.[21]

The Convention on the Rights of the Child outlines these rights in 54 articles and two Optional Protocols, and identifies basic human rights for all children: the right to survival; to develop to the fullest; to protection from harmful influences, abuse and exploitation; and to participate fully in family, cultural and social life. Four core principles of the Convention on the Rights of the Child are also identified: non-discrimination; devotion to the best interests of the child; the right to life, survival and development; and respect for the views of the child.[19]

Particular rights outlined in the Convention on the Rights of the Child pertinent to childhood obesity prevention are the right to develop to the fullest and the right to protection from harmful influences, abuse and exploitation. These can be considered "developmental rights" where the underlying interest is to protect children from circumstances injurious to their well-being and ensure they are not exposed to risks which they do not have the adult capacity to appraise.[5] It has been argued that more effective strategies for addressing childhood obesity can be developed and enacted by articulating the issue as one of children's rights, not just of public health, and that the articles of UNCROC provide a useful template for coordinated interdisciplinary and strategic action.[22]

One way in which this rights-based framework has been used in the context of childhood obesity prevention is in relation to food advertising to children on television.[5] For example, arguments against food advertising to children have been made on the premise that children have less capacity than adults to comprehend completely the intent or persuasive nature of advertising, and consequently are less able to form critical assessments of advertisements.[23]

Framing arguments against food advertising to children using a rights-based discourse has also been suggested to provide a strong rebuttal to counter claims in a number of ways.[5] For example, the assertion that children would suffer from poorly funded television programming due to lost revenue is argued as being far less appealing when it then becomes an argument that the cost of children having television programs made for them is that they are exposed to harm.[5] In a similar vein, contentions from the advertising sector that it would be pointless to ban television advertising to children because they would still be exposed to food advertising in program content, adult time slots and in other media[24] are also claimed to be made irrelevant by a rights-based approach.[5] Furthermore, it is also argued that if food advertising to children is determined to be injurious to their health, and thus counter to their right to protection, bans on such advertising should be made without the need to provide empirical evidence that bans will decrease obesity rates.[5]

A recent practical application of UNCROC and a children's rights approach to childhood obesity prevention has been their use in framing a set of seven principles (The Sydney Principles) to guide action on reducing food and beverage marketing to children through television and other media with the ultimate intent of forming an International Code on Food and Beverage Marketing to Children.[18]

The right to adequate food

The right to adequate food has been considered a human right since it was first articulated internationally in the UDHR in 1948. Article 25 of the UDHR[14] and Article 11 of the IESCR[15] state that

> Everyone has the right to a standard of living adequate for the health and well-being of himself and of his family, including food, clothing, housing …

Historically, this right to adequate food has largely been interpreted and applied in the context of freedom from hunger and undernutrition, the right to food in emergencies and to issues of food access and food security.[25,26] In 2000 the term "food" was identified as covering both solid foods as well as clean drinking water as an essential component of healthy nutrition.[27] It is now argued that a right to food approach encompasses not only these critical issues of freedom from hunger and of food security, but also should require States to respect and protect consumers and to promote good nutrition, including protecting the poor and vulnerable from unsafe food and inadequate diets and helping to address obesity.[28] The Right to Food Voluntary Guidelines produced by the Food and Agriculture Organization (FAO) of the United Nations explicitly places this issue on its right to food agenda with Guideline 10.2:

> States are encouraged to take steps, in particular through education, information and labeling regulations, to prevent overconsumption and unbalanced diets that may lead to malnutrition, obesity and degenerative diseases.[29]

This guideline clearly places obesity and some of its underlying determinants alongside those of malnutrition, and reframes the way in which the right to food is conceptualized. At present, these guidelines are voluntary and non-binding and hence States have no legal obligation to meet them nor are they enforceable. However, they do provide a platform from which to engage and develop further rights-based approaches to childhood obesity prevention and firmly place responsibility on states for the provision of education, responsible food labeling, and the prevention of obesity through poor diet and food consumption. The right of children and adolescents to adequate food was also extended to include a right to be free from obesity and related diseases by the UN System Standing Committee on Nutrition in 2007, along with a call for international regulation of marketing to children of food and beverages.[30] The extent to which action at a legislative and policy level to address these determinants of childhood obesity can be supported and strengthened by a right to food approach is an area for further exploration throughout the international community.

The right to health

The right to health, or in its fullest form, the right to the highest attainable standard of health, was first expressed in the constitution of the WHO in 1946.[31] It was restated in the 1978 Declaration of Alma Ata and again in the World Health Declaration adopted in 1998 by the World Health Assembly.[32] Within international human rights law, the right to the highest attainable standard of health is outlined within the UDHR[14] and subsequently reiterated in Article 12 of UESCR which states that:

> Parties to the present Covenant recognize the right of everyone to the enjoyment of the highest attainable standard of physical and mental health.[15]

This right to health is thus a claim to a set of social conditions, including norms, institutions, laws and an enabling environment that can best secure the realization of this right.[2] The nature of the right to health was further clarified in 2000 with the adoption of a General Comment on the right to health by the Committee on Economic, Social and Cultural rights which monitors the Covenant.[20] This General Comment recognized the close relationship between the right to health and other human rights including, but not limited to, the right to food, housing, work, education, participation, non-discrimination, equality and the prohibition of torture. In this way, the right to health was interpreted as including not only appropriate and timely health care, but also the underlying determinants of health.[2]

The need for the right to health to be universally recognized and understood as a fundamental human right has recently been reiterated with the sixtieth anniversary of UDHR.[1,3] Doing so, it is argued, acknowledges the need for a strong social commitment to good health and thus should be included in national and international health policy.[3] The implications of the right to health, and its expanded focus to include underlying determinants of health, for childhood obesity prevention are yet to be fully explored as the wider public health community grap-

ples with the translation of rights-based frameworks into practice.

Approaches to incorporating human rights into childhood obesity prevention

What then does a rights-based approach mean, in practice, to childhood obesity prevention beyond, as others have said,[4] "having a good heart behind efforts and actions"? It is claimed that one key contribution of human rights to public health is the provision of a persuasive argument for government responsibility to not only provide health services but also to address underlying determinants of health such as poverty, deprivation, marginalization and discrimination.[4] In the context of childhood obesity, this challenges the placing of responsibility for childhood obesity prevention within the family context[33] and clearly makes it an issue of governmental concern. In this way, a rights-based approach to childhood obesity can form the basis for action at a societal level, which is vital, given that childhood obesity is now widely recognized as a "societal rather than a medical problem".[17]

One argument against a human rights approach to health is the lack of binding legislation demanding that they be achieved.[3] While this issue of enforcement does create real challenges, this does not mean that rights-based approaches should be abandoned or dismissed as idealistic and unfeasible. Human rights provide an important overarching framework, or "parent" to guide legislation[34] as well as many other ways of furthering the cause of particular rights.[3] Legislation is not the only requirement for the fulfillment of rights; rather public discussion, social monitoring, investigative reporting and social work all have critical roles to play.[35]

Advocacy using a language of human rights, including those outlined within UNCROC, as well as the right to adequate food and the right to health, is a powerful way of drawing attention to issues related to childhood obesity prevention. This might include mobilizing public opinion and advocating for governmental and institutional changes to implement rights, even if they are not yet legally established.[4] Such advocacy can play an important role in moving such institutions towards a situation where human rights are legally enforceable.[4] Already, within childhood obesity prevention the ongoing work regarding marketing to children using a human rights framework provides an example of such advocacy in action. Similar advocacy is possible using a human rights approach to address other factors contributing to childhood obesity, such as safe spaces for physical activity and access to healthy food alternatives. Using the language of a rights-based approach for protecting children may help to avert the alternative risk-based approach where the health outcomes for children are somehow supposed to be balanced against the profitability of the industries developing and marketing unhealthy foods.

Conclusions

Consideration of human rights as they apply to childhood obesity prevention is an important area of work. Application of rights-based approaches to addressing childhood obesity are emerging internationally, and have so far largely focused on addressing issues of food marketing to children. Advocacy using the language of human rights as it applies to other determinants of childhood obesity prevention is suggested as having much to contribute towards addressing this issue, given that framing childhood obesity within a rights context firmly places responsibility at a governmental level rather than with families or individuals. Further exploration is needed to actualize such approaches in order to achieve positive outcomes for children.

References

1 Editorial. The right to health: from rhetoric to reality. *Lancet* 2008; **372**:2001.
2 World Health Organization: Questions and Answers on Health and Human Rights. Geneva: WHO, 2002.
3 Sen A.: Why and how is health a human right? *Lancet* 2008; **372**(9655):2010.
4 Gruskin S, Tarantola D: Health and human rights: overview. In: Heggenhougen K, Quah S eds. International Encyclopedia of Public Health. San Diego: Academic Press, 2008: 137–146.
5 Ingleby R, Prosser L, Waters E: UNCROC and the prevention of childhood obesity: the right not to have food advertisements on television. *J Law Med* 2008; **16**(1):49–56.
6 Hunt P, Bueno de Mesquita J.: Reducing Maternal Mortality. Colchester UK: University of Essex, 2008.
7 World Health Organization: WHO Resource Book on Mental Health, Human Rights and Legislation, World Health Organization, 2005.
8 Hunt P, Steward R, Bueno de Mesquita J, Oldring L.: Neglected Diseases: A Human Rights Analysis. Colchester Essex: University of Essex, 2007.
9 Pillay N.: Right to health and the Universal Declaration of Human Rights. *Lancet* 2008; **372**(9655):2005–2006.
10 Hunt P, Backman G: Health Systems and the Right to the Highest Attainable Standard of Health. Colchester, UK: Human Rights Centre, University of Essex, 2008.
11 Office of the United Nations High Commissioner for Human Rights: Human Rights Council Resolution 6/29 Special Rapporteur on the Right of Everyone to the Enjoyment of the Highest Attainable Standard of Physical and Mental Health United Nations, 2007.
12 Office of the United Nations High Commissioner for Human Rights and the United Nations Staff College Project: Human Rights: A Basic Handbook for UN Staff. United Nations, 1999.
13 Office of the United Nations High Commissioner for Human Rights: What are human rights? United Nations. www2.ohchr.org (accessed 8 December 2008).
14 United Nations: Universal Declaration of Human Rights. United Nations. 1948 www.unhchr.ch (accessed 8 December 2008).
15 United Nations: International Covenant on Economic, Social and Cultural Rights. United Nations, 1966.
16 United Nations: International Covenant on Civil and Political Rights. Adopted and Opened for Signature, Ratification and Accession by General Assembly Resolution 2200A (XXI) of 16 December 1966 Entry into Force 23 March 1976, in Accordance with Article 49. New York: United Nations, 1966.
17 Swinburn B.: Obesity prevention in children and adolescents. *Child Adolesc Psychiatr Clin N Am* 2009; **18**(1): 209–223.
18 Swinburn B, Sacks G, Lobstein T et al: The "Sydney Principles" for reducing the commercial promotion of foods and beverages to children. *Public Health Nutr* 2008; **11**(9): 881–886.
19 United Nations: Full text of the Convention on the Rights of the Child. United Nations, 1989.
20 United Nations: International Covenant on Economic, Social and Cultural Rights. General Comment 12 on the Right to the Highest Attainable Standards of health. United Nations, 2000.
21 UNICEF. Convention on the Rights of the Child. 2008 (updated). www.unicef.org/crc/index_30160.html (accessed 18 December 2008).
22 Greenway J.: Childhood obesity: bringing children's rights discourse to public health policy. *Community Pract* 2008; **81**(5):17–21.
23 Lobstein T, Dibb S: Evidence of a possible link between obesogenic food advertising and child overweight. *Obes Rev* 2005; **6**(3):203–208.
24 Lavelle P.: Ban junk food ads from kids' TV? 2004. www.abc. net.au/health/thepulse/stories/2004/11/25/1251181.htm (accessed 1 December 2008).

25 Food and Agricultural Organization of the United Nations. The Right to Food in Theory and Practice. Rome: United Nations, 1998.

26 Robinson M.: The Right to Food: Achievements and Challenges—World Food Summit: Five Years Later. United Nations High Commissioner for Human Rights, 2002.

27 United Nations: Report by the Special Rapporteur on the right to food submitted pursuant to Commission on Human Rights resolution 2000/10 (E/CN.4/2001/53). 2000.

28 Mechlem K, Muehlhoff E, Simmersbach F: The Right to Food Brief 5: Nutrition, Food Safety and Consumer Protection, Food and Agricultural Organization of the United Nations 2005.

29 FAO. The Right to Food Guidelines: Information Papers and Case Studies. Rome: Food and Agriculture Organization of the United Nations, 2006.

30 Statement by the Working Groups on Nutrition throughout the Life Cycle and Nutrition Ethics and Human Rights of the United Nations System Standing Committee on Nutrition. The human right of children and adolescents to adequate food and to be free from obesity and related diseases: The responsibilities of food and beverage corporations and related media and marketing industries. Adopted in Geneva, 15 March 2006 and Reiterated at the 34th Session of the SCN, Rome, 26 February to 1 March 2007, 2007.

31 World Health Organization: Constitution of the World Health Organization. Geneva: WHO, 1946.

32 World Health Assembly: WHA51.7. Health-for-all policy for the twenty-first century. Fifty-first World Health Assembly. Agenda Item 19. 16 May, 1998.

33 Birch LL, Fisher JO: Development of eating behaviors among children and adolescents. *Pediatrics* 1998; **101**(3 Pt 2): 539–549.

34 Sen A.: Elements of a theory of human rights. *Philos Public Aff* 2004; **32**:315–356.

35 Sen A.: The limits of law. *Cardozo Law Rev* 2006; **27**: 2913–2927.

PART 2
Evidence synthesis

Bringing together the evidence in the field of child-hood obesity prevention is a challenge. Firstly, at no other stage in history has there been such a thirst for evidence, and at no other time has there been so much. Ensuring that we are building an evidence base that steers us in the right direction for solutions is one that requires a strong practice-evidence-policy partnerships. This challenge coincides with a stronger orientation internationally towards frameworks for public health evidence that suit the context within which we are working, and meet the needs for population health improvements. Organisations like the Cochrane and Campbell Collaboration, the Centers for Disease Control, National Institute for Clinical Effectiveness, international groups such as Equator who are advocating for standards in publications, international trials registers for prospective registering of studies, and methodological working groups such as GRADE, TREND, and CONSORT have enabled developments in high quality standards for generation, reporting and publishing of evidence.

However, significant advancements are still to be made in evaluation standards, common platforms for gleaning the implementation learnings from intervention studies, ensuring that we undertake and extract evidence on distribution of trends by SES and using an 'equity lens'.

The evidence section is extremely comprehensive. It has a predominant focus on the evidence for interventions in settings that children spend time in. It commences with an introductory chapter by Boyd Swinburn that provides a comprehensive framework for evaluation, alternative study designs and components of evaluations that are important in building a useful evidence base, with recommendations for not only the conduct of evidence building, but synthesis of evidence, and then specific areas in which new evidence is required.

With the emergent success of whole of community approaches such as EPODE and the Colac Be Active Eat Well programs, the thirst for whole of community interventions is increasing and compelling. De Silva-Sanigorski and Economos outline the evidence and interface with policy for these approaches, which is all the more useful given their field experience in this area.

The home and family environment, early childhood settings, primary school and secondary school chapters (led by Johannes Brug, Ladda Mo-suwan, Juliana Kain and Lauren Prosser and their international teams) have a lifecourse orientation, providing summaries of what studies have been conducted in these settings and wherever possible, clear recommendations for policy and developments in new programs. As the evidence moves from homeopathic doses over three month time periods to comprehsive, multisectoral, multilevel strategies underpinned by sustainability, the demand for understanding what particular strategies or combination of strategies and partnerships pulled the levers for change is the penultimate question. Demands for this knowledge from practitioners is challenging funders and researchers to evolve more sophisticated and grounded ways of understanding implementation learnings. These chapters provide recommendations for new knowledge and new ways of knowing, understanding. and synthesising.

"What works in primary care" is probably one of the most called for questions of departments of health internationally, given the intuitive sense that primary care practitioners have enormous potential to engage families and individuals and bring about change in behaviours. However, successful solutions still appear intractable, though changes in ways in which primary care practitioners work with other members of community and government agencies remains a magnet and a context within which prevention and management are closely interfaced. Karen Lock and Rebecca Hillier conclude by suggesting that future research should not only tackle the evidence for effective primary care interventions, but also the challenges of translating evidence based guidelines into primary care practice.

The chapter concludes with essential evidence components, though often contested: environmental influences on obesity, food and food marketing, physical activity, and poverty. The section concludes with recommendations and learnings for developing countries. Laura Figuero and Juan Rivera state that whilst the prevalence of childhood obesity continues to rise in developing countries, the experiences of developed countries dominate the prevention literature. However as countries progressively undergo rapid economic growth and urbanisation they face the challenges posed by coexisting undernutrition and obesity. Interventions must be sufficiently flexible in approach to meet the needs of heterogeneous communities.

CHAPTER 6

Evidence framework for childhood obesity prevention

Boyd Swinburn
WHO Collaborating Centre for Obesity Prevention, Deakin University, Melbourne, Australia

Summary and recommendations for practice

- There are complex evidence needs for preventing childhood obesity.
- The International Obesity Taskforce has developed an evidence framework for obesity prevention and it poses five sets of questions that need different types of evidence to answer them.
- The evidence on the burden of obesity is sufficient to warrant action and the evidence on the determinants of obesity is also informative on what to do.
- The priority target groups [*who*] are mainly children and adolescents and high-risk adults, and schools are the favoured setting [*where*] although multiple settings are preferable. The strategies [*how*] also need to be multi-pronged with communications, programs and policies being the main approaches.
- The evidence on effective interventions is quite limited although it is growing rapidly, especially for whole-of-community intervention approaches.
- A priority setting process needs to use all available evidence to define a portfolio of promising interventions.
- There are still very large evidence gaps from too few "solution-oriented" studies.

Introduction

There are enormous evidence needs in obesity prevention but the current evidence base is very nar-

Preventing Childhood Obesity. Edited by
E. Waters, B.A. Swinburn, J.C. Seidell and R. Uauy.
© 2010 Blackwell Publishing.

row in some areas such as intervention effectiveness and cost–effectiveness. In addition, the paradigm of "evidence-based public health" is emerging from its roots in evidence-based medicine and this brings with it the challenge of the complexity of the evidence needed for public health interventions, which are not as susceptible to randomized, controlled trials as clinical interventions.

In an effort to clarify the role of evidence in obesity prevention, the International Obesity Taskforce (IOTF) published a framework[1] that identified the key questions to be answered, the types of evidence needed and outputs produced, and the role of contextual factors (Figure 6.1). In the process of building this framework, a number of general concepts and specific issues emerged about evidence as it applies to obesity prevention.

Definitions and hierarchies of evidence

Evidence, in its widest sense, is information that can provide a level of certainty about the truth of a proposition.[2] This is a very broad definition, more along the lines of the legal, rather than the medical, concept of evidence and implies that this breadth of information is important and valid for decision making. For the purposes of addressing the questions on obesity prevention, the IOTF framework grouped evidence into observational, experimental, extrapolated and experience-based sources of evidence and information.[1] Examples of these are outlined in Table 6.1.[3]

Each type of evidence has its own strengths and weaknesses. Each can be judged on its ability to

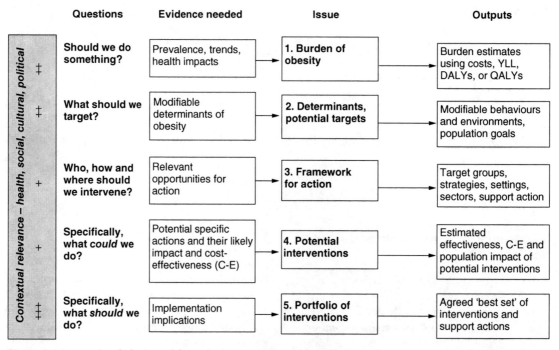

Figure 6.1 International obesity taskforce obesity prevention evidence framework.

contribute to answering the question at hand. In practice, there is wide variation in the quantity and quality of information available in respect of different settings, approaches and target groups for interventions to prevent obesity. There is virtually no evidence concerning the potential effects on obesity of altering social and economic policies, such as agricultural production policies or food pricing policies, while much more evidence is available on localized attempts to influence the consumer through educational and program-based approaches.

Traditional hierarchies of evidence are based on rankings of internal validity (certainty of study conclusions). These tended to be less valuable in the IOTF framework because of the tension between internal validity and the need for external validity (applicability of study findings). The importance of context on evidence and the need for external validity is greater in some areas than others (left-hand bar in Figure 6.1). It is especially important at the priority setting stage (issue 5), and this is where the informed opinions of stakeholders is paramount.

Modeled estimates of effectiveness and informed stakeholder opinion also become important sources

of information where the empirical evidence is complex, patchy and needs to be applied to different contexts. This means that assumptions and decisions must be made explicit and transparent. The acceptance of modeled estimates of effectiveness and informed opinion in the absence of empirical evidence means an acceptance of the best evidence *available* not just the best evidence *possible* (as occurred in systematic reviews with strict inclusion criteria).

Evidence on the burden and determinants of obesity

These are the first two issues in the IOTF framework (Figure 6.1). In general, the size and nature of the obesity epidemic has been well enough characterized to have created the case for action. Of course, many gaps and debates still remain, such as the prevalence and trends in poorer countries, the psycho-social impacts of obesity in children, and the effect of the epidemic on life expectancy.

Evidence on the determinants of obesity is very strong in most areas, although to date, most of it is focused on the more proximal biological and behav-

Table 6.1 Types of evidence and information relevant to obesity prevention.[3]

Type of evidence or information	Description
Observational	
Observational epidemiology	Epidemiological studies that do not involve interventions but may involve comparisons of exposed and non-exposed individuals, for example, cross-sectional, case-control, or cohort studies
Monitoring and surveillance	Population-level data that are collected on a regular basis to provide time series information, for example, mortality and morbidity rates, food supply data, car and TV ownership, birth weights and infant anthropometry
Experimental	
Experimental studies	Intervention studies where the investigator has control over the allocations and/or timings of interventions, for example, randomized controlled trials, or non-randomized trials in individuals, settings, or whole communities
Program/policy evaluation	Assessment of whether a program or policy meets both its overall aims (outcome) and specific objectives (impacts) and how the inputs and implementation experiences resulted in those changes (process)
Extrapolated	
Effectiveness analyses	Modeled estimates of the likely effectiveness of an intervention that incorporate data or estimates of the program efficacy, program uptake, and (for population effectiveness) population reach
Economic analyses	Modeled estimates that incorporate costs (and benefits), for example, intervention costs, cost–effectiveness, or cost–utility
Indirect (or assumed) evidence	Information that strongly suggests that the evidence exists, for example, a high and continued investment in food advertising is indirect evidence that there is positive (but proprietary) evidence that the food advertising increases the sales of those products and/or product categories
Experience	
Parallel evidence	Evidence of intervention effectiveness for another public health issue using similar strategies, for example, the role of social marketing or policies or curriculum programs or financial factors on changing health-related behaviors such as smoking, speeding, sun exposure, or dietary intake. It also includes evidence about the effectiveness of multiple strategies to influence behaviors in a sustainable way, for example, health-promoting schools approach, comprehensive tobacco control programs, or coordinated road toll reduction campaigns.
Theory and program logic	The rationale and described pathways of effect based on theory and experience, for example, linking changes in policy to changes in behaviours and energy balance, or ascribing higher levels of certainty of effect with policy strategies like regulation and pricing compared with other strategies such as education
Informed opinion	The considered opinion of experts in a particular field, for example, scientists able to peer review and interpret the scientific literature, or practitioners, stakeholders, and policy-makers able to inform judgments on implementation issues and modeling assumptions (incorporates "expert" and "lay knowledge")

ioral determinants rather than the more distal, but very important, social and environmental determinants. One poorly researched but very obvious set of determinants are the socio-cultural attitudes, beliefs, values and perceptions that may explain the very large differences in obesity prevalence rates seen across different cultures. These socio-cultural determinants may help to explain why both rich and poor countries have obesity prevalence rates in women of less than 5% (e.g., India, China, Yemen, Ethiopia, Japan and Korea) and greater than 40% (e.g., Samoa, Tonga, Qatar and Saudi Arabia).[4]

Knowing a lot about the determinants of obesity should help to guide interventions but, as Robinson and Sirard point out,[5] "problem-oriented" evidence (what is to blame?) is often quite different to "solution-oriented" evidence (what to do?) It is the solution evidence that decision makers are urgently seeking and it is this evidence that is currently lacking.

Opportunities for action— who, where, how?

This is the third issue on the IOTF framework (Figure 6.1). Many countries have now created strategic plans for action on obesity either as an issue by itself or as part of promoting physical activity or health eating or reducing chronic diseases. Classic frameworks for health promotion specify "who" in terms of target groups (e.g., children, adolescents, pregnant women, minority ethnic groups, those on low incomes), "where" in terms of settings or sectors (e.g., schools, the commercial sector, the health sector), and "how" approaches or strategies (e.g., school education, community development, the use of mass media, environmental change, policy and infrastructure change).[3] These issues are addressed in other chapters in this book but a few brief comments about target groups are warranted.

A potential limitation of identifying target groups is that they become too much the focus of the action (e.g., by encouraging them to make the healthy choices) rather than the players that influence the environments that determine those behaviors (those who can make the healthy choices easier for the target group). In this respect, the definition of target groups may need to be widened to include the providers of the determinants of health, such as the providers of health information—the health services, schools, the media, commercial producers—and widened still further to include those that set the policies which shape access to healthy lifestyles through, for example, pricing, distribution and marketing. In this sense, target groups may include shareholders in companies, professional groups, policy-makers and public opinion leaders, including politicians.

Prevention strategies targeting adults make economic sense (if they work) because the consequences of obesity occurring in middle aged and older adults generate economic costs—especially through Type 2 diabetes and cardiovascular diseases.[6] Adults, especially those with other existing risk factors, are at high absolute risk of these diseases; therefore, they have the potential for high absolute gains. In addition, there is now very strong efficacy evidence that individual lifestyle interventions in high-risk adults prevent diabetes and heart disease.[7,8] However, despite this evidence and logic, children have risen as the priority target group for most action on obesity and this has occurred for a number of reasons—some based on evidence, some based on societal principles, and some based on practicalities.

Excess weight, once gained, is hard to lose but children who are overweight do have a chance to "grow into" their weight. Children's behaviors are also much more environmentally dependent than adults' behaviors and most of the evidence on obesity prevention has been in children. However, far more powerful than the sum of the evidence are two other drivers of children as the priority target group: societal protection of children and access for interventions—especially through schools. Policy-makers have been especially sensitive to children because society has an obligation to protect them from ill-health. For adults, the societal obligation shifts towards protecting personal choice—even if that choice is for unhealthy foods and physical inactivity.

Effectiveness of potential interventions

This is the fourth issue in the IOTF framework (Figure 6.1) and asks: "What are the potential, specific interventions and what is the evidence for their effectiveness?" This question is covered in many other chapters in this book and only some overview comments are be made here.

In general, it is possible to generate quite long lists of potential interventions to help prevent childhood obesity, although some of the intervention areas, such as improved parenting skills, are more readily identified in generalities than in specific interventions. However, adding effectiveness evidence to any more than a few of them is very difficult because of the absence of intervention studie. For the interventions that have been studied, most concern primary school children, most are in school settings, most are short term, most are not sustainable, and most have shown relatively modest effects on anthropometry (although they were often able to show improvements in eating and/or physical activity). The number of reviews in the area is starting to outnumber the number of studies.[9–29]

As interventions move towards more whole-of-community interventions, there is an increased complexity in the study design, the interventions and the evaluations, although some positive results are starting to emerge from these studies, which is very encouraging.[30–32] More sophisticated multi-level modeling will be needed to tease out intervention effects in these more complex interventions.

For policy-makers considering strategy options, the distinction between effectiveness and cost–effectiveness is critical. If a policy objective is to be pursued with no limitation on spending, then effectiveness (the beneficial effect of a strategy in practice) is the primary consideration. But when cost limitations apply (as they inevitably do), an evaluation of cost–effectiveness is essential if rational decisions are to be made.[33]

A remarkable feature of the evaluations and systematic reviews of interventions described above is that they rarely mention the costs of the various programs they examine, and make no estimates of cost–effectiveness. For child obesity prevention, only one study has explicitly examined the costs of an intervention program, the US Planet Health Program.[34] Planet Health's estimated cost–effectiveness ratio gives a value of $4305 per quality-adjusted life year gained, which compares favorably with interventions such as the treatment of hypertension, low-cholesterol-diet therapies, some diabetes screening programs and treatments, and adult exercise programs.[35]

Creating a portfolio of interventions

The evidence for obesity prevention covered thus far has shown: a substantial burden to warrant action; sufficient understanding of the determinants to know *what* to target; a determination of the priority target populations (*who*), the best settings to access (*where*), and the most appropriate strategies to use (*how*), and; a review of the literature about what has been shown to work, or not work. The final challenge in the IOTF framework (prior to actually implementing and evaluating the work) is to create the "portfolio" of interventions to be implemented. And what a challenge in priority setting it is, because the aim of intervention selection is:

to agree upon a balanced portfolio of specific, promising interventions to reduce the burden of obesity and improve health and quality of life within the available capacity to do so.

"Agreement" infers a process with decision makers coming to a joint understanding. "Balanced portfolio" means a balance of content (both nutrition and physical activity), settings (not all school-based), strategies (policies, programs, communications), and target groups (whole population, high risk). Interventions need to be "specific" (not "promote healthy eating") and "promising" rather than proven. The analogy of choosing a balance of products (shares, property, bonds) to create portfolio of financial investments has been used by Hawe and Shiell[36] to conceptualize appropriate investment in health. The best investments are the safe, high-return ones (i.e,. high level of evidence, high population impact) but, inevitably, the choices come down to including some safe, lower-return investments and some higher-risk (i.e., less certainty), potentially higher-return investments while excluding the high-risk, low-return ones. The IOTF framework[1] applies this investment concept to obesity prevention and presents a "promise table", which is a grid of certainty (strength of evidence) versus return (population impact) into which interventions can be placed according to their credentials.

The other key concepts in the priority setting aim are that the interventions reduce the "burden of obesity" and "improve health and quality of life".

These issues are particularly important for obesity prevention because many of the interventions (healthier eating and physical activity) have their own independent effects on health and some interventions have the potential to do harm (such as increase stigmatization and teasing) or increase health inequalities. Fitting the plan of action to the available capacity to achieve it is especially challenging at the community level where the level of health promotion funding is usually very low and the enthusiasm for doing something is usually very high.

Practice-based evidence

Given the challenging aim of intervention selection, how can this be achieved and what role does (or should) evidence play in the process? Certainly, the evidence of effectiveness is not sufficient by itself to guide appropriate decision making, and, indeed, true evidence-based policy-making is probably quite rare.[37] Some major policy decisions are made on the basis of extremely little evidence despite high costs (such as military interventions). A helpful concept to apply is that of "practice/policy-based evidence".[37] Evidence-based practice/policy starts in the library, assesses what has been published and then takes that intelligence to the policy-maker or practitioner to consider for implementation. Practice/policy-based evidence starts at the table with the practitioner or policy-maker and assesses what could be implemented with the ideas coming from many sources: what is already happening here, what is happening elsewhere, what the literature shows, what the politicians want to implement and so on. Then some technical estimates are made using the best evidence available and these are brought back to the table to inform the priority setting. Two examples of this are given below.

Evidence and priority setting processes

The ACE-Obesity project (Assessing Cost–Effectiveness of Obesity Interventions) was funded by the Victorian government in Australia to inform it on the best investments for reducing childhood obesity nationally.[38] The ACE approach (which is also covered in Chapter 20) included extensive economic analyses around agreed, specified interventions to reduce childhood obesity at a state or national level, plus a process that engaged key stakeholders in first selecting the interventions for analysis and then, second, pro-

viding judgements on the modeling assumptions and a number of "second stage filters" (strength of evidence, feasibility, sustainability, acceptability, effects on equity, other positive or negative effects). The definition of evidence was wide and all assumptions in the modeling had to be explicit and have in-built uncertainty estimates. In this way, policies (such as banning food advertisements to children), programs (such as active transport to school) and services (such as gastric banding for very obese teenagers) which lacked trial evidence could still be modeled. The outputs were estimates of total cost, population health gains (BMI units saved or disability-adjusted life years [DALY] saved), cost–effectiveness ($/BMI saved, $/DALY saved), and plus the second stage filter judgements.

The same challenges of defining what *could* be done and then undertaking a priority setting process to determine what *should* be done apply at the community level as much as they apply at a state or national level. Similar principles to ACE-Obesity, but a simplified process, were applied in the formative stages of six demonstration projects in Australia, New Zealand and the Pacific.[39] The details of this process (the ANGELO Process) are covered in Chapter 26.

Evidence needs

There are some major gaps in the evidence base need for sound judgements on preventing childhood obesity. The box outlines some of the key areas of evidence need which have been updated from a WHO meeting on Childhood Obesity in Kobe, Japan in 2005.[40]

Evidence needs for preventing obesity in children and adolescents

- All interventions should include process evaluation measures, and provide resource and cost estimates. Evaluation can include impact on other parties, such as parents and siblings.
- Interventions using comparison groups should be explicit about what the comparison group experiences. Phrases like "normal care" or "normal curriculum" or "standard school PE classes" are not helpful, especially if normal practices have been changing over the years.

- There is a need for more interventions looking into the needs of specific sub-populations, including immigrant groups, low-income groups, and specific ethnic and cultural groups.
- There is a shortage of long-term programs evaluating and monitoring interventions. Long-term outcomes could include changes in knowledge and attitudes, behaviors (diet and physical activity) and adiposity outcomes.
- New approaches to interventions, including prospective meta-analyses, should be considered.
- Community-based demonstration programs can be used to generate evidence, gain experience, develop capacity and maintain momentum.
- There is a need for an international agency to encourage networking of community-based interventions, support methods of evaluation and assist in the analysis of the cost–effectiveness of initiatives.
- There is insufficient evidence on the impacts of cultural values, beliefs, expectations and attitudes around food, physical activity and body size perception to inform interventions in the high-risk ethnic groups.
- Better evidence is needed about the most effective ways of feeding BMI information back to parents and for health professionals to raise the issue of their children's weight with parent.
- Evidence on the most effective and cost-effective monitoring systems and their impacts on national and community actions.

Conclusions

The traditional approaches borrowed from evidence-based medicine need to be adapted to suit obesity prevention—trying to retain the rigour of evidence assessments and uses but trying to incorporate the flexibility and complexity needed for public health intervention research. The IOTF framework attempts to achieve this by articulating the various questions that the evidence needs to address, by expanding the definitions of evidence, by highlighting the need for modeling where there are gaps in the empirical data, by lifting the value of informed stakeholder input for those research questions where contextual factors are important, by taking a "solution-oriented" approach to determining interventions, and by defining how a "policy/practice-based evidence" paradigm can better align evidence with the realities of decision making.

Acknowledgements

Tim Gill, Shiriki Kumanyika, Tim Lobstein, Colin Bell, Andrea Sanigorski, Elizabeth Waters, Rob Carter, Marj Moodie.

References

1 Swinburn B, Gill T, Kumanyika S: Obesity prevention: a proposed framework for translating evidence into action. *Obes Rev* 2005; **6**:23–33.

2 Rychetnik L, Hawe P, Waters E, Barratt A, Frommer M: A glossary for evidence based public health. *J Epidemiol Community Health* 2004; **58**:538–545.

3 Lobstein T, Swinburn BA: Health promotion to prevent obesity: evidence and policy needs. In: McQueen DV, Jones CM, eds. Global Perspectives On Health Promotion Effectiveness. New York: Springer, 2007:125–143.

4 International Association for the Study of Obesity: International Obesity Taskforce database on obesity. www.iotf.org/database/index.asp (accessed December 2008).

5 Robinson TN, Sirard JR: Preventing childhood obesity: a solution-oriented research paradigm. *Am J Prev Med* 2005; **2**(Suppl. 2):194–201.

6 Seidell JC, Nooyens AJ, Visscher TL: Cost-effective measures to prevent obesity: epidemiological basis and appropriate target groups. *Proc Nutr Soc* 2005; **64**(1):1–5.

7 Knowler WC, Barrett-Connor E, Fowler SE et al: Reduction in the incidence of type 2 diabetes with lifestyle intervention or metformin. *N Engl J Med* 2002; **346**(6):393–403.

8 Ornish D, Brown SE, Scherwitz LW et al: Lifestyle changes and heart disease. *Lancet* 1990; **336**(8717):741–742.

9 Summerbell CD, Waters E, Edmunds LD, Kelly S, Brown T, Campbell KJ: Interventions for Preventing Obesity in Children. *Cochrane Database Syst Rev* 2006; 1:(First published online: 20 July 2005 in Issue 3, 2005.).

10 Flynn MA, McNeil DA, Maloff B et al: Reducing obesity and related chronic disease risk in children and youth: a synthesis of evidence with "best practice" recommendations. *Obes Rev* 2006; **7**(Suppl. 1):7–66.

11 Doak CM, Visscher TLS, Renders CM, Seidell JC: The prevention of overweight and obesity in children and adolescents: a review of interventions and programmes. *Obes Rev* 2006; **7**:111–136.

12 Katz DL, O'Connell M, Yeh MC et al: Public health strategies for preventing and controlling overweight and obesity in school and worksite settings: a report on recommendations of the Task Force on Community Preventive Services. *MMWR Recomm Rep* 2005; **54**(RR-10):1–12.

13 Wareham NJ, van Sluijs EM, Ekelund U: Physical activity and obesity prevention: a review of the current evidence. *Proc Nutr Soc* 2005; **64**(2):229–247.

14 Clemmens D, Hayman LL: Increasing activity to reduce obesity in adolescent girls: a research review. *J Obstet Gynecol Neonatal Nurs* 2004; **33**(6):801–808.

15 Carrel AL, Bernhardt DT: Exercise prescription for the prevention of obesity in adolescents. *Curr Sports Med Rep* 2004; **3**(6):330–336.

16 Casey L, Crumley E. Addressing Childhood Obesity: The Evidence for Action. Canadian Association of Paediatric Health Centres: Ottawa, 2004. www.caphc.org/childhood_obesity/obesity_report.pdf.

17 Reilly JJ, McDowell ZC: Physical activity interventions in the prevention and treatment of paediatric obesity: systematic review and critical appraisal. *Proc Nutr Soc* 2003; **62**(3):611–619.

18 Muller MJ, Mast M, Asbeck I, Langnase K, Grund A: Prevention of obesity—is it possible? *Obes Rev* 2003; **2**:15–28.

19 Mulvihill C, Quigley R: The management of obesity and overweight an analysis of reviews of diet, physical activity and behavioural approaches Evidence briefing 1st Edition. October 2003 London, Health Development Agency, 2003.

20 NHS Centre for Reviews and Dissemination (2002) The prevention and treatment of childhood obesity. Effective Health Care Bulletin 7(6).

21 Micucci S, Thomas H, Vohra J: The Effectiveness of School-Based Strategies for the Primary Prevention of Obesity and for Promoting Physical Activity and Nutrition, the Major Modifiable Risk Factors for Type 2 Diabetes: Review of Reviews. Hamilton, Canada: Public Health Research, Education and Development Program, 2002.

22 Schmitz KH, Jeffrey RW: Prevention of obesity. In: Wadden TA, Stunkard AJ, eds. Handbook of Obesity Treatment. New York: Guilford Press, 2002:556–593.

23 Swedish Council on Technology Assessment in Health Care: Obesity—problems and interventions. Stockholm, Sweden, The Swedish Council on Technology Assessment in Health Care, 2002. Report No. 160. www.sbu.se/Filer/Content0/publikationer/1/obesity_2002/obsesityslut.pdf.

24 Dietz W: Gortmaker S Preventing obesity in children and adolescents. *Annu Rev Public Health* 2001; **22**:337–353.

25 Steinbeck K: The importance of physical activity in the prevention of overweight and obesity in childhood: a review and an opinion. *Obes Rev* 2001; **2**:117–130.

26 Hardeman W, Griffin S, Johnston M, Kinmonth AL, Wareham NJ: Interventions to prevent weight gain, a systematic review of psychological models and behaviour change methods. *Int J Obes* 2000; **24**(2):131–143.

27 Story M: School-based approaches for preventing and treating obesity. *Int J Obes* 1999; **23**(Suppl. 2):S43–S51.

28 Goran M, Reynolds KD, Lindquist CH: Role of physical activity in the prevention of obesity in children. *Int J Obes* 1999; **23**(Suppl. 3):S18–S33.

29 NHS Centre for Reviews and Dissemination: The prevention and treatment of obesity. *Eff Health Care* 1997; **3**(2) www.york.ac.uk/inst/crd/ehc32.htm.

30 Economos CD, Hyatt RR, Goldberg JP et al: A community intervention reduces BMI z-score in children. Shape up Sommerville first year results. *Obesity* 2007; **15**(5): 1325–1336.

31 Taylor RW, McAuley KA, Barbezat W et al: APPLE Project. 2y findings of a community-based obesity prevention program in primary school age children. *Am J Clin Nutr* 2007; **86**(3):735–742.

32 SAnigorski AM, Bell AC, Kremer PJ, Cuttler R, Swinburn BA: Reducing unhealthy weight gain in children through community capacity building: results of a quasi-experimental intervention program, be active eat well. *Int J Obes* 2008; **32**(7):1060–1067.

33 Brunner E, Cohen D, Toon L: Cost effectiveness of cardiovascular disease prevention strategies: a perspective on EU food based dietary guidelines. *Public Health Nutr* 2001; **4**(2B):711–715.

34 Wang LY, Yang Q, Lowry R, Wechsler H: Economic analysis of a school-based obesity prevention program. *Obes Res* 2003; **11**:1313–1324.

35 Ganz ML: Commentary: The economic evaluation of obesity interventions: Its time has come. *Obes Res* 2003; **11**:1275–1277.

36 Hawe P, Shiell A: Preserving innovation under increasing accountability pressures: the health promotion investment portfolio approach. *Health Prom Aust* 1995; **5**:4–9.

37 Marmot MG: Evidence based policy or policy based evidence? *BMJ* 2004; **328**:906–907.

38 Haby MM, Vos T, Carter R et al: A new approach to assessing the health benefit from obesity interventions in children and adolescents: the assessing cost-effectiveness in obesity project. *Int J Obes* 2006; **30**(10):1463–1475.

39 Schultz J, Utter J, Mathews L, Cama T, Mavoa H, Swinburn B: The Pacific OPIC Project (Obesity Prevention in Communities)—action plans and interventions. *Pac Health Dialogue* 2007; **14**(2):147–153.

40 World Health Organization: Obesity in Childhood: Report of an Expert Committee. Kobe, Japan, June. Geneva: WHO, 2005.

CHAPTER 7

Evidence of multi-setting approaches for obesity prevention: translation to best practice

Andrea M. de Silva-Sanigorski[1,2] and *Christina Economos*[3,4]

[1] WHO Collaborating Centre for Obesity Prevention, Deakin University, Geelong, Australia
[2] Jack Brockoff Child Health and Wellbeing Program, McCaughey Centre, Melbourne School of Population Health, The University of Melbourne, Melbourne, Australia
[3] Dorothy R. Friedman School of Nutrition Science and Policy, Tufts University, Boston, MA, USA
[4] John Hancock Center for Physical Activity and Nutrition, Tufts University, Boston, MA, USA

Summary and recommendations for practice

- Childhood obesity is a complex issue and both individual efforts and societal changes are needed.
- Multi-setting, community-wide strategies directed at all ages and groups offer a comprehensive, equitable and intergenerational response to the problem.
- Interventions should be developed within an integrated chronic disease prevention model and with a community-based participatory research framework to maximize funding and health impact.
- Interventions that attempt to alter health behaviors must not be developed in isolation from the broader social and environmental context.
- Obesity prevention programs must include rigorous evaluation involving multiple levels and various settings to guide improvements to childhood obesity efforts in a range of contexts.

Method

For this chapter we scanned and reviewed the published literature (e.g., *PubMed* and CINAHL®, The Cumulative Index to Nursing and Allied Health Literature) to select studies that were effective and

Preventing Childhood Obesity. Edited by
E. Waters, B.A. Swinburn, J.C. Seidell and R. Uauy.
© 2010 Blackwell Publishing.

examined the key elements that were consistent across the studies. With input from both authors, the evidence was synthesized and integrated into recommendations. There was no restriction on studies outside the developed countries. However, there is no large representation of studies outside developed countries, which may limit the applicability of the recommendations developed.

Social change models: what can we learn?

Population behavior is influenced by several societal subsystems, including the economy, the political system, social institutions, and culture. To influence behavior on a broad societal level, multiple subsystems must be targeted. To that end, understanding how to prevent a further rise in obesity can been informed through lessons from a range of successful attempts at social change that include increasing breastfeeding rates, seat-belt use, smoking cessation and recycling.[1]

Key elements identified as essential from these past successes include: recognition that there was a crisis; major economic implications associated with the crisis; a science base including research, data and evidence; sparkplugs, or leaders who can work for their cause through their knowledge, competence, talents, skills, and even charisma; coalitions to move the agenda forward and a strategic, integrated media advocacy campaign; involvement of the government at the state level to apply regulatory and fiscal authority, and at the local level to implement change; mass communication that includes consistent positive messages supported by scientific consensus and repeated in a variety of venues; policy and environmental changes that promote healthy lifestyle behaviors; and a plan that includes many components which work synergistically. Applying these social change strategies to the community environment to encourage healthy eating, increased levels of physical activity, and a decrease in sedentary behaviors is emerging as a practical way to address obesity on a large scale.[2,3]

Community approaches to obesity prevention

Communities have their own societal subsystems within a particular geographic area and the way in which an individual often identifies within a community is defined by race, ethnicity, socio-economic status (SES), and group memberships.[4] To conduct research within communities, one must take into account the varied nature of relationships, networks, and how they may all work together synergistically.[5] Community approaches can target components within the population (referred to as community-based interventions or strategies), or they can be implemented on a community-wide basis. Previous community-based approaches to change behavior and prevent disease give promise for the future of community intervention work.[6–13] Furthermore, community-wide strategies directed at all ages and groups offer a comprehensive, equitable and intergenerational response to the problem, and potentially a means of treatment and prevention. The discussion that follows reviews these approaches in the context of social change and their application to obesity prevention.

Evidence in support of health improvement and disease reduction by way of community involvement began gaining ground by the 1970s. The North Karelia Project[14] and the Stanford Three Community Study[11,15] were among the first to break ground in this area. Each proved effective in translating educational messages to significant positive changes and cardiovascular disease risk reduction in the populations that received the interventions, as compared to control populations. The intervention strategies of these projects used mass media, low-cost lifestyle modifications and the involvement of community members. Subsequently, the National Institutes of Health (NIH) financed three major community-based intervention projects: the Stanford Five-City Project,[10] the Minnesota Heart Health Program,[16] and the Pawtucket Heart Health Program.[7]

These trials essentially provided community-wide health education over several years. The Stanford Project provided a comprehensive program using social learning theory, a communication-behavior change model, community organization principles, and social marketing methods.[10] Minnesota's multiple strategy approach provided systematic population screening for hypertension, mass media campaigns, adult and youth education programs, physician and health professional programs and community organization efforts.[17] Pawtucket provided multi-level education, screening and counseling programs throughout the community.[7]

Community-based programs focused on youth have been carried out to increase contraception use,[18] and physical activity.[19] There are very few examples of community-based interventions focused on obesity, owing to the complex nature of both the etiology and the solutions, and we review several of these below.

Community-based obesity prevention interventions in children

The Pathways intervention was a randomized controlled trial conducted within the Native American communities. It was the first of its kind to take into account cultural, theoretical and operational viability in the study population and to operate on a large scale ($n = 1704$) in 41 schools over six years (three years of development and testing and three years of intervention). The aim of the project was to reduce body fat by promoting behavioral change and a holistic view of health among Native American school children in Grades 3–5.[20] Although the intervention was largely carried out within the schools, care was taken to enlist the support of community and tribal leaders, as well as parents. The intervention was developed through a collaboration of universities and American Indian nations, schools and families with a focus on individual, behavioral and environmental factors.

Pathways was successful in reducing the energy density of foods consumed by changing the school food environment.[21,22] While the main outcome of the study, change in the percentage of body fat, produced no significant difference between intervention and control schools, other measurable benefits were demonstrated including a reduction in daily energy intake and percentage of energy from total fat, and increases in physical activity and for intervention verses control schools. The Pathways study demonstrated a successful marriage of theoretical underpinnings, community and family involvement, and cultural and situational appropriateness, and thereby provided an excellent community research framework upon which to build.

Shape Up Somerville (SUS): Eat Smart, Play Hard™, was one of the first community-based participatory research (CBPR) initiatives[23] designed to change the environment to prevent obesity in early elementary school children.[9] Academics were partnered with community members of three culturally diverse urban communities to conduct a controlled trial to evaluate whether an environmental change intervention could prevent a rise in BMI z-scores in young children through enhanced access and availability of physical activity options and healthy food throughout their entire day. The SUS intervention focused on creating multi-level environmental change to support behavioral action and maintenance and to prevent weight gain among early elementary school children through community participation. Specific changes within the before-, during-, and after-school environments provided a variety of increased opportunities for physical activity. The availability of lower-energy-dense foods, with an emphasis on fruits, vegetables, whole grains and low-fat dairy was increased; foods high in fat and sugar were discouraged. Additional changes within the home and the community, promoted by the intervention team, provided reinforcing opportunities to be more physically active and improve access to healthier food. Many groups and individuals within the community (including children, parents, teachers, school food service providers, city departments, policy-makers, health care providers, before- and after-school programs, restaurants and the media) were engaged in the intervention (see http://nutrition.tufts.edu/research/shapeup for details).

These changes were aimed at bringing the overall energy equation into balance, specifically, this intervention was designed to result in an increased energy expenditure of up to 125 kcals per day beyond the increases in energy expenditure and energy intake that accompany growth. A central aim of the intervention was to create a community model that could be replicated nationwide as a cost-effective, community-based action plan to prevent obesity at local levels. After the first school year of intervention (8 months) in the intervention community, BMI z-score decreased by -0.1005 ($P = 0.001$, 95% confidence interval -0.1151 to -0.0859) compared to children in the control communities after controlling for baseline covariates.[9] This approach addressed the complex environmental influences on energy balance and ensured maximal reach within a population of children.

Community-based interventions are also being effectively implemented in other parts of the world. Recently, an Australian intervention program utilizing the socio-ecological model (Be Active, Eat Well)[24] was evaluated and found to be successful in a number of areas. Intervention children had significantly lower increases in body weight, waist, waist/height, and BMI z-score than comparison children. Further, the intervention was shown not to increase health inequalities related to obesity and was also deemed to be safe as changes in underweight and attempted weight loss were not different between the two groups of children.[24]

More interventions that focus on multi-faceted community-based environmental change approaches using key elements of other successful social change models (a recognized crisis, economic impact, evidence based, government involvement) are needed.[1] Advanced community-based research approaches to turn the tide on childhood obesity will require training of future leaders in community research methodology, increased funding to conduct rigorous trials, and acceptance of the study model as viable from the broad scientific community.

The benefits of this approach to obesity prevention

There is broad agreement that, to reduce obesity, priority needs to be given to multi-strategy, multi-setting prevention efforts, particularly in children.[25,26] Controlled obesity prevention trials in childhood are few in number, mostly short term (one year or less), focused on only a single or a few strategies (education or social marketing only) and settings (school-based only) and largely showed little or no impact.[27-29] Until recently, the studies that did show an impact tended to be high-intensity, less sustainable approaches (e.g., extensive classroom time promoting individual behavior change).[27-29] It is clear that innovative approaches that work at multiple levels and are flexible, effective, cost-effective, equitable and sustainable are urgently needed and, as discussed above, multi-setting community-based interventions hold promise as one such option.[2,25,26,29,30]

The success of a multi-setting intervention approach may be the result of a number of factors. An approach such as this works within a framework which recognizes that multiple factors affect a community's function and, in turn, the health of the individuals within it. The socio-ecological model identifies five levels of influence on an individual's health: intrapersonal, interpersonal, organizational, community and environment/policy. This framework also recognizes that these factors (environment, working conditions, economy, education, culture and health systems), affect an individual's health in both direct and indirect ways. Reviews of the intervention literature, particularly in obesity prevention have shown that interventions that use these frameworks to guide their design are more likely to be successful.[29] This also appears to hold true across a number of public health issues, as discussed above.

Behavioral interventions have had limited success at altering individual health outcomes. However, even when shown to have some efficacy, the sustainability of the modest changes in health behavior is low and does not translate to population-level health improvements. Limitations of this type of intervention are that they largely ignore the social context that shapes behaviors and that the complexity of the physiological changes brought about by behavior change is often not recognized. Interventions of this type treat individual behaviors as separate from social context and biology.[31]

Community-based, and community-wide, interventions can also address risk factors that are common to a number of chronic diseases. The integrated chronic disease prevention (CDP) model has developed from a recognition of the preventable risk factors shared by leading chronic diseases.[32] Key concepts in the integrated CDP model include an ecological perspective, intersectoral action, multi-level intervention, and collaborative processes. The multiplicity and complexity of this approach is captured in a definition put forward by Shiell:

> [Integrated chronic disease prevention is an approach] ... that targets more than one risk factor or disease outcome, more than one level of influence, more than one disciplinary perspective, more than one type of research method, or more than one societal sector, and which targets populations—rather than individuals—as a unit.[32]

The influence of the ecological perspective is evident in that integrated CDP frameworks consider the interdependence between individuals and the broader socio-environmental context. For example, a community-wide intervention to improve the delivery of preventative services to children in the United States achieved far-reaching changes.[33] The intervention approach was based on systems theory, which suggests that many opportunities for improvement exist in the interactions between elements of a system. For this intervention, the application of this theory resulted in viewing care delivery as a series of processes extending from the home to the primary care practice and other community health and social services. The intervention activities were directed at the community, practice and family level. At the community level, positive effects were seen in state and community policies, which led to sustainable changes in organization practices and funding approaches. At the practice level, alignment and integration of services delivered by multiple practices resulted in reduced duplication, improved coordination and changes in service delivery. At the family level, the intervention resulted in improved child and maternal health outcomes.[33]

An additional benefit of a multi-setting community-wide approach is its potential to improve the health and development of all children in the community. Interventions that attempt to address at least some of the social determinants of health have the potential to address population-level determinants of ill-health, rather than individual characteristics. They can be equity focused and reduce the socio-economic gradient that currently exists for almost all health outcomes.

This approach can also positively influence individual behaviors through addressing the societal and environmental influences at the community level. Interventions that target multiple aspects of individual environments have the ability to make the more health promoting options easier, and over time can also shift behavioral and cultural norms in a sustainable manner. Targeting environments also represents an upstream approach, as children in low-income families live in environments that limit social and economic opportunities, access to healthy foods and opportunities for physical activity.[34] In the Shape Up Somerville intervention program, a significant reduction in z-BMI was seen after one year in the intervention children.[9] This intervention engaged the community widely and was specifically focused on changing children's environments at school and also enhancing access and availability of healthy eating and physical activity options throughout the entire day for children, including before- and after-school programs.[9] Also, as a result of the intervention, there were changes in the home and community, which provided reinforced opportunities for increased physical activity and improved access to more nutritious food.[9]

Best practice recommendations for intervention activities

In their comprehensive synthesis of the evidence of reducing obesity and related chronic disease risk in children and youth, Flynn et al (2006) present recommendations for a broad range of sectors, organizations and health professionals, which are based on the available evidence and gaps in knowledge identified during the synthesis. With regard to intervention activities, the recommendations[29] can be summarized as follows:

- Population-based interventions should be developed to balance, support and extend the current emphasis on individual-based programs.
- Obesity prevention programs need to be developed with rigorous evaluation components in community and home settings where limited program activity is evident and effectiveness is unknown.

- Interventions need long-term implementation and follow-up to determine the sustainability of program impacts as on body weight.
- To maximize funding and health impact, interventions should be developed within an integrated chronic disease prevention model and with a CBPR framework.
- Program design process should be developed to allow continual incorporation of new elements associated with greater program effectiveness, using an action research model.

Taking this further, Glass and McAtee have developed a multi-level three-dimensional framework to examine health behaviors and disease in social and biological context. They challenge us to develop better theory and data to understand how social factors regulate behaviors, or distribute individuals into risk groups, and how these social factors come to be embodied.[31] This is needed because while we are knowledgeable about the behaviors that lead to ill health and disease, relatively little is known about how these behaviors arise, become maintained and can be changed. By advancing the study of the social determinants, Glass and McAtee suggest that more effective population interventions can be developed. Accordingly, continuing to conduct interventions that attempt to alter health behaviors in isolation from the broader social and environmental context will continue to provide disappointing results. The authors emphasize the need to focus on the health behaviors and the mediating structures that lie between the behavioral sphere and the macro-social context. These mediating structures are termed "risk regulators", and in the obesity context are, for example, cultural norms, area deprivation, food availability, laws and policies, and workplace conditions.[31] These risk regulators influence the two key behaviors related to obesity, nutrition and physical activity, in a way that is dynamic and extends over the life course. Accordingly, population interventions to prevent obesity cannot attempt to influence health behaviors without attempting to address at least some of these risk regulators and a more contextual understanding of health behaviors and health service usage, for example, would increase the effectiveness of obesity prevention interventions and public health policies.[31]

There is growing recognition of the need for a common risk factor approach to public health interventions. This approach is the basis of the integrated chronic disease prevention model, which arose from the need to increase the efficiency and efficacy of traditional, single-disease focused prevention efforts.[32] The best interventions will build on existing collaboration and networking among local health authorities. However, structural factors (e.g., political, financial) must be in place for interventions to be implemented and thoroughly evaluated.[32] Policies and program funding that target all of the determinants of health must be collaboratively developed by government departments such as health, education, and human resources and employment.[32] Findings from the Alberta Heart Health Project show that for an integrated approach to chronic disease prevention to succeed government support is vital and the voluntary, professional, academic, and private sectors must contribute to action on the root causes of health. Effective leadership is important and the public health system, which can be viewed as the embodiment of publicly-funded organized efforts to prevent disease and promote health, must take responsibility for facilitating the inter-sectoral collaborations fundamental to integrated chronic disease prevention.[32]

Summary

Current evidence on obesity prevention and other public health successes demonstrates that early intervention and prevention is more effective and less costly then treatment efforts. Given the complexity of childhood obesity, both individual efforts and societal changes are needed. These changes will require the involvement of multiple sectors and stakeholders, particularly collaboration between community, government and academia. In addition, evaluation needs to occur at multiple levels and settings to guide improvements to childhood obesity efforts and develop initiatives that can be used in a range of contexts.

References

1 Economos CD, Brownson RC, DeAngelis MA et al: What lessons have been learned from other attempts to guide social change? *Nutr Rev* 2001; **59**(3 Pt 2):S40–S56; discussion S7–S65.

2 French SA, Story M, Jeffery RW: Environmental influences on eating and physical activity. *Annu Rev Public Health* 2001; **22**:309–335.

3 Hill JO, Peters JC: Environmental contributions to the obesity epidemic. *Science* 1998; **280**(5368):1371–1374.

4 MacQueen KM, Metzger E, Kegeles DS et al: What is community? An evidence-based definition for participatory public health. *Am J Public Health* 2001; **91**(12):1929–1938.

5 Wellman B, Wortley S: Different strokes from different folks: community ties and social support. *Am J Sociol* 1990; **96**: 558.

6 Community Intervention Trial for Smoking Cessation (COMMIT): Summary of design and intervention. COMMIT Research Group. *J Natl Cancer Inst* 1991; **83**(22): 1620–1628.

7 Carleton RA, Lasater TM, Assaf AR, Feldman HA, McKinlay S: The Pawtucket Heart Health Program: community changes in cardiovascular risk factors and projected disease risk. *Am J Public Health* 1995; **85**(6):777–785.

8 DeMattia L, Denney S: Childhood obesity prevention: succsessful community-based efforts. *Ann Am Acad Pol Soc Sci* 2008; **615**:83.

9 Economos CD, Hyatt RR, Goldberg JP et al: A community intervention reduces BMI z-score in children: shape up somerville first year results. *Obesity* (Silver Spring) 2007; **15**(5):1325–1336.

10 Farquhar JW, Fortmann SP, Flora JA et al: Effects of communitywide education on cardiovascular disease risk factors. The Stanford Five-City Project. *JAMA* 1990; **264**(3): 359–365.

11 Fortmann SP, Williams PT, Hulley SB, Haskell WL, Farquhar JW: Effect of health education on dietary behavior: the Stanford Three Community Study. *Am J Clin Nutr* 1981; **34**(10):2030–2038.

12 Killen JD, Robinson TN, Telch MJ et al: The stanford adolescent heart health program. *Health Educ Q* 1989; **16**(2):263–283.

13 Zahuranec DB, Morgenstern LB, Garcia NM et al: Stroke Health and Risk Education (SHARE) pilot project. Feasibility and need for church-based stroke health promotion in a Bi-ethnic community. *Stroke* 2008; **39**(5):1583–1585.

14 Puska P, Tuomilehto J, Nissinen A et al: The North Karelia project: 15 years of community-based prevention of coronary heart disease. *Ann Med* 1989; **21**(3):169–173.

15 Stern MP, Farquhar JW, McCoby N, Russell SH: Results of a two-year health education campaign on dietary behavior. The Stanford Three Community Study. *Circulation* 1976; **54**(5):826–833.

16 Mittelmark MB, Luepker RV, Jacobs DR et al: Community-wide prevention of cardiovascular disease: education strategies of the Minnesota Heart Health Program. *Prev Med* 1986; **15**(1):1–17.

17 Murray D, Luepker R, Grimm R, Blackburn H: Prevention and treatment of hypertension at the population level: the Minnesota Heart Health Program. *Kardiologiia* 1986; **26**(1): 78–84.

18 Tu X, Lou C, Gao E, Shah IH: Long-term effects of a community-based program on contraceptive use among sexually active unmarried youth in Shanghai, China. *J Adolesc Health* 2008; **42**(3):249–258.

19 Hoehner CM, Soares J, Perez DP et al: Physical activity interventions in Latin America: a systematic review. *Am J Prev Med* 2008; **34**(3):224–233.

20 Davis SM, Going SB, Helitzer DL et al: Pathways: a culturally appropriate obesity-prevention program for American Indian schoolchildren. *Am J Clin Nutr* 1999; **69**(4 Suppl.): 796S–802S.

21 Prevention of obesity in American Indian children: the Pathways study. *Am J Clin Nutr* 1999; **69**(4 Suppl.): 745S–824S.

22 Caballero B: Obesity prevention in children: opportunities and challenges. *Int J Obes Relat Metab Disord* 2004; **28** (Suppl. 3):S90–S95.

23 Leung MW, Yen IH, Minkler M; Community based participatory research: a promising approach for increasing epidemiology's relevant in the 21st century. *Int J Epidemiol* 2004; **33**:499–506;and Minkler M: Community-based research partnerships: challenges and opportunities. *J Urban Health* **82** (Suppl 2) ii3–ii12.

24 Sanigorski AM, Bell AC, Kremer PJ, Cuttler R, Swinburn B: Reducing unhealthy weight gain in children through community capacity building: results of a quasi-experimental intervention program, Be Active Eat Well. *Int J Obes* 2008; **32**:1060–1067.

25 Position of the American Dietetic Association: Individual-, family-, school-, and community-based interventions for pediatric overweigh. *J Am Diet Assoc* 2006; **106**(6): 925–945.

26 Kumanyika S, Jeffery RW, Morabia A, Ritenbaugh C, Antipatis VJ: Obesity prevention: the case for action. *Int J Obes Relat Metab Disord* 2002; **26**(3):425–436.

27 Summerbell CD, Waters E, Edmunds LD, Kelly S, Brown T, Campbell KJ: Interventions for preventing obesity in children. *Cochrane Database Syst Rev* 2005; 3 (Art. No.: CD001871).

28 Doak CM, Visscher TL, Renders CM, Seidell JC: The prevention of overweight and obesity in children and adolescents: a review of interventions and programmes. *Obes Rev* 2006; **7**(1):111–136.

29 Flynn MA, McNeil DA, Maloff B et al: Reducing obesity and related chronic disease risk in children and youth: a synthesis of evidence with "best practice" recommendations. *Obes Rev* 2006; **7**(Suppl. 1):7–66.

30 Sorensen G, Emmons K, Hunt MK, Johnston D: Implications of the results of community intervention trials. *Annu Rev Public Health* 1998; **19**:379–416.

31 Glass TA, McAtee MJ: Behavioral science at the crossroads in public health: Extending horizons, envisioning the future. *Soc Sci Med* 2006; **62**(7):1650–1671.

32 Minke SW, Smith C, Plotnikoff RC, Khalema E, Raine K: The evolution of integrated chronic disease prevention in Alberta, Canada. *Prev Chronic Dis* 2006; **3**(3):1–12.

33 Margolis PA, Stevens R, Bordley WC et al: From concept to application: the impact of a community-wide intervention to improve the delivery of preventive services to children. *Pediatrics* 2001; **108**(3):e42.

34 Economos CD, Irish-Hauser S: Community interventions: a brief overview and their application to the obesity epidemic. *J Law Med Ethics* 2007; **35**(1):131–137.

CHAPTER 8

Evidence of the influence of home and family environment

Johannes Brug[1], *Saskia te Velde*[1], *Ilse De Bourdeaudhuij*[2] and *Stef Kremers*[3]

[1] EMGO Institute for Health and Care Research, VU University Medical Centre, Amsterdam, The Netherlands
[2] Department of Movement Sciences and Sport Sciences, Ghent University, Ghent, Belgium
[3] Department of Health Promotion, NUTRIM School for Nutrition, Toxicology and Metabolism, University of Maastricht, Maastricht, The Netherlands

Summary and recommendations for practice

This chapter explores the influences of the physical, social-cultural and economic environment on children's eating behavior and physical activity. Socialization refers to the process by which a child learns the appropriate behaviors and ways to act in accordance with the cultural and/or societal norms. During childhood, parents are the main socializing agent and can have the biggest influence on their children's food consumption and physical activities. This is where life-long behaviors, habits and routines are learnt. This chapter explores the current research not only on parenting practices and energy-balance behaviors but also the wider determinates such as the environment and economic factors.

We use the ANGELO categories of obesogenic environments[1] to describe evidence on home and family environmental influences on energy-balance behaviors among young people. The home and family are regarded as strong influences on determining children's and adolescents' micro-level social, political, physical, as well as economical nutrition environments, and physical activity environments. We summarize the evidence from recent reviews and original studies which regard the home and family environment as important determinants for healthy eating and physical activities.

Preventing Childhood Obesity. Edited by
E. Waters, B.A. Swinburn, J.C. Seidell and R. Uauy.
© 2010 Blackwell Publishing.

Introduction

In reviewing the evidence base, we used recent systematic reviews that have addressed this topic area.[2–5] The review by Ventura and Birch, comprising 66 articles on associations between parental influences and child eating variables, showed that there is substantial evidence that parenting practices are important.[4] Reviews by Van der Horst et al and Ferreira et al further show that home and family environments are important correlates of nutrition and physical activity behaviors among children and adolescents.[3,5] However, all three reviews conclude that most of the available evidence is based on cross-sectional studies.

The physical home environment determines what is available in terms of food and opportunities for physical activity, the socio-cultural environment determines what is acceptable, and the economic environment what is affordable. Since the home and family micro-political environment cannot really be distinguished from the socio-cultural family environment, we focus here on the physical, socio-cultural and economic environments.

The physical environment

The home is where children spend much of their time, especially at a young age, and it is the place where children and adolescents eat the majority of their meals. The home environment strongly defines what foods and physical activity opportunities are available, especially for younger children.

Food availability

Home availability and accessibility of foods have been found to be associated with consumption among children and adolescents in different studies, especially as related to fruit and vegetable consumption.[3] However, in studies where such associations were adjusted for other potential behavioral determinants such as motivational, ability-related and socio-cultural environmental factors, the association between availability and consumption are reduced, sometimes to insignificance.[6,7]

Haerens et al investigated home environmental correlates of fat, soft drink and fruit consumption among adolescents.[8] In line with findings from other studies,[9] they found that boys with more unhealthy products available at home consumed more fat and more soft drinks. Girls who reported higher availability of healthy products at home ate more fruit.

Physical activity and sedentary behavior

Regarding sedentary behavior, a review by Govely and others[2] indicated that having a TV present in the bedroom was one of the most consistent correlates of TV viewing time among children and adolescents. Haerens et al investigated home and school environmental correlates of physical activity in adolescents.[8] The environmental factors accounted for a significant, but modest 5% of the total 38% explained variance in boys and only 1% of 23% in girls. The availability of sports equipment at home was significantly associated with physical activity among boys only. De Bruijn[10] examined the role of physical environmental factors and individual cognitive determinants in predicting physical activity in adolescents. Availability of local facilities were positively related to physical activity. Modeling these factors with the cognitive motivational factors derived from the theory of planned behavior, revealed that the environmental attributes were fully mediated by perceived behavioral control. In contrast, intention did not play a mediating role in the prediction of future physical activity.

We need to keep in mind that many physical activities and sedentary behaviors among children, such as playing outside after school, watching TV or playing on the computer, are typically routine. They are performed repeatedly, and to a certain extent automatically, in response to (physical) environmental cues. Imagine the child coming home from school,

grabbing a snack, walking directly to the PC, turning it on and immediately starting to play a computer game or to chat with friends. The concept of habit may thus be important in trying to understand environmental influences on these behaviors, in addition to measures of availability and accessibility. A study in 2008[11] provided limited but intriguing early evidence to support the concept of habit as being important in dealing with physical activity and sedentary behavior in children and adolescents. The study showed a high level of habitual engagement in a child's physical activity and sedentary behavior. Additionally, intentions proved to be strongly related to behavior in children with weak habits, but unrelated to behavior in those with strong habits.

The social-cultural environment

The aforementioned review studies clearly indicated that social-cultural environmental factors may be the strongest environmental determinants of children's eating and physical activity behaviors, and family social-cultural factors are of key importance.

Food and eating

Eating is a social behavior, especially for children,[12] and observing the eating behaviors of others, especially parents, influences their own preferences and behavior. Such modeling of eating behaviors can even result in establishing preferences for foods or substances that are inherently disliked. A recent review of the literature on environmental correlates of nutrition behaviors in young people indicates that children's and adolescents' nutrition behaviors are consistently associated with those of their parents,[13] and a second review also concluded that there was substantial evidence, also from experimental studies, that modeling has a significant influence on children's eating behaviors.[4] Parents further influence their offspring by actively encouraging, discouraging or controlling certain behaviors. Restricting children's access to, for example high-fat or sugar-rich, foods may encourage rather than discourage preferences for such foods, especially if these same foods are also used to reward children for good behavior and for celebrations.[12]

However, a study conducted in Belgium indicated that clear restrictive family rules about high-fat foods during childhood were associated with healthier food choices in adolescence,[14] and a recent cross-European study showed that parental demand as well as opportunities to eat fruit and vegetables were associated with higher intake levels in 11-year-old children, while "parental allowance" (i.e., parents allowing children to eat as much as they like), was not.[6,7] Haerens et al[8] also found greater fruit intake in adolescent girls if parents set clear food rules at home. Two recent Dutch studies among adolescents showed that more restrictive parenting practices were associated with lower consumption of sugar-sweetened beverages.[3,15]

The evidence from studies on the association between general parenting styles and children's health behaviors is inconclusive.[4] Some evidence suggests that authoritative parenting, that is, a parenting style characterized by high parental involvement as well as strictness, is associated with more positive health behaviors including higher fruit and vegetable intakes,[16,17] compared to adolescents who reported authoritarian (high strictness, low involvement) or neglectful (low strictness, low involvement) parenting styles. However, results of the Pro Children Study, investigating the relationship between general parenting styles and fruit and vegetable intake in 11-year-olds in four countries (Spain, Portugal, Belgium and the Netherlands) showed no differences in fruit and vegetable intake across parenting styles and only very few significances in social-environmental correlates.[18]

The study by Vereecken et al explored the impact of general parenting style and specific food-related parenting practices on children's dietary habits.[19] They found that general parenting style had no significant impact on dietary habits. In contrast, the food-related parenting encouragement through negotiation showed a significant positive impact, while pressure, catering on demand and permissiveness were practices with an unhealthy impact on the children's dietary habits.[19]

As a result of these parenting practices and rules, as well as parents' own food preferences and choices, parents influence what foods are available and accessible within the home environment. Availability and accessibility of foods have repeatedly been found to be associated with intake levels in children and adolescents.[4,20]

As mentioned, taste preference is perhaps the strongest determinant of food choice. Some specific types of taste-preference learning strategies have been identified, and parents and the home environment are important for the implementation of such strategies. The example of learning to like high-energy foods is referred to as "taste-nutrient learning". Taste-nutrient learning is an example of operant or instrumental conditioning: a stimulus (eating energy-dense, sweet and fatty food) is positively reinforced ("rewarded") by the pleasant feeling of satiety. In the last decades, palatable energy-dense foods have become readily available and accessible for most children in Western countries. This abundance combined with our innate preference for energy-dense foods may be an important cause for the present-day obesity epidemic. Research shows that high-fat and sugar-rich foods are, indeed, among the most preferred foods among children and adolescents.[21] Most fruits and especially vegetables have low-energy densities, and many vegetables have a somewhat bitter taste. Preferences for these foods are, therefore, not so easily learned.

Two other food preference-learning strategies are examples of classical conditioning and are referred to as "taste-taste learning" and "taste-environment learning". If a new, unfamiliar, taste is combined with a taste for which a preference already exists, children will more easily learn to like the new taste. For example, children will more easily learn to like the somewhat bitter taste of tea or the sour taste of yoghurt or grapefruit, if these are first served with sugar. Such taste-taste learning already occurs in very early childhood. Children who are breastfed are introduced to a broader range of tastes than children who are formula-fed, since the taste of breast milk varies, depending on the diet of the mother. Breastfed children are likely to learn to like a wider range of tastes early in life.[22]

Similarly, a liking for tastes that people are exposed to in pleasant physical or social environments are also learned. Foods first encountered as a child in a friendly, pleasant family environment, may become favorite foods for a lifetime. This strategy may indeed be used to teach children to learn to like "new" foods.

A fourth important learning strategy is observational learning or modeling: children learn to like the taste of foods that they see their parents, siblings, friends or other "important others" eat. As mentioned, recent reviews of the literature show that parental modeling is consistently associated with more healthful nutrition behaviors in young people.[23,24]

Physical activity and sedentary behaviors

Similar findings apply to physical activity and sedentary behaviors. A review by Gorely[2] showed that parents TV viewing was a consistent correlate of TV viewing among children and adolescents. Likewise, a recent review by Ferreira and colleagues (2007) showed that parental physical activity and social support from parents were among the most consistent environmental correlates of physical activity in children.[5] A study on the effect of general parenting styles on physical activity and sedentary behaviors conducted in four European countries found some evidence that higher levels of strictness were associated with lower levels of TV viewing during mealtimes and higher levels of physical exercise.[25] However, associations were not present in all countries, suggesting that the impact of parenting styles may be dependent on cultural context. Other studies that specifically looked at TV viewing and parenting, indicate that the "social co-viewing style" in which TV programs are watched together resulted in the highest levels of TV viewing among the children.[26]

Permissive or disengaged parents, particularly, may put their children in front of the television set with food or drinks to distract them, while the parents do other household chores and have minimal interaction with their child. As a result, children may learn to associate television viewing with energy intake from a very early age.[27] Such conditioned relationships between behaviors would imply that television viewing may become an automatic cue for energy intake and that social environmental factors regarding screen-viewing may also influence energy intake. Indeed, in a recent study (2007), Kremers and colleagues, for example, showed that adolescent screen-viewing behavior is associated with consumption of sugar-sweetened beverages.[28] Furthermore, their study indicated that parental norms with regard to screen-viewing was also associated with adolescent sugar-sweetened beverage consumption. By restricting television and computer use, parents appeared to influence their children's consumption. Such "clustering" of behaviors and their social-environmental correlates underlines the importance of an "energy balance-approach" in the study of determinants of weight gain.[29]

The socio-economic environment

The home or family socio-economic position is also of crucial importance. Recent reviews of the literature further confirmed that different indicators of family socio-economic position, including parental education, income and job status, are all associated with less healthy diets and a lower likelihood of sufficient physical activity in children and adolescents.[3,30]

But why is this the case? Is it because people from lower socio-economic positions have less to spend and cannot afford healthier foods and more active lifestyles? Recent research conducted in Australia indicates that perceived differences in price between more and less healthy foods, rather than actual price differences was associated with disparities in healthy eating between lower and higher socio-economic status group.[31] Other studies indicate that healthier eating is not, by definition, more expensive eating. However, Drewnowski and others have argued that foods primarily based on cheap (or more accurately, highly subsidized) high-energy ingredients like palm oil and corn syrup, do provide the best value for money in terms of calories, and that eating such obesogenic foods does make rational sense for people with less money to spend.[32] Drewnowski and others have also published empirical research showing that people choosing diets higher in fats and sugar paid less for food than people choosing healthier diets.[32]

Evidence that knowledge would make a difference

Another possible reason for disparities in healthy eating and physical activity is lack of knowledge. Are the differences there because parents with lower education do not know what is good for their children?

Skills and abilities are, to some extent, dependent on practical knowledge. For example, knowledge of recommended intake levels and healthy alternatives for unhealthy choices help to enable voluntary dietary change. In order to make conscious dietary changes for, for example, better bodyweight maintenance, knowledge is necessary about which dietary changes will be most effective. Some knowledge about which foods are high in calories is helpful to be able to avoid high-calorie foods and for self-monitoring of caloric intake. Knowing why to eat healthily, knowing what healthy foods are, and being aware of the recommended intake levels are important. But knowledge in

67

itself is unlikely to result in healthy food and nutrition choices, and associations between nutrition knowledge and dietary behavior have been found to be weak.[33]

It is also possible that parents from lower socio-economic status groups have different parenting styles or parenting practices, which results in less healthy behaviors in their offspring. Vereecken et al (2004) explored whether differences in children's food consumption by mothers' educational level could be explained by mother's consumption and other eating-related parenting practices.[19] They revealed that SES differences in children's fruit and vegetable consumption were completely mediated by differences in the mothers' food consumption and parenting practices. This was, however, not the case for SES differences in soft-drink consumption. In addition, a recent Australian study showed that adolescents living in lower SES households reported greater availability of unhealthy foods at home and were more likely to be allowed to watch TV during mealtimes, while adolescents from higher SES households reported greater availability and accessibility of fruits.[34]

Neighborhood SES and healthy foods and PA

It may also be that families from lower socio-economic positions live in neighborhoods where healthy foods and physical activity opportunities are less available.

While neighborhood inequalities in food availability have been reported, the evidence on the directions of effects is inconsistent. Some studies showed that there are fewer healthy choices available in stores in more deprived areas,[35–37] but other studies did not find such differences,[38,39] or found evidence that healthier options were better available in the more deprived neighborhoods.[40,41] It appears that the lower availability of healthy foods in the more deprived neighborhoods is especially apparent in US cities,[42] but the majority of individuals in many Western countries— including those with less healthy diets—may have sufficient access to healthy foods.

Regarding physical activity, the review by Feirreira and others showed that neighborhood crime rates are associated with lower levels of physical activity among adolescents,[5] but to date, very few studies have explored the relationship between the built environ-ment and physical activity in youngsters. In contrast to the expectations and the studies in adults, Haerens et al found that participation in moderate to vigorous physical activity (MVPA) measured with accelerometers, was higher among students living further away from facilities that are attractive to adolescents.[8] In line with the findings from Jago et al, no other environmental factors (environmental safety, environmental density, sedentary equipment) were found to be associated with participation in MVPA in adolescents.[43]

Discussion and conclusions

The home and family environment is of key importance for behavioral nutrition and physical activity among children and adolescents. Evidence points out that the home and family physical (what is available), social-cultural (what is appropriate and acceptable), and economic (what is affordable) environments are associated with important nutrition, physical activity and sedentary behaviors that define energy balance.

It should be noticed, however, that the available evidence is mostly based on studies using rather weak research designs. Most studies on potential home and family environmental influences on eating and the physical activities of young people are cross-sectional, and such studies may tell us about associations, but provide no proof of causal relations. An association between, for example, parenting and children's eating habits may indicate that parenting influences eating habits, but it may also mean that a child's eating habits influences parenting practices. If children eat too much, too little, or the wrong things, parents are likely to adjust their parenting practices accordingly. Ventura and Birch presented a conceptual model in which they proposed that parenting, child eating and child weight status all influence each other bidirectionally.[4]

Nevertheless, the associations found in recent studies indicate that obesity prevention for children and adolescents should focus on promoting home and family environments that endorse healthy energy-balance-related behaviors. However, by far the most initiatives for obesity prevention among young people have used school-based approaches, and interventions aiming at home and family environments are scarcer and, thus, less well researched. Results from the process evaluation of the multi-component Pro Children intervention, including activities to get parents involved in the project, showed that a higher level of parental involvement was beneficial for the pupil's fruit and vegetable intake as well as parental fruit and vegetable intake.[25,44] However, only a small proportion of the parents did actually participate in the parental activities.[25] Activities that the pupils and parents had to do together were most popular, such as going to the supermarket together, while very few parents did activities that they had to do on their own, such as parental meetings at school or visiting the Pro Children website. Therefore, more attention should be given towards finding strategies to get parents involved in school-based projects.

In summing up, this chapter has demonstrated the vast influence parent's have on their children's behavior, especially with regard to physical activity and food consumption. It is, therefore, essential for parents to model appropriate behavior in front of their children and encourage a physically active lifestyle rather then promoting sedentary behaviors, such as excessive television viewing and/or computer use. This should stem from the physical home environment (what foods they are providing?), the socio-cultural environment (what is considered acceptable foods?) and the economic environment (are the affordable foods appropriate?). On a wider scale, environmental factors, such as accessible and appropriate parks and footpaths should be available in all suburbs, regardless of the level of disadvantage. Future interventions may look towards dispelling the myth or belief that healthy foods are always more expensive, especially in lower SES areas.

References

1 Swinburn B: Dissecting obesogenic environments: the development and application of a framework for identifying and prioritizing environmental interventions for obesity. *Prev Med* 1999; **29**(6):563–570.

2 Gorley T, Marshall S, Biddle S: Couch kids: correlates of television viewing among youth. *Int J Behav Med* 2004; **11**(3):152–163.

3 Van der Horst K, Kremers S, Ferreira I, Singh A, Oenema A, Brug J: Perceived parenting styles and practises and the consumption of sugar-sweetener beverages by adolescents. *Health Educ Res* 2007; **22**:295–304.

4 Ventura A, Birch L: Does parenting affect children's eating and weight status? *Int J Behav Nutr Phys Act* 2008; **5**(15).

5 Ferreira I, Van der Horst K, Wendel-Vos W, Kremers S, Van Lenthe F, Brug J: Environmental correlates of physical activity in youth—a review and update. *Obes Rev* 2007; **8**:129–154.

6 Wind M, de Bourdeaudhuij I, Te Velde S et al: Correlates of fruit and vegetable consumption among 11-year-old Belgian-Flemish and Dutch schoolchildren. *J Nutr Educ Behav* 2006; **38**:211–221.

7 De Bourdeaudhuij I, Te Velde S, Brug J et al: Personal, social and environmental predictors of daily fruit and vegetable intake in 11-year-old children in nine European countires. *Eur J Clin Nutr* 2007; **62**(7):834–841.

8 Haerens L, Craeynest M, Deforche B, Maes L, Cardon G, De Bourdeaudhuij I: The contribution of psychosocial and home environmental factors in explaining eating behaviours in adolescents. *Eur J Clin Nutr* 2008; **62**(1): 51–59.

9 Lien N, Jacobs D, Klepp K: Exploring predictors of eating behaviour among adolescents by gender and social economic status. *Public Health Nutr* 2002; **5**:671–681.

10 De Bruijn G, Kremers S, De Vries H, Van Mechelen W, Brug J: Modelling individual and physical environmental factors with adolescent physical activity. *Am J Prev Med* 2006; **30**(6): 507–512.

11 Kremers S, Brug J: Habit strength of physical activity and sedentary behaviour among children and adolescents. *Pediatr Exerc Sci* 2008; **20**:5–17.

12 Birch L: Development of food preferences. *Annu Rev Nutr* 1999; **19**:41–62.

13 Brug J, Van Lenthe F, Kremers S: Revisiting Kurt Lewin: how to gain insight into environmental correlates of obesegnic behaviors. *Am J Prev Med* 2006; **31**:525–529.

14 De Bourdeaudhuij I, Van Oost P: De relatie tussen op jonge leeftijd aangeleerde voedingsregels en voedingskeuze in de adolescentie (The relation between in childhood acquired dietary habits and dietary choices in adolescence). *Gedrag en Gezonsheid* 1996; **24**:215–223.

15 De Bruijn G, Kremers S, De Vries H, Van Mechelen W, Brug J: Associations of social-environmental and individual-level factors with adolescent soft drink consumption: results of the SMILE-study. *Health Educ Res* 2007; **22**:227–237.

16 Patrick H, Nicklas T, Hughes S, Morales M: The benefits of authoritative feeding style: caregiver feeding styles and children's food consumption patterns. *Appetite* 2005; **44**: 243–249.

17 Kremers S, Brug J, Vries H, Rcme E: Parenting styles and adolescent fruit consumption. *Appetite* 2003; **41**:43–50.

18 De Bourdeaudhuij I, Te Velde S, Maes L, Perez-Rodrigo C, de Almeida M, Brug J: General parenting styles are not strongly associated with fruit and vegetable intake and social-environmental correlates among 11-year-old children in four countries in Europe. *Public Health Nutr* 2009;**12**(2): 259–266.

19 Vereecken C, Legiest E, De Bourdeaudhuij I, Maes L. Associations between general parenting styles and specific food-related parenting practices and children's food consumption. *Am J Health Promot* 2009; **23**(4):233–240.

20 Cullen K, Baranowski T, Owens E, Marsh T, Rittenberry L, de Moor C: Availability, accessibility, and preferences for fruit, 100% fruit juice, and vegetables influence children's dietary behavior. *Health Educ Behav* 2003; **30**:615–626.

21 Cooke L, Wardle J: Age and gender differences in children's food preferences. *Br J Nutr* 2005; **93**:741–746.

22 Forestell C, Mennella J: Early Determinants of fruit and vegetable acceptance. *Pediatrics* 2007; **120**(6):1247–1254.

23 Van der Horst K, Oenema A, Ferreira I: A systematic review of environmental correlates of obesity-related dietary behaviors in youth. *Health Educ Res* 2007; **22**:203–226.

24 Rasmussen M, Krolner R, Klepp K et al: Determinants of fruit and vegetable consumption among children and adolescents: a review of the literature. Part I: quantitative studies. *Int J Behav Nutr Phys Act* 2006; **3**(22).

25 te Velde S, Wind M, Perez-Rodrigo C, Klepp K, Burg J: Mothers' involvement in a school-based fruit and vegetable promotion intervention is associated with increased fruit and vegetable intakes—The Pro Children study. Under review.

26 Valkenburg P, Krcmar M, Peeters A, Marseille N: Developing a scale to assess three styles of television mediation: "instructive mediation", "restrictive mediation" and "social co-viewing". *J Broadcas Electron Media* 1999; **43**(1):52–66.

27 Lemish D: Viewers in dapers: the early development of television viewing. In: Lindlof T, ed. Natural Audiences: Qualitative Research of Media Uses and Effects. Norwood, NJ: Ablex, 1987:33–57.

28 Kremers S, van der Horst K, Brug J. Adolescent screen-viewing behavior is associated with consumption of sugar-sweetened beverages: the role of habit strength and perceived parental norms. *Appetite* 2007; **48**:345–350.

29 Kremers S, Visscher T, Seidell J, Van Mechelen W, Burg J: Cognitive determinants of energy balance-related behaviors: measurement issues. *Sports Med* 2005; **35**:923–933.

30 Wardle J, Jarvis M, Steggles N et al: Socioeconomic disparities in cancer-risk behaviors in adolescence: baseline results from the Health and Behaviour in Teenagers Study (HABITS). *Prev Med* 2003; **36**:295–304.

31 Giskes K, Van Lenthe F, Brug J, Mackenbach J, Turrell G: Socioeconomic inequalities in food purchasing: the contribution of respondent-perceived and actual (objectively measured) price and availability of foods. *Prev Med* 2007; **45**:41–48.

32 Drewnowski A, Darmon N, Briend A: Replacing fats and sweets with vegetables and fruits—a question of cost. *Am J Public Health* 2004; **94**:1555–1559.

33 Story M, Neumark-Stzainer D, French S: Individual and environemtnal influences on adolescent eating behaviors. *J Am Diet Assoc* 2002; **102**(3):S40–S51.

34 MacFarlane A, Crawford D, Ball K, Savige G, Worsley A: Adolescent home food environments and socioeconomic position. *Asia Pac J Clin Nutr* 2007; **16**(4):748–756.

35 Horowitz C, Colson K, Hebert P, Lancaster K: Barriers to buying healthy foods for people with diabetes: Evidence of environmental disparities. *Am J Public Health* 2004; **94**: 1549–1554.

36 All K, Timperio A, Crawford D: Socioeconomic inequalities in diet: are poor food environments to blame? 9th Behavioral Research in Cancer Control Conference; 2008; Melbourne. 2008.

37 Baker EA, Schootman M, Barnidge E, Kelley C: The role of race and poverty in access to foods that enable individuals to adhere to dietary guidelines. *Prev Chronic Dis* 2006; **3**(3): A76.

38 Winkler E, Turrell G, Patterson C: Does living in a disadvantaged area mean fewer opportunities to purchase fresh fruit and vegetables in the area? Findings from the Brisbane food study. *Health Place* 2006; **12**:306–319.

39 Apparicio P, Cloutier M, Shearmur R: The case of Montreal's missing food deserts: Evaluation of accessibility to food supermarkets. *Int J Health Geogr* 2007; **6**:4.

40 Cummins S, Macintyre S: The location of food stores in urban areas: a case study in Glasgow. *Br Food J* 1999; **101**(7):545–553.

41 Cummins S, Macintyre S: A systematic study of an urban foodscape: the price and availability of food in Greater Glasgow. *Urban Stud* 2002; **39**:2115–2130.

42 McIntyre S: Deprivation amplification revisited; or, is it always true that poorer places have poorer access to resources for healthy diets and physical activity? *Int J Behav Nutr Phys Act* 2007; **4**(34).

43 Jago R, Baranowski T, Zakeri I, Harris M: Observed environmental features and the physical activity of adolescent males. *Am J Prev Med* 2005; **29**(2):98–104.

44 Wind M, Bjelland M, Perez-Rodrigo C et al: Appreciation and implementation of a school-based intervention are associated with changes in fruit and vegetable intake in 10- to 13-year old schoolchildren the Pro Children study. *Health Educ Res* 2007;**23**(6):997–1007.

CHAPTER 9

Obesity prevention in early childhood

Ladda Mo-suwan[1] and *Andrea M. de Silva-Sanigorski*[2,3]
[1] Department of Pediatrics, Faculty of Medicine, Prince of Songkla University, Hat Yai, Songkhla, Thailand
[2] WHO Collaborating Centre for Obesity Prevention, Deakin University, Geelong, Australia
[3] Jack Brockoff Child Health and Wellbeing Program, McCaughey Centre, Melbourne School of Population Health, The University of Melbourne, Melbourne, Australia

Summary and recommendations for practice

- Early childhood is a critical period for obesity prevention. However, prevalence in preschool children is increasing.
- Early childhood settings (home, day care, kindergartens) have an important role in facilitating health promoting behaviors and healthy weight in young children.
- Further evidence is needed to determine the effectiveness of those behavioral interventions during pregnancy, those that promote breastfeeding and those that are family-based on preventing childhood obesity. However, these approaches hold promise.
- Behavioral interventions delivered through child care services have also shown some effectiveness on behaviors. However, reduced unhealthy weight gain was not achieved in most cases.
- The effectiveness of interventions with an environmental focus is also limited. However, these interventions hold great promise for creating environments to support healthy eating and physical activity and to shift social norms related to policies and practices in early childhood services.
- Despite promising results, further trials are needed to determine the best strategies for obesity prevention in the early years of life.

Preventing Childhood Obesity. Edited by
E. Waters, B.A. Swinburn, J.C. Seidell and R. Uauy.
© 2010 Blackwell Publishing.

Introduction

Recent reports from several countries have documented an increase in the prevalence of obesity among preschool children.[1-5] With its associated co-morbid conditions[6] and likelihood of persistence into adulthood,[7] these trends pose a remarkable burden in terms of young children's health and present and future health care costs. Therefore, the need to identify effective prevention of overweight and obesity among young children is urgent before a level of public health crisis is reached.

The importance of early child care settings—home/ family, day care, kindergartens—in shaping children's dietary intake, physical activity and energy balance, and consequently in combating the childhood obesity epidemic has been documented in a recent review[8] and Chapter 30. The role of the home environment and parental dynamics in the development and maintenance of children's healthy behaviors is multifactorial. In addition, parental roles in preventing obesity change as their children move through critical developmental periods from before birth.[9] An unfavorable pre-natal environment (e.g., maternal undernutrition or overnutrition, smoking and diabetes mellitus) increases a future risk of developing obesity in the offspring.[8,10] During infancy, dietary factors such as the extent and duration of breastfeeding,[11-16] and the nutrient content and timing of introduction of complementary foods,[17,18] have been found to be associated with an increased risk of obesity in later childhood. Toshcke et al[19] demonstrated that a combination of low meal frequency, decreased physical activity, watching television >1 h/day, formula feeding and smoking in pregnancy accounted for 48.2% of obese children aged 5–6 years. Modification of these risk factors will potentially yield a maximal achievable prevalence reduction of 1.5% for obesity (3.2% observed prevalence).[19]

As mothers increasingly work outside the home, the percentage of pre-school children being cared for outside the home has also increased. For that reason, parents and child-care providers are sharing responsibility in the formation of children's healthy behaviors during these important early developmental years. Level of physical activity and quality of food in these centers[20,21] has the potential to contribute substantially to the observed acceleration of obesity among preschool children attending day care centers during the past two decades.[22] A recent review of interventions in a variety of locations—home, day care, preschool, and clinic—to prevent or treat obesity among preschool children found seven studies of which four reported significant reduction in weight status or body fat.[23] Showing that interventions to reduce known risk factors from pregnancy through the early years in these settings has a great potential to prevent overweight and obesity in early childhood.

Method

For this chapter we scanned and reviewed the published literature (e.g., PubMed and CINAHL) to select studies that were effective, and examined the key elements that were consistent across the studies. With input from both authors, the evidence was synthesized and integrated into recommendations. Although there is no specific focus on social inequalities, this chapter examines cultural and gender differences in intervention effects and also looks at both behavioral and environmental interventions to find equitable and sustainable solutions.

Interventions during pregnancy

Concerning prenatal factors, a recent review of risk factors for overweight in preschool children found strong evidence for a direct association between childhood overweight and maternal pre-pregnancy body size, maternal weight gain and smoking during pregnancy.[8] On the matter of interventions, there are

currently four published studies on interventions to prevent excessive weight gain during pregnancy[24–27] and more than 50 randomized controlled studies on smoking cessation.[28–31] No studies evaluated the long-term effect on weight status of young children.

Only one of the four studies on gestational weight gain included birth weight as an outcome. Gray-Donald et al[24] based their design on social learning theory, compared 107 control subjects and 112 women who received diet and activity intervention during pregnancy in four Cree communities of James Bay, Quebec. Intervention consisted of regular, individual diet counseling, physical activity sessions and other activities related to nutrition, but did not result in differences in diet measured at 24–30 weeks' gestation, and rate of weight gain over the second half of pregnancy (0.53 ± 0.32 kg per week vs. 0.53 ± 0.27 kg per week). Mean birth weights were also similar (3741 ± 523 g vs. 3686 ± 686 g).

A Cochrane review of interventions promoting smoking cessation published in 2004 shows that smoking cessation programs in pregnancy were effective at reducing the proportion of women who continued to smoke, and also reducing low birth weight and preterm birth.[31] No studies investigated the effect on child obesity later in life.

Together, these studies demonstrate that pregnancy is an important time for intervention. At present, however, there are not enough studies to identify effective interventions during pregnancy for preventing obesity among infants and preschool children. More interventions need to be implemented and evaluated. Future studies should consider a multicomponent approach and have a longer-term follow-up of child anthropometric outcome.

Interventions to promote breastfeeding

Numerous interventions have been conducted to promote breastfeeding.[32] However, only one cluster-randomized trial of a breastfeeding promotion examined the effect on child weight status beyond infancy. From the total of 17,046 healthy breastfed infants enrolled in the Promotion of Breastfeeding Intervention Trial (PROBIT) in the Republic of Belarus, Kramer et al[33] followed 13,889 (81.5%) subjects with measurements of anthropometric variables and blood pressure at 6.5 years. The intervention led to a much greater prevalence of exclusive breast-feeding at three months in the experimental than in the control group (43.3% and 6.4%, respectively; $P < 0.001$) and a higher prevalence of any breastfeeding throughout infancy. At 6.5 years, no significant intervention effects were observed on anthropometric outcomes or blood pressure. This intervention, however, was designed to increase the degree and duration of breastfeeding and as a result of infant feeding supervision, mean weight-for-length z scores of PROBIT infants were well above the Centers for Disease Control and Prevention (CDC) reference throughout the first year.[34] With similar rapid weight gain in both groups, consequently, at 6.5 years no difference of anthropometric indices could be detected.

Home/family-based interventions

There is only one published report of randomized controlled trials using home/family setting to prevent overweight in young children.

Harvey-Berino and Rourke[35] evaluated the result of home visit to overweight Native American mothers (with body mass index >25 kg/m^2) of children aged 9 months to 3 years. Mothers were randomly assigned to receive weekly 1 hour home visits for 16 weeks from an indigenous peer educator who delivered a parenting skills program. For intervention group mothers ($n = 20$), the focus was on using the parenting skills to develop healthy eating and exercise behaviors in their children. Positive changes were reported between baseline and the 16-week follow-up for intervention compared with control group children ($n = 20$) with decreased weight-for-height z-scores (-0.27 vs. 0.31, $P = 0.06$), decreased total energy intake (-39.2 vs. 6.8 kcal/kg/day, $P = 0.06$) and reduced maternal use of restrictive child feeding practices (-0.22 vs. 0.08, $P < 0.05$). No differences were noted for children's fat intake or physical activity, or for maternal BMI, diet or activity behaviors.

This study demonstrates that parents are receptive and capable of behavioral modification and, hence, weight reduction in preschool children. However, a small number of subjects and short duration limits its generalization. A recent review of interventions aimed at positively impacting on weight, physical activity,

diet and sedentary behaviors in children from 0 to 5 years has found a number of family-based behavioral interventions, which showed some level of effectiveness to alter risk behaviors in young children.[36] Yet the interventions were predominately high-intensity, based on social behavioral theory, short term, of small sample sizes and did not include anthropometric assessments or cost–effectiveness analysis.[36] Clearly, more evaluated family-based or parent-based interventions targeting young children with a longer-term follow-up to demonstrate sustainability are needed. In addition, targeting parental behaviors may be more effective than interventions directed solely toward children, suggesting that modification of the child's environment during early development may have a lasting effect.[37]

Interventions in child-care settings

Child-care settings offer untapped opportunities for developing and evaluating effective obesity prevention strategies to reach both children and their parents. Quite a few published obesity prevention studies among preschool children could be located. Among them, an intervention with diet and physical activity components is the common strategy and appears to achieve some level of effectiveness. Interventions to improve food and physical activity environment, curriculum and policies are also examined.

Dietary and/or physical activity/exercise interventions

Five reports have been published, from four child-care-based interventions aiming at healthy diet, increasing physical activity/exercise or reducing sedentary behavior to prevent obesity among preschool children.[38–42]

Dennison et al[38] used a cluster randomized controlled trial to evaluate the efficacy of an intervention program delivered in preschool and day care facilities in rural upstate New York. The 39-week program was designed to change the television viewing, nutrition- and physical activity-related behaviors of the children aged 2.6 to 5.5 years using one-hour weekly sessions and involved eight intervention and eight control preschool and day care facilities. The impacts assessed were behavioral (parent-reported) and anthropometric. It was found that after the intervention period, children in the intervention group ($n = 90$) decreased their television/video viewing by about 3 hours/week, whereas children in the control group ($n = 73$) increased their viewing by 1.6 hours/week, for a significant adjusted difference between the groups of −4.7 hours/week. In addition, the percentage of children watching television/videos more than 2 hours per day also decreased significantly among the intervention group, compared with an increase in the control group. Despite these behavioral changes, no statistically significant differences were found in children's BMI or triceps skin-fold between groups.[38]

Fitzgibbon et al assessed the impact of a randomized controlled trial with culturally proficient dietary/physical activity, the Hip-Hop to Health Jr, on changes in body mass index of 3- to 5-year-old minority children from schools randomized to a weight control intervention or to a control group that received a general health intervention.[39,40] Two cohorts of children participated in the trial: the first group of children attended 12 predominantly black preschools,[39] whereas the second cohort attended 12 predominantly Latino preschools.[40] Children in the six intervention schools received thrice-weekly lesson plans that incorporated two major components: (1) a 20-minute lesson that introduced a healthy eating or exercise concept with an activity, and (2) 20 minutes of ongoing physical activity for 14 weeks. Their parents received weekly newsletters with information mirroring the children's curriculum. The control children in the other six centers received a general health intervention that did not address either diet or physical activity. The intervention children (99% Black) had significantly smaller increases in BMI compared with control children (80.7% Black, 12.7% Latino) at 1-year follow-up, 0.06 vs. 0.59 kg/m^2; difference −0.53 kg/m^2 (95% CI −0.91 to −0.14), $P = 0.01$; and at 2-year follow-up, 0.54 vs. 1.08 kg/m^2; difference −0.54 kg/m^2 (95% CI −0.98 to −0.10), $P = 0.02$, with adjustment for baseline age and BMI. The only significant difference between intervention and control children in food intake/physical activity was the Year 1 difference in percentage of calories from saturated fat, 11.6% vs. 12.8% ($P = 0.002$). In the second cohort, with Latino children, there were no significant differences between intervention and control schools high-lighting the need to modify intervention activities to the cultural context.

Mo-suwan et al[41] examined the effect of a school-based aerobic exercise program on overweight indices of preschool children in Thailand. Half of the classes of second-year pupils of two schools were randomized into the intervention (mean age 4.5 ± 0.4 years, $n = 145$) or control (mean age 4.5 ± 0.4 years, $n = 147$) group. The intervention program included an extra 15-minute walk in the morning and a 20-minute aerobic exercise session in the afternoon three times per week. The exercise program was led by trained personnel and lasted about 30 weeks. This intervention program was provided in addition to the usual practices of the schools. At the initial evaluation at 29.6 weeks, a reduction of the prevalence of obesity in the intervention preschool children reached near statistical significance ($P = 0.057$). The study showed that intervention girls had a lower likelihood of having an increased BMI slope than control girls (odds ratio 0.32; 95% CI 0.18 to 0.56), while the opposite was true for boys (odds ratio 1.08; 95% CI 0.62 to 1.89). The significant difference may be related to gender roles and expectations in Thailand. At six months post-intervention, the prevalence of obesity in the control group decreased from 12.2% at baseline to 9.4% after the intervention, and was 10.8% at 29.6 weeks plus six months. In the exercise intervention group, the prevalence of obesity was 12.9% at baseline, 8.8% at 29.6 weeks and 10.2% six months later.[43]

A randomized control trial carried out by Reilly et al[42] examined the effect of an enhanced physical activity program implemented in nurseries in Scotland. The program consisted of three 30-minute sessions a week over 24 weeks, delivered by trained personnel, with additional home-based health education aimed to increase children's physical activity through play and reduce sedentary behaviors. The total of 545 children from 36 nurseries in Glasgow, Scotland were randomized to either intervention (mean aged 4.2 ± 0.3 years, $n = 268$) or control group (mean aged 4.1 ± 0.3 years, $n = 277$). The evaluation found that the program had no significant effect on physical activity, sedentary behavior or body mass index. The only significant effect of the physical activity program was enhanced fundamental movement skills for intervention children compared to children in the control group at the six-month follow-up ($P = 0.0027$) after adjustment for sex and baseline performance.

These interventions achieved significant behavioral changes, yet only two produced some effects on prevention of obesity—one had a directed exercise program,[41] the other included both diet and exercise components.[39] However, the effect was significant only among girls and not sustainable after six months post intervention in one study,[41] while it was effective and sustainable only among Blacks[39] not the Latinos[40] in the other, suggesting that gender and cultural difference should be addressed in designing the intervention activities. The two studies that did not report significant reductions in weight status had similar intervention approaches and intensity, and a comparable number of participants in one study (but less in the other). However, the duration of follow-up was shorter. These equivocal results highlight the need for more studies to provide further evidence on effectiveness of these promising strategies.

Innovative educational program

For a young child, health and education are inseparable. There is no published evaluation of an educational program for young children on preventing obesity. The only published report, the "Color Me Healthy" intervention, evaluated program acceptability and implementation and children's knowledge and some behaviors.[44] This educational program was implemented widely in North Carolina and was designed to increase physical activity and promote healthy eating in 4–5-year-old children through the development of fun, colorful and innovative educational materials. The content development was guided by social cognitive theory and the socio-ecological model. Trained child-care providers (1338 participants in 53 training sessions) delivered the program in a range of care settings and the eight-week follow-up evaluation showed that over 90% of providers reported increases in children's physical activity, knowledge about movement and knowledge about healthy eating.[44] The train-the-trainer model in this intervention holds promise as a way of improving the child-care environment on a large scale and in a range of child-care settings. It will be important to determine the sustainability of the program and its ability to positively influence children's risk and protective behaviors related to childhood obesity.

Interventions with an environmental focus

Child-care settings should provide an environment in which young children are offered nutritious foods and regular physical activity through structured and unstructured play, so that they learn these healthy lifestyle behaviors at an early age.[20] Thus child care plays a critical role in laying a foundation for healthy weight. Currently, there are four published studies of environmental interventions in child care.[45–48] One study reported self-assessment of the nutrition and physical activity child-care environment and its implementation, feasibility and acceptability; and found a variety of environmental improvements post-intervention.[45] Food and nutrition environments were the focus of interventions in the other studies.[46–48] Leahy et al[46] altered the energy density of a lunch entrée and determined the effect on 2- to 5-year-old children's subsequent *ad libitum* intake of lunch. This intervention was found to be effective in reducing children's energy intake from the entrée and total lunch energy intake. Matwiejczyk et al[47] evaluated an incentive initiative—the "Start Right Eat Right" award—that aimed to improve the nutrition provided to children attending child-care centers in South Australia. Substantial changes were reported in the food policies of the child-care centers and there was a resulting improvement in food provision and nutrition practices in these settings.

Children's anthropometric measurement was included as the outcome in only one study. Williams et al[48] examined how a change in the school food service aimed at reducing saturated fat intake, without compromising energy intake or nutrient content of the available diet, modified serum cholesterol and weight status. The intervention was based on the Piaget Stage 2 Model, Social Learning Theory and High/Scope Active Learning. Nine Head Start Centers, which served predominantly minority children from families with incomes below the US poverty level. Children were assigned to one of the three study groups: a control group with a safety education curriculum but without food service modification (350 children aged 49.3 ± 6.1 months), an intervention group with food service modification plus a child/family nutrition education program (242 children aged 48.3 ± 6.9 months), or an intervention group with food service modification plus a safety curriculum (195 children aged 47.9 ± 6.4 months). Behavioral changes regarding participation either in the school meals program or in the take-home activities included in this program were not measured. At the end of the school year, there was a statistically significant difference in the change in weight–height ratio between the intervention and control groups among white children ($n = 130$), mean difference 0.034 (95% CI 0.023 to 0.045). However, no differences were observed for Black or Latino children. Despite some limitations, these results are encouraging in that a relatively simple intervention aimed at changing an important environmental component of school health (the food service) can have direct effects on energy intake and promote a healthier rate of weight gain as well as reduce a major CVD risk factor in a young minority population.

These approaches hold promise for creating communities that promote healthy weight for young children. They have the ability to shift social norms with regards to the policies and practices in child-care centers and subsequently affect individual behavior change in a way that is meaningful and sustainable. These studies now need to go further to evaluate the effectiveness of these environmental changes themselves, in order to reduce unhealthy weight gain in the children attending these centers over time.

Conclusion and implication

The early childhood period holds promise as a time in which obesity prevention may be most effective. Interventions during pregnancy to promote optimum birth weight and interventions during early childhood to promote healthy eating and physical activity have a great potential to prevent childhood obesity.

Despite ample evidence on modifiable risk factors of overweight in early childhood which are amenable to effective prevention programs, relatively few published interventions focused on changes in weight status among infants and preschool children. In addition to the paucity of current published studies, the heterogeneous nature of the settings, methodologies, intervention strategies, definitions of obesity and outcome measures make it difficult to determine the most effective strategy or make recommendations on how to prevent obesity in the early childhood period.

Despite the limitations of the available evidence, findings from these interventions provide a basis for further development of effective intervention strategies. Two of the four effective interventions included parent education programs[33,39] and another sent materials home to parents on a weekly basis.[48] As supported by the recent review of Bluford et al,[23] it seems sensible to recommend that interventions for children include parents and other adult role models (e.g., teachers) rather than children alone. However, more work is needed to examine how active parental involvement needs to be in intervention programs for young children.

Diet and exercise are the common strategies used. Gender and cultural differences were found to influence the effectiveness of the interventions,[39–41] thus an intervention program should be designed in a way to appropriately address inequalities, gender, ethnic and cultural aspects. Moreover, given the dynamicity of child development abilities during the early years, the nutrition and the physical activity components of the interventions also need to be tailored to age-specific abilities.[23]

Consideration also needs to be given to the duration of intervention programs as the evidence demonstrates the need for a longer follow-up period of 1–2 years to assess change in weight status and increase the likelihood of adequately evaluating program impacts and sustainability.[23]

In conclusion, given the potential for early intervention to have long-lasting impacts on individual and population health, more interventions need to be implemented and comprehensively evaluated to determine their effectiveness on reducing the prevalence of childhood obesity. A focus on interventions that involve the family and create sustainable environmental changes to promote quality nutrition and physical activity should be a priority.

References

1 Bundred P, Kitchiner D, Buchan L: Prevalence of overweight and obese children between 1989 and 1998: population based series of cross-sectional studies. *BMJ* 2001; **322**:313–314.

2 Herpertz-Dahlmann B, Geller F, Böhle C, Khalil C, Trost-Brinkhues G, Ziegler A, et al: Secular trends in body mass index measurements in preschool children from the City of Aachen, Germany. *Eur J Pediatr* 2003; **162**:104–109.

3 Ogden CL, Troiano RP, Briefel RR, Kuczmarski RJ, Flegal KM, Johnson CL, et al: Prevalence of overweight among preschool children in the United States, 1971 through 1994. *Pediatrics* 1997; **99**:e1.

4 Reilly JJ, Dorosty A, Emmett PM: Prevalence of overweight and obesity in British children: cohort study. *BMJ* 1999; **319**: ••–1039.

5 Sherry B, Mei Z, Scanlon KS, Mokdad AH, Grummer-Strawn LM: Trends in state-specific prevalence of overweight and underweight in 2- through 4-year-old children from low-income families from 1989 through 2000. *Arch Pediatr Adolesc Med* 2004; **158**:1116–1124.

6 Baker S, Barlow S, Cochran W, Fuchs G, Klish W, Krebs N, et al: Overweight children and adolescents: a clinical report of the North American society for pediatric gastroenterology, hepatology and nutrition. *J Pediatr Gastroenterol Nutr* 2005; **40**:533–543.

7 Freedman DS, Srinivasan S, Valdez RA Williamson DF, Berenson GS: Secular increase in relative weight and adiposity among children over two decades: the Bogalusa heart Study. *Pediatrics* 1997; **99**:420–426.

8 Hawkins SS, Law C: A review of risk factors for overweight in preschool children: a policy perspective. *Int J Pediatr Obes* 2006; **1**(4):195–209.

9 Lindsay AC, Sussner KM, Kim J, Gortmaker S: The role of parents in preventing childhood obesity. *Future Child* 2006; **16**:169–186.

10 Whitaker RC, Dietz WW: Role of the prenatal environment in the development of obesity. *J Pediatr* 1998; **132**: 768–776.

11 Arenz S, Ruckerl R, Koletzko B, von Kries R: Breast-feeding and childhood obesity—a systematic review. *Int J Obes* 2004; **28**:1247–1256.

12 Agras SW, Kraemer HC, Berkowitz RI, Hammer LD: Influence of early feeding style on adiposity at 6 years of age. *J Pediatr* 1990; **116**:805–809.

13 Gilman MW, Rifas-Shiman SS, Camargo CA, Jr., Berkey CS, Frazier AL, Rockett HR, et al: Risk of overweight among adolescents who were breastfed as infants. *JAMA* 2001; **285**: 2461–2467.

14 Hediger ML, Ooverpeck M, Kuczmarski RJ, Ruan WJ: Association between infant breastfeeding and overweight in young children. *JAMA* 2001; **285**:2453–2460.

15 von Kries R, Koletzko B, Sauerwald T, von Mutius E, Barnert D, Grunert V, et al: Breast feeding and obesity: cross sectional study. *BMJ* 1999; **319**:147–150.

16 Owen CG, Martin RM, Whincup PH, Davey-Smith G, Gilman MW, Cook DG: The effect of breastfeeding on mean body mass index throughout life: a quantitative review of published and unpublished observational evidence. *Am J Clin Nutr* 2005; **82**:1298–1307.

17 Owen CG, Martin RM, Whuncup PH, Smith GD, Cook DG: Effect of infant feeding on the risk of obesity across the life course: a quantitative review of published evidence. *Pediatrics* 2005; **115**:1367–1377.

18 Toschke AM, Kuchenhoff H, Koletzko B, von Kries R: Meal frequency and childhood obesity. *Obes Res* 2005; **13**: 1932–1938.

19 Toschke AM, Ruckinger S, Bohler E, Von Kries R: Adjusted population attributable fractions and preventable potential of risk factors for childhood obesity. *Public Health Nutr* 2007; **10**(9):902–906.

20 Story M, Kaphingst KM, French S: The role of child care settings in obesity prevention. *Future Child* 2006; **16**(1): 143–168.

21 Vasquez F, Salazar G, Andrade M, Vasquez L, Diaz E: Energy balance and physical activity in obese children attending day-care centres. *Eur J Clin Nutr* 2006; **60**(9):1115–1121.

22 Velasquez MM, Salazar G, Vio F, Hernandez J, Rojas J: Nutritional status and body composition in Chilean preschool children attending day care centers. *Food Nutr Bull* 2002; **23**(3 Suppl.):250–253.

23 Bluford DA, Sherry B, Scanlon KS: Interventions to prevent or treat obesity in preschool children: a review of evaluated programs. *Obesity* 2007; **15**(6):1356–1372.

24 Gray-Donald K, Robinson E, David K, Renaud L, Rodrigues S: Intervening to reduce weight gain in pregnancy and gestational diabetes mellitus in Cree communities: an evaluation. *Can Med Assoc J* 2000; **163**:1247–1251.

25 Kinnunen TI, Pasanen Fogelholm M, Aittasalo M, et al: Preventing excessive weight gain during pregnancy—a controlled trial in primary health care. *Eur J Clin Nutr* 2007; **61**(7):884–891.

26 Olson CM, Strawderman MS, Reed RG: Efficacy of an intervention to prevent excessive gestational weight gain. *Am J Obstet Gynecol* 2004; **191**(2):530–536.

27 Polley BA, Wing RR, Sims CJ: Randomized controlled trial to prevent excessive weight gain in pregnant women. *Int J Obes Relat Metab Disord* 2002; **26**(11):1494–1502.

28 Panjari M, Bel R, Bishop S, Astbury J, Rice G, Doery J: A randomized controlled trial of a smoking cessation intervention during pregnancy. *Aust N Z J Obstet Gynaecol* 1999; **39**(3):312–317.

29 Polanska K, Hanke W, Sobala W, John B, Lowe JB. Efficacy and effectiveness of the smoking cessation program for pregnant women. *Int J Occup Med Environ Health* 2004; **17**(3):369–377.

30 Wisborg K, Henriksen T, Jespersen LB, Secher NJ: Nicotine patches for pregnant smokers: a randomized controlled study. *Obstet Gynecol* 2000; **96**:967–971.

31 Lumley J, Oliver SS, Chamberlain C, Oakley L: Interventions for promoting smoking cessation during pregnancy. *Cochrane Database Syst Rev* 2004; 4 (Art. No.: CD001055). doi: 10.1002/14651858.CD001055.pub2

32 Dyson L, McCormick FM, Renfrew MJ: Interventions for promoting the initiation of breastfeeding. *Cochrane Database Syst Rev* 2005; 2 (Art. No.: CD001688). doi: 10.1002/14651858. CD001688.pub2

33 Kramer MS, Matush L, Vanilovich I et al: Effects of prolonged and exclusive breastfeeding on child height, weight, adiposity, and blood pressure at age 6.5 y: evidence from a large randomized trial. *Am J Clin Nutr* 2007; **86**(6): 1717–1721.

34 Kramer MS, Guo T, Platt RW, Sevkovskaya Z, Dzikovich I, Collet J-P, et al: Infant growth and health outcomes associated with 3 compared with 6 mo of exclusive breastfeeding. *Am J Clin Nutr* 2003; **78**:291–295.

35 Harvey-Berino J, Rourke J: Obesity prevention in preschool native-american children: a pilot study using home visiting. *Obes Res* 2003; **11**(5):606–611.

36 Campbell KJ, Hesketh KD: Strategies which aim to positively impact on weight, physical activity, diet and sedentary behaviours in children from zero to five years. A systematic review of the literature. *Obes Rev* 2007; **8**(4):327–338.

37 Golan M, Crow S: Targeting parents exclusively in the treatment of childhood obesity: long-term results. *Obes Res* 2004; **12**(2):357–361.

38 Dennison BA, Russo TJ, Burdick PA, Jenkins PL: An intervention to reduce television viewing by preschool children. *Arch Pediatr Adolesc Med* 2004; **158**(2):170–176.

39 Fitzgibbon ML, Stolley MR, Dyer AR, VanHorn L, KauferChristoffel K: A community-based obesity prevention program for minority children: rationale and study design for Hip-Hop to Health Jr. *Prev Med* 2002; **34**(2):289–297.

40 Fitzgibbon ML, Stolley MR, Schiffer L, Van Horn L, KauferChristoffel K, Dyer A: Hip-Hop to Health Jr. for Latino preschool children. *Obesity* (Silver Spring) 2006; **14**(9):1616–1625.

41 Mo-suwan L, Pongprapai S, Junjana C, Puetpaiboon A: Effects of a controlled trial of a school-based exercise program on the obesity indexes of preschool children. *Am J Clin Nutr* 1998; **68**:1006–1011.

42 Reilly JJ, Kelly L, Montgomery C, Williamson A, Fisher A, McColl JH, et al: Physical activity to prevent obesity in young children: cluster randomised controlled trial. *BMJ* 2006; **333**:1041.

43 Summerbell CD, Waters E, Edmunds LD, Kelly S, Brown T, Campbell KJ: Interventions for preventing obesity in children. *Cochrane Database Syst Rev* 2005; 3 (Art. No.: CD001871).

44 Dunn C, Thomas C, Ward D, Pegram L, Webber K, Cullitan C: Design and implementation of a nutrition and physical activity curriculum for child care settings. *Prev Chronic Dis* 2006; **3**(2):A58.

45 Benjamin SE, Ammerman A, Sommers J, Dodds J, Neelon B, Ward DS, et al: Self-assessment for child care (NAP SACC): results from a pilot intervention. *J Nutr Educ Behav* 2007; **39**(3):142–149.

46 Leahy KE, Birch LL, Rolls BJ: Reducing the energy density of an entree decreases children's energy intake at lunch. *J Am Diet Assoc* 2008; **108**(1):41–48.

47 Matwiejczyk L, Colmer K, McWhinnie J-A: An evaluation of a nutrition intervention at childcare centres in South Australia. *Health Promot J Austr* 2007; **18**:159–162.

48 Williams CL, Strobino B, Bollella M, Brotanek J: Cardiovascular risk reduction in preschool children: the "Healthy Start" project. *J Am Coll Nutr* 2004; **23**(2):117–123.

CHAPTER 10

Obesity prevention in primary school settings: evidence from intervention studies

Juliana Kain,[1] *Yang Gao,*[2] *Colleen Doak*[3] *and Simon Murphy*[4]

[1] Institute of Nutrition and Food Technology (INTA), University of Chile, Santiago, Chile
[2] School of Public Health, The Chinese University of Hong Kong, Hong Kong SAR, China
[3] Department of Health Sciences, Faculty of Earth and Life Sciences, VU University, Amsterdam, The Netherlands
[4] Cardiff Institute of Society and Health, School of Social Sciences, Cardiff University, Cardiff, UK

Summary and recommendations for practice

- Interventions should be complex and ecological in nature, addressing the multiple and interactive influences on obesity, of which the primary school is one part.
- Interventions within schools should be multifaceted covering curriculum, policy and social and physical environments.
- School interventions should be developed and implemented with community involvement.
- Interventions within schools should address multiple rather than single risk behaviors.
- Interventions should be implemented within a rigorous evaluation framework to develop an adequate evidence base and to assess their impact on health inequalities.

Method

References were searched and retrieved from international databases, including MEDLINE, EMBASE, PsycINFO, and Cochrane databases from 1991 to February 2008. Effective interventions were recommended mainly based on findings in systematic reviews.

Rationale/importance of primary setting

Childhood obesity has increased rapidly over the past two decades, both in developing and industrialized countries.[1] Interventions targeted at primary school-aged children are considered critical to prevent and control this disease since food and physical activity related behaviors are established early in life and persist into adulthood.[2] The life-course approach to public health suggests that interventions in early life may define lifelong behaviors and protect children from developing unhealthy dietary habits. Children aged 5–11 have been identified as the optimal group to target for interventions on physical activity and healthy food preferences.[3] School settings are the prime focus for preventive actions since they cover most children in a country. Most children attend school approximately 180 days/year for six or more hours per day.[4] Children can easily be reached to assess their health needs, receive tailored interventions such as health education and physical activity promotion, be provided with healthy school meals, and be affected by environmental factors that

Preventing Childhood Obesity. Edited by
E. Waters, B.A. Swinburn, J.C. Seidell and R. Uauy.
© 2010 Blackwell Publishing.

condition obesity in children.[2] This is well recognized in the Health Promoting Schools (HPS) program, launched by World Health Organization (WHO). This presents a collaborative, interactive and participatory model for health promotion in the school by strengthening and enriching, the curriculum, developing a supportive environment reinforcing health enhancing behaviors, and creating strong links and access to community resources.[5]

Defining the primary school settings

This chapter examines the need for interventions in light of current trends in overweight and obesity in children as a global concern. In this context, the significance of school-based interventions goes beyond the opportunity to address the determinants that exist in the school environment; schools also provide an opportunity to reach individual children, families and the wider community.

It is difficult to estimate the true extent of the obesity problem among children, because diverse classifications of childhood obesity have been used across study populations. However, using current International Obesity Task Force (IOTF) estimates, one out of ten school- aged children in the world is overweight or obese, with the highest prevalence occurring in the Americas (Figure 10.1).[2]

As economies grow, obesity shifts from the more affluent to less affluent groups. Social and economic

development, modernization, urbanization and globalization collectively nurture unhealthy eating patterns and physical inactivity and constitute the main causes of obesity. Figure 10.2 draws on a socio-ecological perspective[6–8] to illustrate how determinants of childhood obesity at different levels—namely, at individual, family-school-neighbourhood (community), national, and global—may interact and contribute to the current epidemic of obesity.

As shown in Figure 10.2, schools play a key role in determining a child's immediate environment. Meals and snacks at schools form part of the child's overall diet, and the physical environment of the school, together with school policy, determine activity patterns. Furthermore, curriculum helps to form children's knowledge and behaviors both in nutrition and physical activity. Public primary schools in some countries provide meals (breakfast and/or lunch) to the children, either at no cost or subsidized in a significant way; in most cases the programs are designed with the objective of meeting established nutritional standards. Unfortunately, these programs do not always offer fresh vegetables and fruits and other healthy foods (lean meats and fish) as part of the menu. School meals are an important source of total daily energy intake and, especially for low-income children, may mitigate hunger and serve to prevent undernutrition.

Both state-funded and private schools in developed countries, and private schools in developing countries, may have a cafeteria inside the school offering

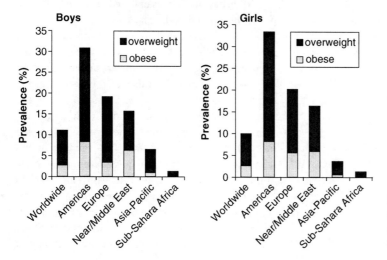

Figure 10.1 Prevalence of overweight and obesity among school-age boys and girls by global region.[5]

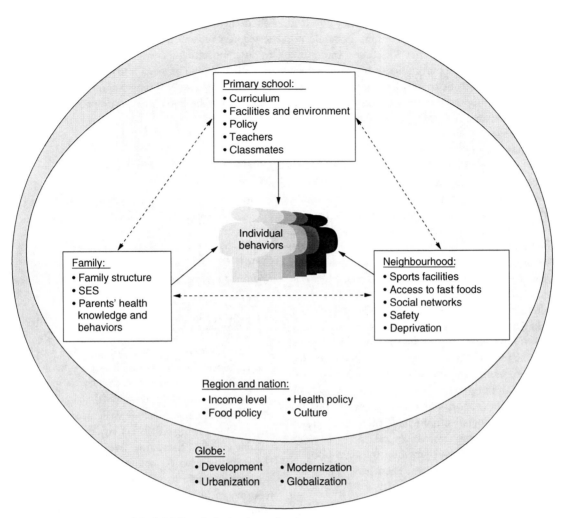

Figure 10.2 A macro model of childhood obesity determinants.

meals à la carte, which generally comply with nutritional standards. In addition, food items can be sold in vending machines and/or tuck shops and, in general, are not regulated. In some cases, unhealthy foods cannot be sold during meal periods in the food service areas; nevertheless, they can be sold anywhere else in the school. The kinds of foods sold in school vending machines are mostly high-fat and high-sugar nutrient poor foods and beverages that promote weight gain. Because the sale of these foods can generate revenue to the school to support different types of activities, regulating the sale of these items can be quite difficult. Furthermore, offering this type of

foods for sale inside the school contradicts the health messages that children receive in the classroom or in health promotion efforts.[4]

Schools also influence children's level of physical activity. School-based physical activity or physical education programs help primary school children to remain active. Schools should have good quality physical education classes (PE) (a minimum of three times a week to total 135 minutes), health education, sufficient recess time and an intramural sports program.[9] Unfortunately, PE classes are often undervalued despite their importance in achieving fitness, skills and health. Because playtime is a necessary activity for the release of energy and stress and it may also help children concentrate in the classroom. It should not be scheduled before or after PE classes. Intramural activities can offer opportunities to increase physical activity, but mostly better-off children take advantage of them, because even though the school may offer them, lower-income students may have transportation problems.[10]

Health education including formal instruction in healthy eating and promotion of physical activity is needed in all grades in order to improve children's knowledge and encourage children to adopt a healthy lifestyle. Research supports the use of behavioral techniques to achieve effectiveness in this task.[11] Aspects of health education can also be integrated into the lesson plans of other subjects such as mathematics, language, art, and so on. In addition to health education, school health centers can play an important role offering students, primary care or referral services to other health centers. Such centers can be found in state-funded and private schools in developed countries and private schools in developing countries, and may provide screening as well as information on prevention and treatment of obesity. In addition, schools can provide opportunities to implement obesity-prevention programs through after-school programs. In the United States there are several large-scale federally funded after-school programs to prevent obesity among low- income children. These may include academic enrichment, physical activity and free snacks.[12]

School-based obesity prevention programs can also provide a means of reaching the family. Family involvement and active participation by parents in obesity prevention is crucial; nevertheless, this can be quite difficult. Some programs that have achieved high rates of recruitment and retention have used incentives such as food, transportation and rewards. A promising initiative to involve parents may be to open school facilities such as gyms and swimming pools after school and at weekends. Another strategy of family involvement is parental notification of the child's BMI. Kubik et al[13] reports that parents of elementary school children are generally supportive of BMI reporting, but they want assurance about student privacy, respect and to know that overweight children will not be stigmatized. The US Institute of Medicine endorses BMI reporting and making it available once a year to parents with appropriate indications in cases

where the child is overweight. This activity should be tested in other societies so as to assess its effectiveness in different settings. The box below lists some of the issues that should be taken into account before deciding whether to use BMI reporting, and the chapter on ethics within this book provides more detail on ethical considerations.

Parental notification of children's BMI

- Which parents are going to be notified?—all of them, or only parents of overweight children.
- What will the parents be told when notified?
- Will they be advised to seek medical guidance or will they receive other recommendations? Are these readily available?

Finally, schools and school-based prevention programs can help to provide links with communities and families. For example, some schools have programs that link local farmers as suppliers for school meals. These programs have the advantage of providing high-quality produce and supporting local agriculture. Other initiatives include walking and cycling to school which, being a daily activity, can provide substantial energy expenditure over the school year.[14] Unfortunately, active commuting to schools has declined dramatically in recent decades. The reasons reported include long distances, traffic danger and crime. A final means by which schools can involve the larger community is through School Wellness Programs. Because schools are large employers, they become ideal places for health promotion for teachers and staff. This could encourage them to value the importance of healthy eating and physical activity and eventually to become role models for their students and their families

Type of Interventions

Interventions in primary school settings may be grouped together by aspects such as the aim, target population, intervention levels, extent of stakeholders involved, determinants addressed, specific intervention components, duration of the intervention and the outcomes measured. The intervention aim can be focused primarily on reducing obesity, or this can be a component of an intervention with another main goal (e.g., interventions for preventing childhood diabetes). Furthermore, the targeting can be primary prevention (addressing the general population), secondary prevention (addressing the population at risk of obesity), tertiary prevention (treating the obese population), or integrated/comprehensive (combination of the three level preventions).

Intervention programs may take place only in one school (single level), or multiple schools at the community, region, national, and even international levels (multiple levels). The intervention may engage any combination of stakeholders including individual participants or organizations from the health sector, non-health sector, policy-makers, teachers, school nurse, parents and grandparents. A number of determinants can be addressed, including one or any combination of the determinants as described in Table 10.1. In general, interventions lasting less than one year are defined as short-term, while those lasting one year or more are long term.[15] Considering that behavior change is central to preventing obesity, the effectiveness of short-term interventions may be biased and even regressive whereas effective long-term interventions are more promising. Commonly used outcomes can be divided into the following categories: body composition (e.g., BMI, fat distribution, prevalence of obesity/overweight, skin-fold thicknesses); nutrition/dietary habits (e.g., food choice, food consumption, energy intake and sources); physical activity (e.g., frequency, duration, intensity, sedentary behaviors); psycho-social factors (e.g., self-esteem, body image, stress level, feelings of support); knowledge (e.g., knowledge of chronic disease risk factors, nutrition and physical activity requirements for optimal health); and policy options (e.g., using a panel of experts and an appropriate framework such as a socio-ecological model/life-course/social model of health.[16]

In the absence of other evidence, experts suggest that these should be multi-component in nature. It is important to take into consideration that schools are faced with multiple curricular obligations with limited financial and staff resources. Even well-intentioned and motivated teachers have reported limited classroom time to address health education adequately.

Table 10.1 Intervention components.

Level of determinants	Components
Individual determinants	
	Substantial dietary modifications
	Substantial physical activity modifications
	Psycho-social interventions focusing on self-esteem, body image, peer support and stress management
	Behavior modifications focusing on motivational reinforcement
	Health education on diet and physical activity
	Tailored individually
	Subject-directed (subjects actively engaged in the programs)
Familial determinants	
	Health education
	Dietary modifications
	Physical activity modifications
	Knowledge and attitude
	Support from family members
Environmental determinants	
	Create or advocate for healthy social environments
	Physical environments (e.g., sports equipment, time and place, transport, canteen, snack shop, vending machines)
	Cultural environments (e.g., media and culture)

What has been proven effective

The primary focus of this chapter is interventions that include a primary prevention approach at the school-based level on which a number of reviews have been conducted.[15–24] The aim of the intervention is a key inclusion/exclusion criterion used by various reviews. The Cochrane review series, most recently updated by Summerbell et al,[15] aimed to examine the effectiveness of interventions on overweight/obesity prevention, whereas Flynn et al[25] and De Mattia et al[22] included aims other than obesity prevention. Interventions struggle to achieve changes in BMI despite finding effectiveness on some behavioral and other outcomes.[26] In addition to intervention aim, another critical issue is whether interventions are carried out at a single school or within the same small community (single level) or at multiple schools in multiple communities or districts. Doak et al[25] found that effective interventions had, on average, fewer participating schools, in particular, single-level interventions that were carried out in only a few schools. This may be due to the ability of such interventions to target the specific needs of the children. Although interventions have found sub-group differences in intervention effect,[25,27] Flynn et al[25] found that only four interventions addressed the health concerns of special needs populations. In addition, Flynn et al[25] confirmed the preliminary findings[15,24] of earlier reviews that boys require special targeting for intervention.

Comparisons of specific elements of study design show some consistent trends but, unfortunately, there are not enough interventions for statistical comparisons. Reviews have identified that interventions that target physical activity through compulsory physical education[19] or reduced TV viewing or soft drinks interventions[20,24,28] are the most promising. A meta-analysis that pooled results from 12 interventions showed that interventions with both nutrition and physical activity resulted in significant reductions in body weight compared to controls,[21] with a stronger effect for interventions that involved parents. In contrast, Summerbell et al[15] concluded that studies combining diet and physical activity did not significantly improve BMI. Likewise, Doak et al[24] also identified multiple component interventions as less likely to be effective. However, evidence shows that school-based interventions should target only a few behaviors and that these require an "environmental-behavioral" synergy: that is, food and physical activity environments should echo and support the targeted behaviors. This includes the type of foods offered in schools, infrastructure for physical activity and good quality PE classes.[29]

If interventions are to provide long-term solutions, they must not only be shown as effective, but must also be sustainable. Whereas early reviews had too few studies to compare results, more recent reviews show consistent evidence for short-term rather than long-term benefits of interventions.[15,24,25] While few studies have been shown as effective a year or more after the initial intervention, fewer still continue outcome evaluation a couple of years after the intervention. Unfortunately, in one such example,[28] the intervention effect at one year was lost after three years of follow-up. Sharma[18,26] argues that intervention length can be shortened if the intervention is based on behavior theory. However, sustainable interventions effective over a long time frame are needed to reverse rising trends of overweight and obesity.

In a review of interventions specifically focused on physical activity, DeMattia et al[22] were only able to assess outcomes using BMI because of a lack of comparable outcomes. Although these authors found the majority (4 out of 6 interventions) to be effective, adiposity measures would have been more appropriate. Many reviews have also chosen to focus on BMI-based measures where multiple and/or conflicting results are presented. The review by Lissau[30] argues that focusing on BMI outcomes is likely to produce a false negative if used to assess physical activity interventions. In fact, the literature provides evidence of interventions that show no reduction in BMI outcomes, but reductions in skin-folds, indicating improvements in body composition. Existing evidence illustrates the need to ensure the quality of interventions and to develop systematic methods for evaluating multiple, conflicting outcomes in a manner that is unbiased and appropriate to the study design.

Future perspectives

The school setting is subject to a number of barriers in implementing sustainable obesity prevention programs[31–33] with programs requiring infrastructure and resources that may well not exist in poor schools. It is also clear that there is a need to develop our understanding of the multiple, interactive and cumulative obesogenic influences on primary school pupils within the "obesity system". Recognizing and addressing this complexity highlights that schools "definitely cannot counteract all the stressors and tensions originating in other life spheres such as unfavorable economic conditions, dysfunctional families or lack of supportive friends"[34] and "that schools are only one component and probably quite small in their influence in altering a person's health status".[35]

Given these reservations, a number of recommendations can be made regarding obesity prevention in primary schools, not least of these is the need to develop the evidence base. Achieving change is hampered by a lack of robust scientific evidence about how to intervene effectively in ways that reduce, rather than exacerbate, health inequalities.[36] Systematic reviews have highlighted the need for improved evaluation designs that draw on mixed methods in particular (e.g., Norton et al).[37] There is also a need to increase the number of comparative studies outside Europe and North America, in countries where problems of undernutrition still exist but where obesity is rapidly emerging.[38,39]

Study methods also require development, with a need to develop standardized self-report measures and to assess their relationship to changes in BMI in large-scale trials. Indeed, the measurement of obesity in children continues to be controversial, with epidemiological evidence demonstrating that measures of BMI are sensitive to population differences in age of puberty[40] and height.[41,42] More worrisome is the potential bias in the error in weight-based measures, as evidence indicates that effectiveness differs based on the outcome used. It also noted that a number of systematic reviews to date have not provided information on costs or cost–effectiveness,[35,43] presumably because this was not addressed in the primary studies.

Given this lack of evidence, a number of tentative suggestions for future policy can be made. Even though there has been a tendency for initiatives to focus on single risk behaviors,[14,44,45] emerging evidence indicates that such behaviors cluster, suggesting a need for complex interventions to address multiple behaviors simultaneously. It has also been argued that "a multifaceted approach is likely to be most effective, combining a classroom program with changes to the school ethos and/or environment and/or with family/ community involvement".[46] The importance of such multi-factorial interventions was clearly set out in the 1986 Ottawa Charter and was reiterated in the WHO's more recent Bangkok Charter in 2005.[47] While providing the impetus for a growth in settings-based interventions, many such interventions have been criticized for focusing on the most accessible setting and groups and for conceptualizing setting as a channel of delivery rather than a dynamic context that both shapes and is shaped by those within it.[48]

This is compounded by a lack of understanding of the *interactive* effect of interventions, both within and across such contexts. Indeed, a recently published synthesis of evidence indicated mixed evidence of effectiveness and concluded that "there is a lack of evidence on all the elements that contribute to an effective health promotion program or to the health promoting schools approach as a whole".[49] This suggests that mono-behavior interventions that fail to address behavioral contexts are unlikely to reduce health inequalities or develop sustainable health improvement. Evaluating such an approach highlights particular challenges relating to causal attributions of effects and the time required for intervention implementation. Such an approach may require long-term evaluation designs that address the intervention as a complex adaptive system. As Hawe et al[50] state, there is a need to reverse current custom and to begin to theorize about "complex systems and how the health problem or phenomena of interest is recurrently produced by that system".

References

1 Popkin B: The nutrition transition and obesity in the developing world. *J Nutr* 2001; **131**:871S–873S.

2 Lobstein T, Baur L, Uauy R: IASO International Obesity TaskForce. Obesity in children and young people: a crisis in public health. *Obes Rev* 2004; **5**(Suppl. 1):4–104.

3 Brown T, Kelly S, Summerbell C: Prevention of Obesity: a review of interventions. *Obes Rev* 2007; **8**: (Supp. 1): 127–130.

4 Peterson K, Fox M: Addressing the epidemic of childhood obesity through school-based interventions: what has been done and where do we go from here? *J Law Med Ethics* 2007; **35**:113–130.

5 WHO Health Promoting Schools. Global School Initiative. www.who.int/school_youth_health/gshi/en/ (accessed 22 February 2008).

6 Kumanyika S: Environmental influences on childhood obesity. Ethnic and cultural influences in context. *Physiol Behav* 2007. doi: 1016/j.physbeth.2007.11.019

7 McLeroy K, Bibeau D, Steckler A, Glanz K: An ecological perspective on health promotion programs. *Health Educ Behav* 1988; **15**:351–377.

8 Bauer G, Davies K, Pelikan J: The EUHPID Health Development Model for the classification of public health indicators. *Health Promot Int* 2006; **21**:153–159.

9 Cawley J, Meyerhoefer C, Newhouse D: The impact of state physical education requirements on youth physical activity and overweight. *Health Econ* 2007; **16**:1287–1301.

10 Floriani V, Kennedy C: Promotion of physical activity in children. *Curr Opin Pediatr* 2008; **20**:90–95.

11 Baranowski T: Advances in basic behavioral research will make the most important contributions to effective dietary change programs at this time. *J Am Diet Assoc* 2006; **106:** 808–811.

12 Story M, Kaphingst KM, French S: The role of schools in obesity prevention. *Future Child* 2006; **16:**109–142.

13 Kubik M, Story M, Rieland G: Developing school-based BMI screening and parent notification programs: findings from focus groups with parents of elementary school students. *Health Educ Behav* 2007; **34:**622–633.

14 Reilly J, McDowell Z: Physical activity interventions in the prevention and treatment of paediatric obesity: systematic review and critical appraisal. *Proc Nutr Soc* 2003; **62:** 611–619.

15 Summerbell C, Waters E, Edmunds L, Kelly S, Brown T, Campbell K: Interventions for preventing obesity in children. *Cochrane Database Syst Rev* 2005; 3 (Art. No. CD001871).

16 McNeil D, Flynn M: Methods of defining best practice for population health approaches with obesity prevention as an example. *Proc Nutr Soc* 2006; **65:**403–411.

17 Mueller M, Asbeck I, Mast M, Lagnaese L, Grund A: Prevention of Obesity—more than an intention. Concept and first results of the Kiel Obesity Prevention Study (KOPS). *Int J Obes Relat Metab Disord* 2001; **25**(Suppl. 1): S66–S74.

18 Stevens J, Alexandrov A, Smirnova S et al: Comparison of attitudes and behaviors related to nutrition, body size, dieting, and hunger in Russian, Black-American, and White-American adolescents. *Obes Res* 1997; **5:**227–236.

19 Connelly J, Duaso M, Butler G: A systematic review of controlled trials of interventions to prevent childhood obesity and overweight: a realistic synthesis of the evidence. *Public Health* 2007; **121:**510–517.

20 Sharma M: School-based interventions for childhood and adolescent obesity. *Obes Rev* 2006; 7261–7269.

21 Katz D, O'Connell M, Njike V, Yeh M, Nawaz H: Strategies for the prevention and control of obesity in the school setting: systematic review and meta-analysis. *Int J Obes (Lond)* 2008; **32**(12):1780–1789.

22 DeMattia L, Lemont L, Meurer L: Do interventions to limit sedentary behaviours change behaviour and reduce childhood obesity? A critical review of the literature. *Obes Rev* 2007; **8:**69–81.

23 Campbell K, Waters E, O'Meara S, Summerbell C: Interventions for preventing obesity in childhood. A systematic review. *Obes Rev* 2001; **2:**149–157.

24 Doak C, Visscher T, Renders C, Seidell J: The prevention of overweight and obesity in children and adolescents: a review of interventions and programmes. *Obes Rev* 2006; **7:** 111–136.

25 Flynn M, McNeil D, Maloff B et al: Reducing obesity and related chronic disease risk in children and youth: a synthesis of evidence with "best practice" recommendations. *Obes Rev* 2006; **1:**7–66.

26 Doak C, Heitman BL, Summerbell C, Lissner L: Prevention of childbood obesity—what type of evidence should we conside relevant: *Obes Rev* 2009; May **10**(3):350–356.

27 Webber L, Osganian S, Feldman H et al: Cardiovascular risk factors among children after a 2 1/2-year intervention-The CATCH Study. *Prev Med* 1996; **25:**432–441.

28 Sharma M: International school-based interventions for preventing obesity in children. *Obes Rev* 2007; **8:**155–167.

29 Committee on Prevention of Obesity in Children and Youth. FNB, IOM, Preventing Childhood Obesity: Health in the Balance. Washington, DC: National Academy of Sciences, 2004.

30 Lissau I: Prevention of overweight in the school arena. *Acta Paediatr Suppl* 2007; **96:**12–18.

31 Hesketh K, Crawford D, Salmon J, Jackson M, Campbell KInt J: Associations between family circumstance and weight status of Australian children. *Pediatr Obes* 2007; **2:**86–96.

32 Dwyer J, Stone E, Yang M et al: Prevalence of marked overweight and obesity in a multiethnic pediatric population: findings from the Child and Adolescent Trial for Cardiovascular Health (CATCH) study. *J Am Diet Assoc* 2000; **100:**1149–1156.

33 Francis CC, Bope AA, MaWhinney S, Czajka-Narins D, Alford BB: Body composition, dietary intake, and energy expenditure in nonobese, prepubertal children of obese and nonobese biological mothers. *J Am Diet Assoc* 1999; **99:** 58–65.

34 Hurrelmann K, Laaser U: Health sciences as an interdisciplinary challenge: the development of a new scientific field. *Int J Occup Med Environ Health* 1995; **8:**195–214.

35 St Leger L: What's the place of schools in promoting health? Are we too optimistic? *Health Promot Int* 2004; **19:** 405–408.

36 Viner RM, Barker M: Young people's health: the need for action. *BMJ* 2005; **16**(330):901–903.

37 Norton I, Moore S, Fryer P: Understanding food structuring and breakdown: engineering approaches to obesity. *Obes Rev* 2007; **8**(Suppl. 1):83–88.

38 Kain J, Uauy R, Albala Vio F, Cerda R, Leyton B: School-based obesity prevention in Chilean primary school children: methodology and evaluation of a controlled study. *Int J Obes Relat Metab Disord* 2004; **28:**483–493.

39 Gao Y, Griffiths S, Chan E: Community-based interventions to reduce overweight and obesity in China: a systematic review of the Chinese and English literature. *J Public Health* 2007; **11:**1–13.

40 Cameron N: The biology of growth. *Nestle Nutr Workshop Ser Pediatr Program* 2008; **61:**1–19.

41 Rush E, Plank L, Chandu V et al: Body size, body composition, and fat distribution: a comparison of young New Zealand men of European, Pacific Island, and Asian Indian ethnicities. *N Z Med J* 2004; **117:**U1203.

42 Nooyens A, Koppes L, Visscher T et al: Adolescent skinfold thickness is a better predictor of high body fatness in adults than is body mass index: the Amsterdam Growth and Health Longitudinal Study. *Am J Clin Nutr* 2007; **85:**1533–1539.

43 Stewart-Brown S: Promoting health in children and young people: identifying priorities. *J R Soc Health* 2005; **125**: 61–62.

44 Thomas R, Perera R: School-based programmes for preventing smoking. *Cochrane Database Syst Rev* 2006; 3 (Art. No. CD001293).

45 Foxcroft D, Ireland D, Lister-Sharp D, Lowe G, Breen R: Primary prevention for alcohol misuse in young people. *Cochrane Database Syst Rev* 2002; 3 (Art. No. CD003024).

46 Lister-Sharp D, Chapman S, Stewart-Brown S, Sowden A: Health promoting schools and health promotion in schools: two systematic reviews. *Health Technol Assess* 1999; **3**: 1–207.

47 World Health Organization: The Bangkok Charter for health promotion in a globalized world. *Health Promot J Austr* 2005; **16**:168–171.

48 Bolam B, Murphy S, Gleeson K: Individualization and inequalities in health: a qualitative study of class identity and health. *Soc Sci Med* 2004; **59**:1355–1365.

49 Stewart-Brown SL: What is the evidence on school health promotion in improving health or preventing disease and, specifically what is the effectiveness of the health promoting schools approach. Copenhagen, WHO Regional Office for the Europe Health Evidence Network (HEN). 2006.

50 Hawe P, Shiell A: Use of evidence to expose the unequal distribution of problems and the unequal distribution of solutions. *Eur J Public Health* 2007; **17**:413.

CHAPTER 11

Obesity prevention in secondary schools

Lauren Prosser,[1] *Tommy L.S. Visscher,*[2] *Colleen Doak*[2] and *Luis A. Moreno*[3]
[1] Jack Brockoff Child Health and Wellbeing Program, McCaughey Centre, Melbourne School of Population Health, The University of Melbourne, Melbourne, Australia
[2] Institute of Health Sciences, VU University, Amsterdam, The Netherlands
[3] Department of Public Health, University of Zaragoza, Zaragoza, Spain

Summary and recommendations for practice

- Stakeholders such as parents, schools, teachers and peers can be involved in stimulating activity and improving dietary patterns.
- Communities are a strong advocates in leading and implementing government initiatives and developing their own policy changes.
- School-driven initiatives combined with policy change are the most effective in changing eating habits and physical activity patterns in adolescents.
- Parents motivated to change their own behavior will influence a change in behavior in adolescents.
- Efforts are required to increase active transport in adolescents and move away from reliance on cars.

Method

The evidence provided in this chapter on obesity prevention for the adolescent population has been comprehensively searched using the Medline database, researching available systematic reviews for obesity in children and adolescents and identifying papers from experts in the field of adolescent research. The available literature has then been synthesized and integrated into this chapter with the aim of capturing

Preventing Childhood Obesity. Edited by
E. Waters, B.A. Swinburn, J.C. Seidell and R. Uauy.
© 2010 Blackwell Publishing.

best available evidence for obesity prevention in adolescents.

Adolescence and overweight and obesity

To implement effective health promotion and disease prevention programmes it is necessary to establish an environment that supports positive health behavior and a healthy lifestyle. Most nutrition-related diseases have their origin during childhood and adolescence, but the relationship between their development and adolescence is poorly understood. Adolescence is a crucial period in life and implies multiple physiological and psychological changes that affect lifestyle habits.

Adolescents have particular food habits and their meal choices may differ from both adults and children.[1] They also differ in other respects, having irregular eating patterns and indulging in frequent snacking and/or skipping meals, particularly breakfast.[2] At this stage of the lifespan, adolescents are confronted with body weight problems and pressure concerning eating (both with respect to the type of food they are eating and the amounts of food). Despite the irregular food patterns for adolescents, it is still a crucial time as dietary patterns established during childhood and adolescence continue into adulthood and have implications for the development of chronic disease, both at present and in the future.[3] Irregular food habits, such as snacking, have increased over the last 25 years across all age groups but particularly in adolescents.

Snacks now account for a substantially larger percentage of total daily energy and macronutrient intake than they did in the late 1970s.[3]

Physical activity in adolescents is on the decrease and low levels of activity seem to persist into adulthood. Not only does lack of physical activity increase a young person's risk for overweight and obesity but may contribute to cardiovascular disease, cancer and osteoporosis in later life. The increasing lifestyle of sedentary behaviors means the development and evaluation of physical activity interventions is, therefore, a priority for the promotion of adolescent health.

Sedentary behavior in adolescence is often mentioned as risk factor in obesity development and may have a link to its increasing prevalence and severity. The increase in playing digital games, using computers and especially watching television, have been associated with obesity. The link between obesity and television viewing has suggested that there is a delayed effect of TV viewing on body fatness.[4] This suggestion resulted from longitudinal studies, specifically focusing on girls who exceeded two hours of television viewing per day.[4] During adolescence, boys generally tend to spend more time playing videogames than watching television. Videogames contribute more to energy expenditure than watching television.[5] This increase in energy is very minimal and does not diminish the risk of overweight and obesity. Computer use is also a major contributor to increasing sedentary behavior but at this stage there is no evidence to suggest a link with overweight and obesity in adolescence. There is a real lack of research in this area.[4] Overall, with screens increasingly taking up adolescents' leisure time it is still unclear from the research whether or not sedentary behavior replaces physical activity[4] and what the impacts are on obesity development. There is sufficient evidence to recommend that adolescents have limits placed on their time spent watching television, that video game playing should be carefully monitored, and ensure that time spent on computers does not reduce physical activity levels.[4]

A diverse variety of settings have an impact on children's and adolescents' behavior. Many environments and numerous stakeholders, including parents, teachers, peers and many more, can or should be involved to stimulate activity and/or improve dietary patterns. The counteracting factors are difficult for all of those involved in the prevention of overweight and obesity

in adolescents. Children and adolescents are of particular focus for obesity prevention because overweight adolescents are at elevated risk for obesity in adulthood.[5] The evidence suggests there is a role to play from many different parties including: schools, family, individual and policy.[6] From the evidence, it is difficult to conclude what are the best strategies to reduce overweight and obesity in adolescents. However, it is possible to suggest from those studies that have effective outcomes which strategies might have the most success in reducing overweight and obesity. The way that information and interventions are delivered will vary and also counter cultural barriers.

There are also potential differences from effects such as gender, age and ethnicity (e.g., Doak et al)[7] and the effect of gender has been suggested to be linked to physical activity focus.[8] The evidence is unclear with regard to age and ethnicity as the studies that focus on these determinants are few and often low on quality.[7] Further studies are required to cross-compare ethnicity groups and stratify age groups in order to make any conclusions. This chapter provides an overview of what the key learnings are for beginning the process of reducing obesity in adolescents.

School, family and community approaches

As discussed in Chapter 10 (Obesity prevention in primary school settings: evidence from intervention studies) the associated determinants that influence overweight and obesity are complex and vary across communities and cultures. The link between community and the individual is in itself an important part of obesity prevention. Communities will often have to lead and may even implement government initiatives—therefore, it is important for teachers, schools, parents, families and adolescents to be provided with the knowledge and skills that may assist in the prevention of overweight and obesity (e.g., Sluijs et al).[9] When identifying potential strategies for what may work at community, school or home levels, it is important to remember that strategies which may be more effective are those which build on ideas for appropriate interventions derived from children's views and experiences.[10] The building of knowledge translation (see Chapter 22, Knowledge translation and exchange for obesity prevention) is the notion that there needs to be an exchange between all stakeholders. Therefore adolescents should be consulted on matters concerning the promotion of their healthy eating and physical activity behaviors.

School-based approach

A "whole school" approach (i.e., one involving all members of the school community) can be effective in promoting healthy eating.[11] If schools make changes to the availability of foods within their canteens/ tuck-shops, complemented by classroom activities, providing information on nutrition can be effective.[11] Classroom-based activities that promote healthy eating have been most successful when working in small group discussions and peer-led activities. These activities can also be complemented by learning about the environmental influences on food as this has been judged effective for reported healthy eating, particularly among young women in secondary schools. It is important that teacher preparation time must be kept to a minimum in order to ensure successful implementation within classrooms.[10]

Currently, there is limited evidence for the effectiveness of single component interventions, such as classroom lessons alone or providing fruit-only tuck-shops.[10] However, in South Wales and South-west England one particular study provided promising results, finding that children who attend schools that run fruit tuck shops are much more likely to eat fruit if they and their friends are also banned from bringing unhealthy snacks on to the school premises.[12] This parallel between school-driven initiatives and policies seems to have more impact on students than those who do not implement joint strategies. For example, changing attitudes and perspectives about what comprises a "normal" school lunch can be accelerated through school food policies.[13]

Despite the lack of evidence for implementing single component strategies, it is still important that schools continue to work towards these initiatives. Overall, school-based interventions will lead to, on average, an increase in children's intake of fruit and vegetables equivalent to one fifth of a portion of fruit per day, and a little less than one fifth of a portion of vegetables per day.[10] Strategies such as these do raise concerns that parents are no longer providing fruit and vegetables within the home or in school lunch boxes when children are being given "free" fruit or attend a school with a fruit-only tuck-shop. This is yet to be evaluated across countries, but may be an anecdotal caution when implementing such initiatives. The offering of fruit and vegetables in schools needs to be examined in more depth and for longer follow-up periods, and its effectiveness and cost–effectiveness (e.g., Pomerleau et al)[14] needs to be evaluated. However, it is important to understand that a single component strategy in weight gain prevention will never do on its own. Weight gain prevention in general will have to deal with multiple determinants of obesity, targeting multiple stakeholders. Therefore, portfolios are needed with different available strategies.

Three studies evaluated school travel interventions aimed at changing the mode of children's travel to school. Only one—a small non-randomized trial of an active commuting pack—found a significant net increase in self-reported walking on the school journey.[15]

Family-based approach

Parental involvement in obesity prevention is a very important factor. Parents who are motivated to change their own behavior will have a large influence on changing the behavior of their adolescent children.[10] The complex make-up of families makes it difficult to provide large-scale strategies that will be effective in reducing overweight and obesity, hence, the lack of evidence for family-based approaches.

A large-scale study found that counseling and lectures on prevention by trained instructors was effective in reducing body mass index[31]. This same study also found reduced body mass index among children with risk factors for overweight and obesity who were invited with their parents to a single individual counseling session. Also, when the primary setting is not the family setting, parental involvement is important and is among the few clear determinants for success of weight gain prevention in the young.[16]

Further research into this area should include family-based interventions and link to theory, research and clinical practice. Health promotion programs should include one or both parents or siblings, should use different interventions for parents, children and adolescents, and should assess outcomes using valid and reliable measures (e.g., McCallum et al, 2004).

Individual approach

Accumulating 30 minutes of moderate-intensity physical activity on most days of the week substantially reduces the risk of many chronic diseases.[15] Walking is a popular, familiar, convenient, and is a free form of exercise, from which many sedentary people could gain the health benefits of moderate-intensity physical activity.[15] Walking may be influenced by environmental and societal conditions as well as by interventions targeted at individuals.[15] The Ogilvie et al (2007) review found that interventions tailored to people's needs, targeted at the most sedentary, or at those most motivated to changes, and delivered either at the level of the individual or household or through groups can increase walking by up to 30–60 minutes a week on average, at least in the short term.

Children's, young peoples and parents' views about what helps and hinders their walking and cycling involves the strong culture of car use, the fear and dislike of local environments, children as responsible transport users, and parental responsibility for their children. "Cultures of transport" vary by age, sex and location (urban, suburban or rural).[17]

Studies of people's views have several implications for intervention. The most important is the need to reduce the convenience of car travel and simultaneously increase the safety of pedestrians and cyclists in residential areas and around schools. According to the research evidence, this would encourage children, young people and parents to walk and cycle, and to use public spaces more, which would strengthen overall community environments. Furthermore, this could lead to more opportunities to nurture children's and young people's independence in a safer environment. In the adolescent population, there is a notion of car as "cool".[17] Future strategies will need make car use appear less attractive for effectiveness in active transport to become practice in communities.

Evidence for obesity prevention in adolescence

When considering studies that assess the means for overweight and obesity reduction, primary school interventions dominate the literature.[13] Existing reviews of overweight and obesity prevention interventions generally include primary school, and even preschool, children.[7,18–21] Even with comprehensive age inclusion, these reviews are limited by the small numbers of existing interventions. For example, applying the Cochrane criteria to a review as recently as 2005 gave only 22 studies[19] and more recently the 2008 update found 18 studies.[22] A more inclusive set of criteria, used by another review published in 2005 resulted in only 24 interventions.[7] An ongoing update of this review has resulted in additional information (Solerno, personal communication) with 18 new studies fitting the original criteria for the Doak et al review. However, most of these additional interventions focus on primary school children.

While age was identified as a key concern in earlier reviews, even updated numbers are insufficient for a comprehensive study of interventions in secondary schools. Some key general conclusions found in the earlier reviews, based on a pooling of results for all children, are especially relevant to the adolescent age group. The Doak et al[7] review identified the issue of measuring overweight and obesity as a concern in assessing interventions as effective. Namely, there are discrepancies in conclusions about intervention effectiveness depending on whether heights and weights or skin-fold measures are used to assess effective outcomes. A recently submitted commentary[23] pooled the results of two reviews[7,19] to further explore the importance of outcome assessment. One key difference in the conclusions of the two reviews relates to differences in how discrepant height/weight based results were assessed for 10 studies included by both reviews. Based on height and weight results only, three of the 10 studies were assessed as effective by Summerbell et al[19] whereas six were assessed as effective by the Doak et al review[7]. These differences could be explained by the focus of the Summerbell et al[19] review on mean BMI over prevalence change,[24] effect on slope,[25] or an effective skin-fold measure.[26]

The criteria, references and definitions to be used for overweight and obesity outcomes in adolescents is a challenging issue.[6] While the review results illustrate the importance of this issue, it is as yet unclear which measures are most valid. It is long known that the stage of maturation matters in assessing overweight and obesity risk (Wang, 2002[33]) Furthermore, additional evidence shows that there are clear population differences in onset of puberty.[27] There is evidence supporting the need for adjustment for maturation with height as a proxy,[28] or using population specific references.[2] Evidence from the literature indicates that skin-folds, but not BMI, track from adolescence into adulthood.[29] This evidence supports the need for further clarification of measures used to assess overweight and obesity, and that skin-fold measures may provide better information in relation to long-term risks. In particular, where interventions focus on physical activity, BMI may not be appropriate as these interventions are likely to increase muscle mass even while skin-folds are reduced.[16]

Sustainability should become more important in future strategies to combat the obesity epidemic. It has been recently suggested[23] that weight gain prevention programs should at least take six months. Evaluations should take place long thereafter, but such long term evidence is scarce.[16,19] It is for this reason, therefore, that the International Obesity Task Force has put a strong focus on contributing factors and points of interventions, and in the range of opportunities for weight gain prevention.[30]

Interventions are available to reduce overweight and obesity in adolescence; and it is important to understand which of them are effective for the population group. Interventions often aim to reduce BMI or skin-fold thickness. However, there are also interventions that are effective in increasing physical activity and healthy eating and decreasing sedentary behaviors. Many of these strategies require the support and involvement of several community sectors, including schools. A majority of interventions for this population group are school-based. The following evidence recommendations are from WHO (2005) KOBE expert reported in Lobstein and Swinburn.[13] These recommendations may assist in the future direction of intervention studies:

- All interventions should include process evaluation measures and provide resources and cost estimates. Evaluation can include impact on other parties such as parents and siblings.
- Interventions using control groups should be explicit about what the control group experiences.

Phrases like "normal care" or "normal curriculum" or "standard school PE classes" are not helpful.
- There is a need for more interventions looking into the needs of specific sub-populations, including immigrant groups, low-income groups, and specific ethnic and cultural groups.
- There is a shortage of long-term programs monitoring interventions. Long-term outcomes could include changes in knowledge and attitudes, behaviors (diet and physical activity) and adiposity outcomes.
- New approaches to interventions, including prospective meta-analyses, should be considered.
- Community-based demonstration programs can be used to generate evidence, gain experience, develop capacity and maintain momentum.
- There is a need for an international agency to encourage the networking of community-based interventions, support methods of evaluation and assist in the analysis of the cost–effectiveness of initiatives.
- Monitoring of activities and monitoring of an increased number of outcome-measures is urgently needed and will contribute importantly to childhood and adolescence obesity prevention.

References

1 Moreno LA, Kesting M, de Henauw S et al: How to measure dietary intake and food habits in adolescence: the European perspective. *Int J Obes* 2005; **29**:S66–S77.

2 Moreno LA, Rodríguez G: Dietary risk factors for development of childhood obesity. *Curr Opin Clin Nutr Metab Care* 2007; **10**:336–341.

3 Sebastian R, Cleveland L, Goldman J: Effect of snacking frequency on adolescents' dietary intakes and meeting national recommendations. *J Adolesc Health* 2008; **42**(5): 503–511.

4 Rey-Lopez JP, Vicente-Rodriguez G, Biosca M, Moreno LA: Sedentary behavior and obesity development in children and adolescents. *Nutr Metab Cardiovasc Dis* 2008; **18**: 242–251.

5 Wang X, Perry AC: Metabolic and physiologic responses to video game play in 7–10 year old boys. *Arch Pediatr Adolesc Med* 2006; **160**(4):411–415.

6 Flodmark CE, Lissau I, Moreno LA, Pietrobelli A, Widhalm K: New insights into the field of children and adolescents' obesity: the European perspective. *Int J Obes Relat Metab Disord* 2004; **28**:1189–1196.

7 Doak C, Visscher T, Renders C, Seidell JC: The prevention of overweight and obesity in children and adolescents: a review of interventions and programmes. *Obes Rev* 2006; **7**:111–136.

8 Sallis J, Buono M, Roby J, Micale F, Nelson J: Seven-day recall and other physical activity self-reports in children and adolescents. *Med Sci Sports Exerc* 1993; **25**(1):99–108.

9 Sluijs E, McMinn A, Griffin S: Effectiveness of interventions to promote physical activity in children and adolescents: systematic review of controlled trials. *BMJ* 2007; **335**(7622): 703.

10 Thomas J, Sutcliffe K, Harden A et al: Children and Healthy Eating: A Systematic Review of Barriers and Facilitators. London: EPPI-Centre, Social Science Research Unit, Institute of Education, University of London, 2003.

11 Shepherd J, Harden A, Rees R et al: Young People and Healthy Eating: A Systematic Review of Research on Barriers and Facilitators. London: EPPI-Centre, Social Science Research Unit, Institute of Education, University of London, 2001.

12 Moore L, Tapper K: The impact of school fruit tuck shops and school food policies on children's fruit consumption: A cluster randomised trial of schools in deprived areas. *J Epidemiol Community Health* 2008; **62**:926–931.

13 Lobstein T, Swinburn B: Health promotion to prevent obesity. In: McQueen D, Jones C eds. Global Perspectives on Health Promotion Effectiveness. New York: Springer New York, 2007:125–150.

14 Pomerleau KC, Lock K, McKee M: Getting children to eat more fruit and vegetables: a systematic review. *Prev Med* 2006; **42**(2):85–95.

15 Ogilvie D, Foster CE, Rothnie H et al: Interventions to promote walking: a systematic review. *BMJ* 2007; **334**: 1204.

16 Doak C, Adair LS, Bentley M, Monteiro C, Popkin B: The dual burden household and the nutrition transition paradox. *Int J Obes* 2005; **29**:129–136.

17 Brunton G, Oliver S, Oliver K, Lorenc T: A Synthesis of Research Addressing Children's, Young People's and Parents' Views of Walking and Cycling for Transport. London: EPPI-Centre, Social Science Research Unit, Institute of Education, University of London, 2006.

18 Campbell K, Waters E, O'Meara S, Summerbell C: Interventions for preventing obesity in childhood. A systematic review. *Obes Rev* 2001; **2**:149–157.

19 Summerbell CD, Waters E, Edmunds LD, Brown KS, Campbell KJ: Interventions for Preventing Obesity in Children (Review). 3. The Cochrane Collaboration. Wiley Interscience, 2005.

20 Flynn MA, McNeil DA, Maloff B et al: Reducing obesity and related chronic disease risk in children and youth: a synthesis of evidence with "best practice" recommendations. *Obes Rev* 2006; **7**(Suppl. 1):7–66.

21 Bluford D, Sherry B, Scanlon KS: Interventions to prevent or treat obesity in preschool children: A review of evaluated programs. *Obesity* 2007; **15**(6):1356–1372.

22 Waters E, Brown KS, Campbell KJ et al: Interventions for Preventing Obesity in Children and Adolescents (Review). The Cochrane Collaboration. John Wiley & Sons Ltd Publishers, 2009, in press.

23 Doak C, Heitmann BL, Summerbell C, Lissner L. Prevention of childhood obesity—what type of evidence should we consider relevant? *Obes Rev* 2009 May;**10**(3):350–6.

24 James J, Thomas P, Cavan D, Kerr D: Preventing childhood obesity by reducing consumption of carbonated drinks: cluster randomised controlled trial. *BMJ* 2004; **328**:1237.

25 Kain J, Uauy R, Albala Vio F, Cerda R, Leyton B: School-based obesity prevention in Chilean primary school children: methodology and evaluation of a controlled study. *Int J Obes* 2004; **28**(4):483–493.

26 Mueller MJ, Asbeck I, Mast M, Lagnaese L, Grund A: Prevention of Obesity—more than an intention. Concept and first results of the Kiel Obesity Prevention Study (KOPS). *Int J Obes* 2001; **25**(Suppl. 1):S66–S74.

27 Wang Y, Adair L: How does maturity adjustment influence the estimates of overweight prevalence in adolescents from different countries using an international reference? *Int J Obes Relat Metab Disord* 2001; **25**(4):550–558.

28 Seidell J: Dietary fat and obesity: an epidemiologic perspective. *Am J Clin Nutr* 2007; **67**:546S–550S.

29 Nooyens A, Koppes L, Visscher T et al: Adolescent skinfold thickness is a better predictor of high body fatness in adults than is body mass index: the Amsterdam Growth and Health Longitudinal Study. *Am J Clin Nutr* 2007; **85**(6):1533–1539.

30 Swinburn B, Gill T, Kumanyila S: Obesity prevention: a proposed framework for translating evidence into action. *Obesity* 2005; **6**:23–33.

31 Alexandrov AA, Maslennikova GY, Kulikov SM, Propirnij GA, Perova NV. Primary prevention of cardiovascular disease: 3-year intervention results in boys of 12 years of age. *Prev Med.* 1992 Jan;**21**(1):53–62.

32 McCallum Z, Wake M, Gerner B, et al: Outcome date from the LEAP (Live, Eat and Play) trial: a randomized controlled trial of a primary care intervention for childhood overweight/mild obesity. *Int J Obes (Lond)* 2007; **31**:630–636.

33 Wang Y. Is obesity associated with early sexual maturation? A comparison of the association in American boys versus girls. *Pediatrics.* 2002 Nov;**110**(5):903–910.

The prevention of childhood obesity in primary care settings: evidence and practice

Karen Lock and *Rebecca Hillier*
Department of Public Health and Policy, London School of Health and Tropical Medicine, London, UK

Summary and recommendations for practice

- The current evidence base for childhood obesity prevention in primary care is poor, and no clear effective approach can be advocated from the literature.
- Evidence from the wider literature suggests that multi-component interventions (e.g., including combinations of diet and physical activity advice, behavior change approaches) are the most effective approach in the clinical setting, although there is limited evidence on which intervention components are essential.
- Most national guidelines recommend the use of "BMI percentiles for age" for assessment and monitoring of overweight in children.
- There is little research on the differential impacts of different primary care practitioners in obesity prevention.
- Parental involvement is recommended by many national guidelines, although there is little conclusive evidence for the role of parents in primary care.
- There are a number of barriers for primary care providers implementing obesity prevention and management interventions. Future research should not only tackle the evidence for effective primary care interventions, but also the challenges of translating evidence-based guidelines into primary care practice.

Preventing Childhood Obesity. Edited by
E. Waters, B.A. Swinburn, J.C. Seidell and R. Uauy.
© 2010 Blackwell Publishing.

Introduction

The majority of research into childhood obesity interventions, including prevention, has focused on school and community prevention, or tertiary care. This chapter explores the evidence for preventive approaches in primary care settings.

What is primary care?

Since the Alma Alta conference in 1978, there has been worldwide acceptance of the importance of primary health care (PHC) as the key factor for attainment of the goal of "health for all".[1] The World Health Organization defines primary health care as "essential health care made universally accessible to individuals and families in the community by means acceptable to them, through their full participation and at a cost that the community and country can afford. It forms an integral part both of the country's health system of which it is the nucleus and of the overall social and economic development of the community."[2]

In more developed countries, PHC is the term for the health services that play a central role in the local community; including general practitioners, pharmacists, dentists and midwives. It provides integrated, accessible health care services by clinicians who are accountable for addressing a large majority of personal health care needs, developing a sustained partnership with patients, and practising in the context of family and community.[3]

Besides appropriate treatment of common diseases and injuries, provision of essential drugs, maternal and child health, and prevention and control of locally endemic diseases and immunization, it should ideally include measures to promote public health, including education of the community on prevalent health problems and delivering approaches to prevent them. In this chapter we aim to take a broad approach to defining PHC including general practice, community pediatrics and other community health services and primary-care led public health.

Is childhood overweight and obesity seen as an important issue for primary care?

Only two settings, schools and primary care, see children regularly enough to offer an effective secondary prevention program for obesity.[4] However, in most countries worldwide the involvement of primary care has been limited.

Studies by general practitioners (GPs) in the UK, USA and Australia have found that childhood overweight and obesity was recognized as an important health problem.[5-9] However, a number of barriers were perceived in tackling the issue in primary care including lack of time and resources, and a lack of practical, effective approaches. In the UK, GPs and practice nurses felt that their role in obesity management was centered on raising the issue of a child's weight, and providing basic diet and exercise advice.[5] There was concern that the clinician–patient relationship could be adversely affected by discussing what was often seen as a sensitive topic. GPs and practice nurses felt ill-equipped to tackle childhood obesity, given a lack of evidence for effective interventions, and many were skeptical that providing diet and exercise advice would have any impact upon a child's weight.

What is prevention of obesity in children?

There is some ambiguity in the terminology for obesity prevention. Are we concerned with the prevention of increased incidence of obesity? Or is the goal preventing weight gain among those overweight to prevent progression to more severe levels of obesity?

The traditional public health classification system designates three types of prevention: primary, secondary and tertiary.[10] The goal of primary prevention is to decrease the number of new cases (incidence) of a disorder. In secondary prevention, the goal is to lower the rate of established cases of the disorder in the population (prevalence). Tertiary prevention seeks to

reduce the amount of disability associated with an existing disorder. For obesity, tertiary prevention could refer to decreasing the likelihood of associated diseases (e.g., diabetes).

When this prevention classification system was introduced, the implicit disease model was one of an acute condition with a uni-factorial cause. It was assumed that mechanisms linking the cause of a specific disease to its subsequent occurrence could be identified. However, obesity is recognized as having multi-factorial etiologies and research is still identifying high-risk and protective factors for the development of obesity, and determining which key factors can be effectively targeted by preventive interventions. This had led to greater emphasis on risk reduction in disease prevention.

The US Institute of Medicine (IOM) has recommended an alternative terminology for disease prevention, which identifies three types of prevention: universal, selective and indicated prevention.[11] Universal preventive measures or interventions are designed for everyone in the eligible population. Selective preventive measures are directed toward a subgroup of the population who have a higher risk of developing the disorder. Indicated preventive interventions are targeted to high-risk individuals identified as having minimal but detectable signs or symptoms of the disorder, or exhibiting biological markers indicating predisposition.

Universal prevention programs are aimed at the general public. Such programs can have advantages particularly as they are usually cost-effective and the intervention is acceptable and of low risk for the population involved. Universal obesity programs can be classified into two broad categories: (1) preventive education and skills for all individuals (e.g., programs in various settings designed to improve diet and increase physical activity in a population); and (2) modification of social, environmental and economic policies in an attempt to reduce the population's exposure to the environmental causes of obesity (e.g., regulating food marketing). Programs in the first category are often based on a model of individual behavior change, which for obesity are usually delivered in a range of non-clinical settings, including schools. There is currently little evidence for the effectiveness of universal childhood obesity prevention programs or policies.[12]

Selective prevention programs are designed for groups at high risk of obesity or who are already overweight but not yet obese. Personal high-risk factors for obesity include individual level factors, such as a family history of obesity or non-insulin-dependent diabetes mellitus and low resting metabolic rate: personal eating habits and physical activity (e.g., a high-fat diet, a sedentary lifestyle), developmental periods associated with weight gain (e.g., pre-puberty), and critical life events (e.g., illness). A recent systematic review showed that such high-risk prevention strategies have been poorly tested and have no currently confirmed beneficial effects.[13]

In the past, **indicated prevention** has sometimes been referred to as secondary prevention or early interventions. These can be designed for individuals (in contrast to entire groups) who show biological markers for obesity, or who are already overweight but do not meet the diagnostic criteria for obesity. Risk factors for such individuals include a family history of obesity as well as biological markers and the development of early symptoms. Although research is still in the preliminary stages of identifying reliable biological markers for obesity, interventions that target individuals who are already overweight (or whose health risks are increased owing to their weight and/or a sedentary lifestyle) have proved to be effective in a number of settings, including primary care.

Many approaches to prevent obesity have been proposed, although as discussions in other chapters show, few studies have shown long-term, sustained reductions in weight. The emphasis on working with high-risk individuals with interventions that are matched or targeted to specific risk factors (as in selective and indicated prevention strategies) appears to have considerable value, and is a particular focus of interventions in primary care.

In this chapter, we consider that the primary aim of obesity prevention in primary care is to reduce the number of new cases. An important secondary aim is to delay the onset of obesity in those who are overweight. Consistent with the IOM definition of prevention (i.e., interventions that occur before onset), we do not include a discussion of weight maintenance to prevent the exacerbation of obesity or its complications in those in whom the condition is established. Neither do we cover the treatment of obesity, although it is worth mentioning that there are research trials

and national guidelines for use of drugs and surgery in obese adolescents. At least four national guidelines have already issued recommendations with regard to bariatric surgery in adolescents: National Health and Medical Research Council (NHMRC) Australian guidelines for the management of overweight and obese children and adolescents,[14] the Singapore Ministry of Health clinical guidelines,[15] and guidelines from the Institute for Clinical Systems Improvement (ICSI),[16] and the UK Institute for Health and Clinical Excellence (NICE).[17]

This chapter is based on a literature review of published and unpublished studies in English, conducted in June 2008, of obesity prevention and treatment interventions based in primary care settings worldwide. The review considered the impact of interventions in children of all main age-groups: preschool (0–4), early school years (5–11) and adolescents (12–18). We included clinical and non-clinical services provided by health professionals, or associated primary care staff, who may or may not have received special training to manage obese children. In some clinical programs, an individual professional provider may work alone; in others, a multi-disciplinary group of professional providers works together and systematically coordinates their efforts.

Evidence and guidelines for obesity prevention interventions in primary care

Evidence from all clinical settings

There is limited evidence on the essential components of effective health sector interventions for childhood obesity. However, throughout the literature it appears that a multi-disciplinary approach is most commonly advocated. Programs normally include one or several of the following components:

- nutritional and physical activity advice
- behavioral treatment components
- decreasing sedentary activities and increasing lifestyle-related physical activity
- social and/or psychological support involving families.

There have been several extensive literature reviews of the evidence for management and treatment of childhood obesity including a 2003 Cochrane review,[18] which was updated in 2006 for the UK

NICE guidelines.[17] Other reviews for national guidance include the Australian Clinical Practice Guidelines for the Management of Overweight and Obesity in Children and Adolescents (NHMRC),[14] the Scottish Intercollegiate Guidelines Network (SIGN),[19] recommendations of a US expert committee convened by the American Medical Association, Department of Health and Human Services and the CDC,[20] as well as a large number of other academic literature reviews.[13,21–32]

The 2006 NICE review resulted in evidence-based guidance on obesity prevention and management for a range of sectors in the UK. Its main conclusions for the health sector, which are echoed in several national guidelines (see Table 12.1), were that multi-component interventions were the "treatment of choice", and that weight management strategies should include behavior change to increase children's physical activity and improve eating behavior or quality of the diet.[17] These conclusions were based on a review of 42 randomized and non-randomized controlled trials of more than six months follow-up in clinical settings. However, only one of these studies was based in primary care, with the majority of study findings from tertiary care consisting of specialist outpatient weight reduction programs in university obesity research clinics (mostly in the USA). The review also commented on the poor methodological quality of the studies, including high drop-out rates, which would have impacted on the robustness of the evidence.

Summarizing the evidence of obesity management from specialist weight management programs, the review suggests that physical activity and diet combined are more effective in weight management in children aged 4–16 years, than diet alone.[33]

There was no evidence of effectiveness for physical activity interventions alone, and no clear evidence of which dietary interventions are most effective. Targeting sedentary behavior, including TV viewing, was shown to be as effective as promoting physical activity in managing weight in obese children.[34–36] Lifestyle-related activity was shown to be more effective than organized aerobic exercise in maintaining weight loss in obese children aged 8–12 years.[37] In specialist weight management programs, behavioral treatment combined with physical activity and/or diet is also effective in the treatment of obese children and

adolescents aged 3–18 years. Behavioral treatment can be more effective if parents, rather than children (aged 6 to 16 years), are given the main responsibility for behavior change. However, there is no evidence on which components of behavioral treatment are the most effective for childhood and adolescent obesity.

Despite the lack of robust research evidence, many countries have published national guidelines for the prevention and management of childhood obesity. In September 2005, the National Guideline Clearinghouse synthesized the recommendations on the assessment and management of obesity and overweight in children from six published guidelines. This information has been summarized in Table 12.1, with the addition of more recent guidelines. Most of the guidelines do not make specific recommendations for primary care providers.

Evidence from primary care interventions

Since many of the guidelines were published, four childhood obesity intervention trials in primary care have been completed.

The Live, Eat and Play (LEAP) RCT was a secondary prevention intervention nested within a baseline cross-sectional study of 2112 overweight children aged 5–10 years attending 29 general practices in Melbourne, Australia. A total of 82 children and their parents were randomized to receive the intervention of four standard GP consultations over 12 weeks targeting nutrition, physical activity and sedentary behaviors with supplementary personalized family materials. The control group families were notified of BMI status by letter but with no further follow-up, although GP attendances in this group were audited. There were no statistically significant differences between the two groups at nine and 15 month follow-up, although there was some evidence of an increase in nutrition measures and daily physical activity in the intervention group.[38,39]

One US trial also involved a multi-component primary care intervention for overweight adolescents: 44 overweight adolescents were randomized either to a four-month behavioral weight control program, which was initiated in a primary care setting and extended through telephone and mail contact, or to the control group, which received a single session of physician weight counseling. At end of intervention

Table 12.1 Recommendations on the prevention and management of childhood overweight and obesity from selected national guidelines.

Guideline reference	Target audience	Recommendations
National Health and Medical Research Council (NHMRC), Australia 2003 (6)	Health care providers	• Recommends that BMI should be used as the standard measure of overweight and obesity for 2–18-year-olds in Australia, making use of CDC BMI for age percentile charts (BMI > 85th percentile = overweight; BMI > 95th percentile = obese).
		• Advocates breastfeeding promotion as infant feeding method of choice for prevention.
		• In young children weight maintenance is an acceptable goal.
		• Recommends multi-component intervention approach until further evidence is gained (states that relative contributions of diet, exercise and behavioral modification are unknown). Approaches to include assessment of physical activity and television viewing levels and family eating styles.
		• Recommends medium- to long-term intervention.
		• Recommends the involvement of parents in the management of overweight and obesity in children and adolescents, especially in primary school age.
Registered Nurses Association of Ontario (RNAO), Canada 2005 (74)	Aimed at advanced practice nurses	• No specific primary care recommendations.
		• Recommends monitoring BMI changes over time using US CDC percentiles (BMI 85th–95th percentile = overweight; BMI > 95th percentile = obese).
		• Recommends general promotion of healthy eating and physical activity at all levels of society.
Canadian Clinical Practice Guidelines, Obesity Canada (NFP organization), Canada 2007 (27)	Designed to provide evidence-based recommendations to health care providers involved in obesity prevention and management	• Recommends the creation of a national surveillance system incorporating measurement of BMI in all children and adolescents aged 2 years and over.
		• Discussion of prevention of childhood obesity with the pregnant mother and encouragement of exclusive breastfeeding until 6 months.
		• General childhood obesity prevention advice: reduction of sedentary pursuits, with a reduction in TV viewing time to <2 hours per day; a recreational approach to activity, appropriate to the family context; limiting energy-dense snack foods high in sugar and fat.
		• For overweight and obese children recommends comprehensive multi-component healthy lifestyle interventions with a focus on lifestyle, diet and physical activity and incorporating an element of family oriented behavior therapy.
		• Recommends ongoing follow up by a health professional for 3 months.
		• Advocates a multi-sectoral and multi-professional approach and specifically recommends involvement of dietary specialist aiming towards the reduction of energy intake within the context of a balanced diet.

Continued

Table 12.1 *Continued*

Guideline reference	Target audience	Recommendations
National Institute for Health and Clinical Excellence (NICE), England and Wales 2006 (9)	The first national guidance for England and Wales on prevention, identification, assessment and management of overweight and obesity. Aimed at all health professionals who provide interventions in primary or secondary care	• Recommends use of BMI at the clinician's discretion as an identification and assessment tool (not advocating universal monitoring or screening). Advises caution in interpretation in children. Recommends to consider tailored intervention if BMI at 91st percentile or above. • Recommends targeting of at risk children with one or both parents obese. • Encourages health professionals to reinforce messages regarding regular family meals, reducing sedentary behaviors and encouraging active games and sports within daily lives and as structured activities. • Recommends multi-component, tailored interventions in both children and young adults, aiming to address lifestyle within the family and in social settings with a focus on dietary improvement and increasing physical activity. Recommends the inclusion of behavior change techniques. • Recommends long term rather than brief interventions with ongoing regular support from a trained professional. • Recommends involvement of the parents in interventions with family based as well as individual level programs depending on the age and maturity of the child. Encourage parental responsibility for lifestyle changes in children under 12 years.
Scottish Intercollegiate Guidelines Network (SIGN) 2003 (12)	Aimed at all health professionals who provide interventions in primary or secondary care	*Recommendations for weight maintenance* • In most obese children (BMI > 98th percentile) weight maintenance is an acceptable goal (recommendation grade: D). • Weight maintenance and/or weight loss can only be achieved by sustained behavioral changes, for example healthier eating, increasing physical activity. In healthy children, 60 minutes of moderate vigorous physical activity/day has been recommended. • Reducing physical inactivity (for example, watching television, playing computer games) to <2 hours/day on average or the equivalent of 14 hours/week (recommendation grade: D). • In overweight children (BMI > 91st percentile) weight maintenance is an acceptable goal. Annual monitoring of BMI percentile may be appropriate to help reinforce weight maintenance and reduce the risk of children becoming obese.
Singapore Ministry of Health 2004 (7)	Aimed at all health professionals who provide interventions in primary or secondary care	• Focus on increasing physical activity, decreasing sedentary time and dietary change (although comments that less restrictive diets should be used compared with adults). • Behavior treatment programs recommended for weight loss. • Interventions for obesity in children should be directed at both parents and the child, rather than the child alone.
US Preventive Services Task Force (USPSTF), USA 2005 (59)	Aimed at all health professionals who provide interventions in primary or secondary care	• Insufficient evidence is available on the effectiveness of interventions for overweight children and adolescents that can be conducted in primary care settings or to which primary care clinicians can make referrals. • No specific recommendations are given concerning management of overweight and obesity.

Continued

Table 12.1 *Continued*

Guideline reference	Target audience	Recommendations
American Academy of Pediatrics (AAP), USA 2003 (75)	Aimed at health care providers, physicians	• Calculating and plotting BMI once a year in all children and adolescents (BMI 85th–95th percentile considered at risk of overweight. BMI > 95th percentile is considered overweight or obese).
	Targets all children	• Health care providers advised to encourage breastfeeding, healthy eating, physical activity in multiple settings and the limitation of television viewing to <2 hrs per day.
		• Combination of dietary and physical activity interventions for an optimal approach. Families to be educated with regards to the impact they can have on their children's development of physical activity and eating habits.
American Medical Association (AMA), USA 2007 (13)	Aimed at clinicians to offer practical guidance and recommendations in all areas of childhood obesity care	• Recommends documentation of BMI at each well child visit (In children over 2 years BMI 85th–94th percentile = overweight; BMI > 95th percentile = obese. In youths obesity defined as BMI > 30 kg/m^2. In children <2 years weight for height values >95th percentile categorized as overweight).
		• Recommends targeting of at risk children with one or both obese parents.
		• Role of universal assessment and evidence-based preventive recommendations including limited consumption of sugary drinks, appropriate levels of fruit and vegetables in diet, no television before 2 years of age and thereafter <2 hrs per day, breakfast, limiting portion size and regular family meals.
		• Three treatment stages according to BMI and other risk factors: (i) prevention; (ii) prevention plus structured weight management; (iii) comprehensive multi-disciplinary intervention with a consistent focus on dietary factors and eating and physical activity behaviors.
		• Emphasizses the importance of parental involvement, relevant to the age and level of independence of the child.
American Heart Association (AHA), USA 2005 (76)	Aimed at health care providers, physicians	• Recommends yearly screening of BMI percentiles (BMI 85th–95th percentile considered at risk of overweight; BMI > 95th percentile considered overweight or obese).
		• Recommends age specific prevention advice including breast feeding, healthy home environments, 5-a-day fruit and vegetables, family meals, 1 hour of active play per day, <2 hrs television per day.
		• The principal intervention strategies for children are similar to those for adults (dietary modification and increased physical activity), but stress that family involvement was critical and the interventions had to be age-specific and tailored to degree of overweight.

NB: all BMI reference values cited are percentiles for age and sex unless stated.

and at three-month follow up, the intervention group had greater improved BMI scores than controls.[40]

The patient-centered assessment and counseling for exercise and nutrition (PACE+) is a RCT of a joint primary care and home-based intervention of 878 adolescent boys and girls aged 11–15 years, recruited through primary care providers in California, USA.[41]

This was a primary prevention intervention focused on improving physical activity and dietary behaviors. It had two stages: primary care based computer-assisted diet and physical activity assessment and goal setting followed by brief counseling, and then 12 months of monthly mail and telephone counseling at home. The comparison group received an intervention addressing sun exposure protection, which followed the same approach and intensity as the intervention. The intervention group significantly reduced sedentary behaviors, and showed some improvements in daily physical activity (boys) and dietary saturated fat intake (girls), but there were no differences between the two groups in BMI.

An Italian controlled trial investigated the management of children age 3–12 years in family pediatric practices,[42] where 186 obese children were recruited from the 18 practices that agreed to participate. The children were randomized to two different treatment groups: routine counseling approach (group A) and enhanced counseling approach (group B), and followed for 12 months. A reduction in overweight in both groups resulted but the enhanced intervention group showed significantly greater decrease in BMI as well as changes in dietary behavior and higher parental involvement.

Thus, the evidence base for primary care based interventions is currently extremely poor, and there is no clear effective approach that can be advocated from the literature. Although many interventions are occurring in primary care practice, most have not been formally evaluated in terms of effectiveness and cost–effectiveness. This paucity of evidence from both research and practice is extremely surprising, given the primary care obesity workload.

Is there evidence for the role of other primary care practitioners?

Although primary care and professional health care literature discusses the roles of primary care practitioners in obesity management, there have been few studies comparing differences between the different professional groups, or interventions focusing on specific practitioners other than GPs.

Health visitors and child care nurses perceive that childhood obesity is an important issue and that they have a role in prevention including giving physical activity advice,[43] although one study reported that they devote less clinical activity to childhood obesity than practice nurses.[44] A pilot study showed that a specialist health-visitor-led weight management clinic in primary care can reduce BMI and improve dietary behavior in adults.[45] We have found two ongoing cluster randomized trials of early childhood interventions that may prove promising for health visitors or

community nurses—one targeting parents during the first 18 months of a child's life based in the community child health centres,[46] and a second using specially trained community nurses undertaking multiple home visits to prevent overweight.[47]

The role of nurses in public health is well recognized. Several studies show that practice nurses are comfortable about routinely giving lifestyle advice on diet and physical activity, but many are not necessarily aware of the correct recommendations.[43] Although nurses also recognize childhood obesity as an important health issue, one study found that primary care nurses were not necessarily clear or happy with their roles, feeling that GPs were offloading the obesity workload onto nurses.[48] One US study found that although family nurse and pediatric nurse practitioners recognized the seriousness of being overweight and were educating parents, they were not consistently using BMI age index. Those aware of BMI and health lifestyle guidelines were more likely to do preventive work with families.[49]

The role of parents

Why involve parents in obesity prevention?

Many reviews of obesity interventions highlight the role of the family and the importance of parental involvement in preventing childhood obesity.[20,21,50–52] Inevitably, with a paucity of trial data focused on primary care interventions, much of the evidence is drawn from school and community-based programs. Even then, authors note that relatively few and often poor quality studies exist, which look at the effectiveness of obesity preventions with a parental focus.[21,50]

Golan et al demonstrated in a US-based behavioral change study of 6 to 11-year-olds that a focus on parents as exclusive agents of change significantly improved the outcome of mean percentile weight reduction in children.[51] A seven-year follow-up of this study showed that mean reduction of overweight was still significantly improved in the parent-only, compared to the children-only, group.[52]

Four ten year follow-up studies conducted by Epstein et al, again in the USA, targeted children aged 6–12 years with family-based behavioral obesity interventions. They demonstrated that the direct involvement of at least one parent as a participant improved short- and long-term outcomes as regards weight regulation in the children.[53,54]

Further supporting the involvement of parents in obesity interventions, there is a growing body of evidence from studies on child nutrition and growth detailing the impact that parent choices and behaviors can have on child nutrition and physical activity habits.[50]

A recent meta-analysis, however, has found conflicting evidence regarding the benefits of parental involvement in obesity interventions. When interventions of all age groups were considered together, there was no significant difference comparing those with and without parental involvement.[55]

What barriers may exist to parental involvement in primary care interventions?

In primary care, an effective universal approach will rely on the motivation of the health care provider. Although perhaps not the view of most primary care providers, several UK based qualitative studies have demonstrated that primary health care professionals, including GPs and practice nurses, felt that obesity prevention was an inappropriate use of their time and was a problem of the family and child.[5,7,48]

A more targeted approach, however, perhaps aimed at secondary prevention of obesity in already overweight children, starts to rely more on parental involvement for successful initiation and implementation. It is the parent who might initiate contact with primary care services in this situation, even if initially prompted through BMI measurement in other settings such as schools. Evidence suggests that an important barrier in this scenario is parents' inability to recognize overweight or obesity in their children, or see it as a problem.[56,57] Health professionals (pediatricians, nurse practitioners and dieticians) felt that lack of parental involvement was a major barrier.[8]

Parenting styles are discussed in some obesity intervention reviews,[58] focusing on the authoritative parenting style as having been shown to be the most successful in effecting behavioral change in relation to smoking behaviors, and also in increasing physical activity in adolescent girls.[59,60] Some behavior change research has also focused on the parents, rather than the children's, stage of readiness to accomplish lifestyle changes,[61] particularly given that parents can influence the outcome of obesity interventions in different ways, according to their child's developmental stage, though parental involvement seems to have most impact in younger children.[55]

How are primary care interventions involving parents?

We see several levels of parental involvement in child obesity interventions. The parent may simply be required to offer a supportive role at home, for example, getting children to activities; or they they may receive education during clinic attendance, participate in education sessions without the specific aim of getting them to to adopt a behavioralist role, or receive information packs.[38,39,41] The parent may be trained in behavioral techniques and required to take a very active role in the intervention. The parent may be a subject themselves in family intervention programs where nutrition and activity behaviors or parent BMI may be a trial outcome.

Conclusions

The role of primary care will be expected to increase in the coming years as the incidence and prevalence of overweight and obesity in children prevails, and programs are introduced that highlight the issue for parents, schools and the health care system.

Most effective obesity prevention programs have been carried out through comprehensive approaches that include a combination of dietary and behavioral modification, physical activity and parental involvement. They have mostly been based in preschool, school, community, family or tertiary care settings. It is clear that virtually no evidence of effectiveness and cost–effectiveness exists about interventions tackling overweight and obesity in primary care. The continued identification of effective prevention and weight reduction strategies for children, and the clarification of the role of primary care in this, must be research priorities.

It is clear that there are many barriers for GPs, nurses and other primary care professionals in addressing childhood overweight and obesity, many of which relate to lack of time, resources, appropriate skills and training. However, the challenges of translating evidence-based guidelines into health systems practice must also be addressed.[62] The evidence base for future obesity prevention interventions can be improved by reporting of contextual environmental, cultural and other issues,[63] which may be useful in both helping explain variability in outcomes of different approaches, but also for practitioners in adopting future research into practice.

References

1 World Health Organization, UNICEF: Primary Health Care: Report of the International Conference on Primary Health Care. Alma-Ata USSR: Geneva: WHO. 1978.

2 World Health Organization: Primary Health Care. In: www.who.int/topics/primary_health_care/en/ ed. World Health Organization, Geneva, 2008.

3 Vanselow N, Donaldson M, Yordy K: From the Institute of medicine. *JAMA* 1995; **273**(3):192.

4 Wake M, McCallum Z: Secondary prevention of overweight in primary school children: what place for general practice? *Med J Aust* 2004; **181**(2):82.

5 Walker O, Strong M, Atchinson R, Saunders J, Abbott J: A qualitative study of primary care clinicians' views of treating childhood obesity. *BMC Fam Pract* 2007; **8**(50): Published online 3 September 2007. doi: 10.1186/1471-2296-8

6 Waters E, Haby M, Wake M, Salmon L: Public health and preventative healthcare in children: current practices of Victorian GPs and barriers to participation. *Med J Aust* 2000; **173**:68–71.

7 Epstein L, Ogden J: A qualitative study of GPs' views of treating obesity. *Br J Gen Pract* 2005; **55**(519):750–754.

8 Story MT, Neumark-Stzainer DR, Sherwood NE et al: Management of child and adolescent obesity: Attitudes, barriers, skills, and training needs among health care professionals. *Pediatrics* 2002; **110**(1):210–214.

9 King LA, Loss JH, Wilkenfeld RL, Pagnini DL, Booth ML, Booth SL: Australian GPs' perceptions about child and adolescent overweight and obesity: the Weight of Opinion study. *Br J Gen Pract* 2007; **57**(535):124–129.

10 Commission on Chronic Illness: Chronic Illness in the United States, vol. 1. Cambridge: MA Harvard University Press, 1957.

11 Thomas P, ed. Weighing the Options: Criteria for Evaluating Weight-Management Programs. Washington: Institute of Medicine, 1995; pp. 152–162.

12 Summerbell CD, Waters E, Edmunds LD, Kelly S, Brown T, Campbell KJ: Interventions for preventing obesity in children. *Cochrane Database Syst Rev*: Reviews 2005, Issue 3 John Wiley & Sons, Ltd Chichester, UK, 2005;3. doi: 10.1002/14651858.CD001871.pub2

13 Flodmark CE, Marcus C, Britton M: Interventions to prevent obesity in children and adolescents: a systematic literature review. *Int J Obes (Lond)* 2006; **30**(4):579–589.

14 National Health and Medical Research Council: Clinical practice guidelines for the management of overweight and obesity in children and adolescents. 2003. www.health.gov.au/internet/wcms/publiching.nsf/content/obesityguidelines-guidelines-children.htm.

15 Singapore Ministry of Health: Obesity. Singapore: Agency for Healthcare Research and Qulaity, 2004.

16 Institute for Clinical Systems Improvement: Prevention and Management of Obesity (Mature Adolescents and Adults). ICSI, 2005.

17 Institute for Health and Clinical Excellence: CG43 Obesity: Full Guideline, Section 5a—Management of Obesity in Clinical Settings (Children): Evidence Statements and Reviews. London: NIHCE, 2006.

18 Summerbell CD, Ashton V, Campbell KJ, Edmunds L, Kelly S, Waters E: Interventions for treating obesity in children. *Cochrane Database Syst Rev* 2003; 3 (Art. No. CD001872).

19 Scottish Intercollegiate Guidelines Network: Management of Obesity in Children and Young People: A National Clinical Guideline. Edinburgh: SIGN, 2003.

20 Barlow SE: Expert committee recommendations regarding the prevention, assessment, and treatment of child and adolescent overweight and obesity: summary report. *Pediatrics* 2007; **120**(Suppl. 4)S164–S192.

21 McLean N, Griffin S, Toney K, Hardeman W: Family involvement in weight control, weight maintenance and weight-loss interventions: a systematic review of randomised trials. *Int J Obes Relat Metab Disord* 2003; **27**(9): 987–1005.

22 Jelalian E, Saelens BE: Empirically supported treatments in pediatric psychology: pediatric obesity (structured abstract). *J Pediatr Psychol* 1999; **24**(3):223–248.

23 Fulton JE, McGuire M, Caspersen C: Interventions for weight loss and weight gain prevention among youth: current issues. *Sports Med* 2001; **31**:153–165.

24 Reilly JJ: Obesity in childhood and adolescence: Evidence based clinical and public health perspectives. *Postgrad Med J* 2006; **82**(969):429–437.

25 Haddock CK, Shadish WR, Klesges RC, Stein RJ: Treatments for childhood and adolescent obesity. *Ann Behav Med* 1994; **16**:235–244.

26 Epstein L, Myers MD, Raynor HA, Saelens BE: Treatment of pediatric obesity. *Pediatrics* 1998; **101**:554–570.

27 Epstein L, Goldfield GS: Physical activity in the treatment of childhood overweight and obesity: current evidence and research issues. *Med Sci Sports Exerc* 1999; **31**:S553–S559.

28 Maziekas M, LeMura LM, Stoddard NM et al: Follow up exercise studies in paediatric obesity: implications for long term effectiveness. *Br J Sports Med* 2003; **37**:425–429.

29 Berry D, Sheehan R,. Heschel R, Knafl K, Melkus G, Grey M: Family-based interventions for childhood obesity: a review (Structured abstract). *J Fam Nurs* 2004; **10**(4):429–449.

30 Herrera E, Johnston CA, Steele RG: A comparison of cognitive and behavioral treatments for pediatric obesity. *Child Health Care* 2004; **33**:151–167.

31 Bautista-Castano I, Doreste J, Serra-Majem L: Effectiveness of interventions in the prevention of childhood obesity. *Eur J Epidemiol* 2004; **19**(7):617–622.

32 Connelly JB, Duaso MJ, Butler G: A systematic review of controlled trials of interventions to prevent childhood obesity and overweight: a realistic synthesis of the evidence. *Public Health* 2007; **121**(7):510–517.

33 Woo KS, Chook P, Yu CW: Effects of diet and exercise on obesity-related vascular dysfunction in children. *Circulation* 2004; **109**(16):1981–1986.

34 Robinson TN: Reducing children's television viewing to prevent obesity: a randomized controlled trial. *JAMA* 1999; **282**(16):1561–1567.

35 Epstein L, Valoski AM, Vara LS et al: Effects of decreasing sedentary behavior and increasing activity on weight change in obese children. *Health Psychol* 1995; **14**:109–115.

36 Epstein L, Paluch RA, Gordy CC et al: Decreasing sedentary behaviors in treating pediatric obesity. *Arch Pediatr Adolesc Med* 2000; **154**:220–226.

37 Epstein L, Wing RR, Koeske R et al: A comparison of lifestyle exercise, aerobic exercise and calisthenics on weight loss in obese children. *Behav Ther* 1985; **16**:345.

38 McCallum Z, Wake M, Gerner B et al: Can Australian general practitioners tackle childhood overweight/obesity? Methods and processes from the LEAP (Live, Eat and Play) randomized controlled trial. *J Paediatr Child Health* 2005; **41**(9–10):488–494.

39 McCallum Z, Wake M, Gerner B et al: Outcome data from the LEAP (Live, Eat and Play) trial: a randomized controlled trial of a primary care intervention for childhood overweight/mild obesity. *Int J Obes (Lond)* 2007; **31**(4): 630–636.

40 Saelens BE, Sallis JF, Wilfley DE, Patrick K, Cella JA, Buchta R: Behavioral weight control for overweight adolescents initiated in primary care. *Obes Res* 2002; **10**(1):22–32.

41 Patrick K, Calfas KJ, Norman GJ et al: Randomized controlled trial of a primary care and home-based intervention for physical activity and nutrition behaviors: PACE+ for adolescents. *Arch Pediatr Adolesc Med* 2006; **160**(2):128–136.

42 Nova ARASE: Long-term management of obesity in paediatric office practice: experimental evaluation of two different types of intervention. *Ambul Child Health* 2001; **7**(3–4): 239–247.

43 Douglas F, van Teijlingen E, Torrance N, Fearn P, Kerr A, Melonia S: Promoting physical activity in primary care settings: health visitors' and practice nurses' views and experiences. *J Adv Nurs* 2006; **55**(2):159–168.

44 Brown I, Stride C, Psarou A, Brewins L, Thompson J: Management of obesity in primary care: nurses' practices, beliefs and attitudes. *J Adv Nurs* 2007; **59**(4):329–341.

45 Jackson C, Coe A, Cheater FM, Wroe S: Specialist health visitor-led weight management intervention in primary care: Exploratory evaluation. *J Adv Nurs* 2007; **58**(1):23–34.

46 Campbell K et al: The infant feeding activity and nutrition trial (INFANT) an early intervention to prevent childhood obesity: cluster randomised controlled trial. *BMC Public Health* 2008; **8**:103.

47 Wen L, Baur LA, Rissel C, Wardle K, Alperstein G, Simpson JM: Early intervention of multiple home visits to prevent childhood obesity in a disadvantaged population: a home-based randomised controlled trial (Healthy Beginnings Trial). *BMC Public Health* 2007; **7**(76).

48 Mercer SW, Tessier S: A qualitative study of general practitioners' and practice nurses' attitudes to obesity management in primary care. *Health Bull (Edinb)* 2001; **59**(4):248–253.

49 Larsen L, Mandleco B, Williams M, Tiedeman M: Childhood obesity: prevention practices of nurse practitioners. *J Am Acad Nurse Pract* 2006; **18**(2):70–79.

50 Lindsay AC, Sussner KM, Kim J, Gortmaker S: The role of parents in preventing childhood obesity. *Future Child* 2006; **16**(1):169–186.

51 Golan M, Weizman A, Apter A, Fainaru M: Parents as the exclusive agents of change in the treatment of childhood obesity. *Am J Clin Nutr* 1998; **67**(6):1130–1135.

52 Golan M, Crow S: Targeting parents exclusively in the treatment of childhood obesity: long-term results. *Obes Res* 2004; **12**(2):357–361.

53 Epstein LH, Valoski A, Koeske R, Wing RR: Family-based behavioral weight control in obese young children. *J Am Diet Assoc* 1986; **86**(4):481–484.

54 Epstein LH, Valoski A, Wing RR, McCurley J: Ten-year follow-up of behavioral, family-based treatment for obese children. *JAMA* 1990; **264**(19):2519–2523.

55 Stice E, Shaw H, Marti CN: A meta-analytic review of obesity prevention programs for children and adolescents: the skinny on interventions that work. *Psychol Bull* 2006; **132**(5):667–691.

56 Etelson D, Brand DA, Patrick PA, Shirali A: Childhood obesity: do parents recognize this health risk? *Obes Res* 2003; **11**(11):1362–1368.

57 Wake M, Salmon L, Waters E, Wright M, Hesketh K: Parent-reported health status of overweight and obese Australian primary school children: a cross-sectional population survey. *Int J Obes Relat Metab Disord* 2002; **26**(5):717–724.

58 Davis MM, Gance-Cleveland B, Hassink S, Johnson R, Paradis G, Resnicow K: Recommendations for prevention of childhood obesity. *Pediatrics* 2007; **120**(Suppl. 4): S229–S253.

59 Jackson C, Bee-Gates DJ, Henriksen L: Authoritative parenting, child competencies, and initiation of cigarette smoking. *Health Educ Q* 1994; **21**(1):103–116.

60 Schmitz KH, Lytle LA, Phillips GA, Murray DM, Birnbaum AS, Kubik MY: Psychosocial correlates of physical activity and sedentary leisure habits in young adolescents: the Teens Eating for Energy and Nutrition at School study. *Prev Med* 2002; **34**(2):266–278.

61 Rhee KE, De Lago CW, Arscott-Mills T, Mehta SD, Davis RK: Factors associated with parental readiness to make changes for overweight children. *Pediatrics* 2005; **116**(1):e94–e101.

62 Saelens BE, Liu L: Clinician's comment on treatment of childhood overweight meta-analysis. *Health Psychol* 2007; **26**(5):533–536.

63 Klesges LM, Dzewaltowski DA, Glasgow RE: Review of external validity reporting in childhood obesity prevention research. *Am J Prev Med* 2008; **34**(3):216–223.

CHAPTER 13

Links between children's independent mobility, active transport, physical activity and obesity

Carolyn Whitzman,[1] *Vivian Romero,*[2] *Mitch Duncan,*[3] *Carey Curtis,*[4] *Paul Tranter*[5] and *Matthew Burke*[6]

[1] Faculty of Architecture, Building and Planning, University of Melbourne, Melbourne, Australia
[2] Faculty of the Built Environment, University of New South Wales, Sydney, Australia
[3] Central Queensland University, Rockhampton, Australia
[4] School of Built Environment, Curtin University, Bentley, Australia
[5] School of Physical, Environmental and Mathematical Sciences, University of New South Wales, Australian Defence Force Academy, Canberra, Australia
[6] Urban Research Program, Faculty of Environment, Planning, and Architecture, Griffith University, Brisbane, Australia

Summary and recommendations for practice

- Internationally, the past 40 years have seen a number of inter-related trends in developed Anglo-American countries, including radically declining levels of children's independent mobility (CIM), increased parental use of cars to transport children to school and play, decreasing everyday physical activity of both children and adults, and increasing child obesity rates.
- The level of children's everyday physical activity is influenced by gender, household income, parental and societal fears, the physical design of neighborhoods, and broader social policies that discourage "risk".
- Several promising practices can have an impact on improving children's active transport, everyday physical activity and autonomy:
    - traffic calming, lowering speed limits, improving access to destinations, and other physical environment modifications
    - social planning and marketing interventions, including school travel plans and walking school bus schemes
    - rights-based participatory planning approaches such as Child Friendly Cities projects.

Introduction

Children's independent mobility means the freedom of those under 18 years to move around in public spaces without adult accompaniment.[1] The phrases "battery reared" and "free range" refer to two diametrically opposed approaches to children's upbringing.[2,3] "Free range" children have traditionally been allowed, and indeed expected, to walk, cycle, or take public transport on their own for everyday trips between home, school, parks, shops and friends' houses. They have also been allowed, in previous generations, to independently explore their immediate neighborhood and the broader city with increasing confidence as they mature. Internationally, the past 40 years have seen a number of inter-related trends: radically declining levels of CIM, increased parental use of cars to transport children to school and play, decreasing everyday physical activity of both children and adults, and increasing child obesity rates.

Preventing Childhood Obesity. Edited by
E. Waters, B.A. Swinburn, J.C. Seidell and R. Uauy.
© 2010 Blackwell Publishing.

There is a relatively small and recent interdisciplinary research on children's independent mobility, primarily reflecting the disciplines of transportation planning, social geography, environmental psychology and public health. The purpose of this chapter is to explore the links between these various phenomena, to detail the complex factors behind these trends, and to examine policy changes that show promise in addressing these interrelated problems. It draws on research published in English, most of which has been conducted in Western Europe, North America and Australasia. Research websites (e.g., Active Living Research, health-evidence.ca, UNESCO Child Friendly Cities) were searched for additional literature regarding promising policies and practices.

Battery-reared children: the extent of the problem

Most research on levels of CIM focuses on the journey to school, for two reasons. First, the majority of children must enact a journey to and from school each weekday. Second, the journey to and from school has often been a springboard for children to exercise their initial acts of independent mobility.

Studies in several developed countries show a radical shift from children walking to school on their own in the 1970s, to children being driven, mostly by parents, in the 1990s and 2000s. For instance, Hillman et al[1] found that in 1971, 80% of 7–8-year-olds in the UK were allowed to travel to school on their own, but in 1990, this had fallen to 9%. In Perth, Western Australia, the percentage of children walking or cycling to school fell from 66% in 1974 to 9% in 2005.[4] Successive UK National Travel Surveys show car trips taken by children aged 5–16 have increased 37% from 1985/86 to 1997/99, with a corresponding decrease of 31% in the number of trips walked by children.[5]

The radical reduction of CIM increases children's reliance on adults and their health risks, and establishes a car-addicted lifestyle that may continue to adulthood.[4] Children who are dependent upon vehicular transport may miss out on the incidental accumulation of physical activity that walking and cycling, as well as hopping, climbing and exploring, provide.[6,7] Although debates persist about whether the journey to school constitutes the most important source of physical activity for most children, it can be a part of a daily physical routine that can increase activity levels.[8] For example, regular walking to and from school was associated with greater energy expenditure than school organized physical education.[9]

There are also mental health impacts from adult dependent mobility. Opportunities for talking with friends and neighbors are reduced when children are transported via automobiles, with implications for social connectedness and community well-being.[10] Childhood experiences may determine adult behaviors. Walking, cycling and public transport may not even be considered as possible forms of transport when children become accustomed to being driven.[11–13] When Malone[14] asked 50 children aged 4 to 8 in the regional Victorian city of Bendigo to take photographs of their typical week, over half included a picture of the back seat of the family car. In Perth Australia, children living in low-density suburbs were found to travel predominantly by car for all trip purposes in 2006. For those aged less than 10, 80% of all trips were by car. While there was a reduction in car trips to around 55% of total journeys in the adolescent years 10 to 17, once they obtained drivers' licences 80% of trip-making reverted to car journeys.[15]

The confinement of children: possible causes

The most commonly cited reason for declining children's independent mobility is child and parental fears of traffic safety and stranger danger (the latter connoting children getting abducted or molested). A recent Australian survey found that 80% of children aged 10–12 and 84% of children aged 5–6 said they were concerned about road safety, with even higher self-reported fears about stranger danger.[16] Fear of cars and strangers were also the two most common reasons given for limiting children's independent mobility in a large-scale study of parents in Italy,[17] and in the UK.[1] Such fears can be provoked by media coverage of relatively rare incidents.[2]

In addition to the perception of fear, there is a growing pressure to be a "good" parent, protecting children from all potential risks while providing them with the best opportunities.[18–20] Social interactions between parents play an important part in establishing local norms about children's trips to school, with peer pressure that all parents *should* drive their children to school.[21] Conversely, those parents engaged in practices out of line with the local norm claim that they are stigmatized and marginalized by other parents.[22]

The chauffeur role of parents is reinforced when they drive their children to school, based on the convenience of dropping off their children on the way to work, in what transport researchers call trip-chaining behaviour. The location of a parent's workplace has a strong bearing on whether or not a child's school journey will be taken on foot.[19,23,24] Journeys to school are "bound up with other activities and this affects both the nature of the journey and mode of transport used".[25]

Some of the factors influencing parental choices to limit children's active and independent travel are intrinsic to the particular community, while others are related to the culture of the broader society. Some countries such as Germany and Japan have an ethos of collective responsibility for looking out for children, and also have large numbers of people of all ages using outdoor public space, owing to built environment and socio-cultural factors. This contrasts with more individualistic societies such as the USA, UK, Australia and New Zealand, which have lower levels of children's independent mobility.[1,11,14]

Socio-economic status (SES), both of families and of areas, is another factor, although the evidence is somewhat contradictory. Timperio et al[26] found that children from lower SES areas were less likely to be physically active than children from high SES areas, even though low SES households are less likely to own vehicles. Another Australian study found that a higher proportion of children living in low SES areas reported being able to travel to more destinations over larger distances than those living in high SES areas.[27] In their study of four neighborhoods in Christchurch, New Zealand, Tranter and Pawson[11] found that traffic levels were greater determinants of active transport than household income.

In addition to parental regulations and socio-economic status, children's active transport is contingent upon the physical planning and design features of their neighborhoods. Studies of the environmental attributes of particular areas in relation to children's mobility have found that key factors include the age, density, and proximity of the neighborhood to the central city (with older, denser neighborhoods tending to encourage independent mobility); a set of traffic danger signifiers including amount of traffic, width of roadway, presence or absence of footpaths, dangerous crossings and lots of cars parked on the street; and a set of stranger danger signifiers, including visible signs of incivilities and alcohol/drug use (dog mess, broken bottles, used drug paraphernalia); and local air and noise pollution.[17]

Promising policies and practices

Several studies have shown that children prefer active transport over driving to destinations. A UK survey of 800 children aged 7 to 11 found that 38% of children who are at present driven to school would prefer to walk or cycle.[28] In Melbourne, where 72% of children are driven to school, 61% say that they would prefer to walk, given the choice.[29] Many children also prefer independent over dependent travel. A recent study of Sydney primary school pupils found that while 70% from the inner city and 80% from the outer suburb traveled with a parent or guardian to school, 33% of inner-city children and 44% of outer-suburb children would prefer to walk to school with a friend or sibling, with 24% of inner-city children and 14% of outer-suburb children preferring to walk alone.[7]

Given children's preferences, and the negative physical and mental health consequences of adult dependent mobility, there are surprisingly few policies or programs in the English-speaking developed countries most affected to address these interrelated issues. More recently, researchers have begun to address the interaction between environmental, interpersonal and social barriers and enablers. For instance, Timperio et al[16] studied 235 children aged 5 to 6 years and 677 children aged 10 to 12 years, and found that parental perceptions of few other children walking in the neighborhood and no safe road crossings were negatively correlated with walking or cycling to school, while for children, distance and (for younger children) steep inclines were negatively correlated with wanting to walk or cycle to school. Creating supportive environments for children's independent mobility and physical activity thus requires overcoming both social and built environment barriers at the neighborhood level, as well as creating opportunities to listen to the children themselves.

Modifying the built environment

Built environment modifications (e.g., traffic calming and home zones) seek to promote the safe passage and increased visibility of child pedestrians. Traffic-calming measures endeavor to reduce the negative effects of vehicles, alter driver behavior, and enhance overall conditions for pedestrians. Posted travel speed, street alignments, vehicular obstacles and other design tactics act to lower travel speeds. In some cases, streets are closed off to through traffic, particularly in residential areas.[17,30–33]

Traffic calming measures have been shown to be successful in a number of countries. For instance, up until the 1970s, Denmark had the highest rate of child road deaths in western Europe. In 1976, the Danish national government passed legislation requiring local authorities to reduce the speed on roads to a norm of 30 km/h and to invest in greater walking and cycling infrastructure. Today, Denmark has much higher levels of walking and cycling than the UK and much lower casualty rates.[34] In the UK, where introduction of 30 km/h zones has met with much more limited acceptance by local traffic engineers, the zones have proved successful in terms of speed reduction, accident rates and increased resident perceptions of safety, although traffic calming and enforcement are still necessary in these areas.[32]

The UK Home Zone projects, introduced in 1999, usually involve a shared surface for cars and pedestrians (no grade or other separation of roadway and footpath), tree planting, improved lighting, use of colored and textured surface treatments, and sometimes other design aspects such as a symbolic "gateway" entrance to the street.[35] Possible benefits of Home Zones, apart from reducing road traffic accidents, include engendering greater social interaction and a sense of symbolic ownership, reducing the fear of crime, and providing places for children's informal recreation close to home. They are the opposite of the more traditional "Radburn" approach to transportation planning, which stressed complete separation of vehicle and pedestrian pathways, since the isolated subways and footbridges that resulted from the Radburn approach were widely perceived as being unsafe in terms of stranger danger,[36] and remained unpopular for walking.[35]

An evaluation of seven home zones indicated the development of stronger communities in all sites as a result of their establishment. Adult residents reported knowing more neighbors afterwards, and an increased ability to resolve neighborhood disputes through discussion rather than bringing in the authorities.[33] Lower speeds and reduced traffic resulted at all sites, and in five sites there were measurable increases in CIM. However, implementation has been slow and some researchers contend that traffic speeds may need to be as low as 12 km/h to encourage greater child pedestrian use.[33]

New research between planning, transport and health is also articulating the importance of accommodating children's incidental physical activity through accessible facilities and interesting environments. Approximately 150 children aged 10 in three Melbourne schools were asked to map and photograph neighborhood attractions that they could walk or cycle to. Common destinations included playgrounds and sports fields as well as less elaborate recreational possibilities such as a target painted on a wall for ball playing.[37] Other studies provide encouraging evidence of associations between children's activity levels and the proximity of parks.[38–40] Gill[33] suggests that amenities such as children's mosaics and other public art may increase symbolic control of streets (see Engwicht),[41] while Prezza et al[17] suggest that greenery in road dividers and along streets may mitigate immediate air pollution, reduce traffic noise and create a degree of amenity. Unlike the evaluation literature on traffic calming, no studies have been located to either prove or disprove that policies aimed at increasing the number and types of neighborhood amenities increase children's autonomous and active movement.

Finally, a set of larger-scale built environment interventions, including "smart growth" and "new urbanism" projects, have developed "a persuasive hypothesis attributing the change in travel behaviour … to the urban form of our communities".[42] Yet the evidentiary support for built environment changes influencing children's (as opposed to adult's) travel behaviour is not well advanced.

Social planning and marketing: school travel plans and the walking school bus

In contrast to the built environment emphasis on the community level, much public health literature is focused on individual level social determinants of children's modal choice, such as self-confidence in one's abilities (known as "self-efficacy"), time, interest, perceived health and encouraging parents to allow their children to walk or cycle.[42]

A number of policies and programs combining built environment changes with social marketing have been implemented, particularly in relation to the journey to school. Safe Routes to School programs were pioneered in Denmark in the 1980s as part of the national road safety initiative described above.[42] The program has been adopted in several different countries, including the USA,[42] the UK,[43] and Australia.[44] According to McMillan,[42] Safe Routes to School involve "3Es":

1. education of both children and drivers on road safety
2. enforcement of traffic laws around schools
3. engineering of the street environment along the routes to school.

Evaluations of School Travel Plans have found mixed results. Evaluations in the UK show that schools were successful in producing plans, but unsuccessful in changing travel behavior, which was generally due to the long-term commitment necessary from both the school and parents.[26] An intensive US School Travel Plan initiative that included walk/bike to school days, a "frequent rider miles" competition, classroom education, walking school buses and bike trains resulted in a 64% increase in walking, a 114% increase in cycling, and a 91% increase in car-pooling to the school, along with a 29% reduction in driving alone after two years.[45] However, there was no comparison with a control group, changes in independent mobility were not tested, and a limited number of the same children were tested both before and after the changes. A more general criticism is that while school travel plans involving extensive activities over a number of years can be successful, children's needs go well beyond traveling in the same way to a fixed destination repeatedly, and attempts to restrict children to "safe" routes and designated play areas may be both socially undesirable and impractical.[32]

There is a similar controversy related to another school-based program, the walking school bus (WSB). The idea was for walking bus drivers, who would "walk a set route, much like a school bus, collecting children along the route and delivering them safely to school".[30] The idea rapidly diffused through at least five countries—Canada, the UK, the USA, Australia

and New Zealand—to the point where thousands of local initiatives have been established in the past 10 years.[5,9,46] Along the way, the informal basis of the idea has been lost. Engwicht, who in 2003 unequivocally stated that "in many cases, WSB has outlived its usefulness and in some circumstances has become counterproductive", gives an example of over 100 volunteers showing interest in one program in his home town of Brisbane; but by the time compulsory training and exhaustive background checks had been completed, only three potential volunteers were left.[47]

Mackett et al,[48] in the UK, found that children are twice as likely to report positive social aspects of WSB initiatives than parents, although both report greater friendships with neighbors as a result of these programs. Yet evaluations indicate no decrease in local car traffic. Parents may walk their children to school and then return to drive their car.[43] School teachers report mixed results in lessening car congestion near school entrances as a result of WSB, and also a loss of parent volunteers over time, particularly since child interest in WSB declines in senior primary grades.[9]

An evaluation of WSB schemes in New Zealand suggests that WSB may result in increased physical activity, but actually reinforces adult-dependent mobility, since it relies on adult supervision and adult-imposed rules on group travel that is inimical to independent exploration.[46] However, children and adults are both highly articulate on the benefits, reporting enjoying talking as they walk, meeting neighbors, and enjoying the daily exercise.[46] A criticism of the Auckland, New Zealand WSB initiative is the prevalence of WSB in higher SES areas, while child pedestrian injuries are more likely to occur in low SES areas.[49] Another New Zealand study agreed that parents report new and better friendships and acquaintances, leading to other get-togethers on the street.[5] Kingham and Ussher[5] also suggested that the WSBs may increase independent mobility. Children say that they want to walk to other places as a result of improved fitness and knowing their neighborhood better, and children do "graduate" from WSB,[9] presumably to independent walking, at the age of 9 or 10.[5]

A rights-based approach: Child-Friendly Cities and participatory planning

Child-Friendly Cities (CFCs) is a UNICEF-sponsored program that aims to improve local governance capacity to support children's rights, among them the right to "participate freely and fully in city life", including walking safely on the street.[50–52] The UN Convention on the Rights of the Child, adopted by all member states in 2000, includes "the child's right to live in a safe, clear, and healthy environment and to engage in free play, leisure and recreation in the environment".[50] It sees children as "the future contributors, decision makers, and citizens of the world", and children's well-being and quality of life as prime indicators of a healthy environment, good governance and sustainable development.[50]

There are a plethora of child assemblies, consultation processes with children and youth, and child-empowering activities taking place, including many that are directly related to active transport and independent mobility. Dozens of European and Latin American cities have child assemblies where children regularly co-plan developments.[53,54] In the USA, there is a Community-Based Education Resource (CUBE) manual on child-oriented communities: the Dutch Institute of Design has published design guidelines for children, and the Canadian Institute of Planners has *A Kid's Guide to Building Great Communities*.[55] However, the Child Friendly Cities commitment from local governments is often limited to vision and consultation rather than implementation, and a review of the Child Friendly Cities database has found very limited information on outcomes arising from projects.[53]

Despite such limitations, the Italian projects, in particular, have led to substantial changes in both the physical and the social environment. In Fano, the Children's City project combines letting children plan urban renewal through creative laboratories, children's councils that entrench participatory planning practices, and initiatives to encourage autonomy. Certain streets have been closed to traffic, access to sports installations and equipment has been improved, and there has been increased redevelopment of public squares and semi-public areas within condominium areas as play spaces. In Pistoia, the project "Safe Routes round the school C. Collodi" has led to increases in children walking to the school by themselves since its inception in 2000, although exact figures are not provided, and children have also reclaimed a square near the school that was previously used as a car park.[52] Identifying the concerns and/or

neighborhood improvements important to children may increase their interests in using such spaces actively and autonomously.

Conclusion

There is a clear interrelationship between declines in CIM, reduced everyday physical activity and increased obesity rates. However, the evidence base on what might work to increase children's independent mobility is still poor, partly because it is still not recognized as a policy priority, and partly because the mechanisms to include children in evaluating and changing their urban environments are so poor. Traffic calming is promising at the very local level of the individual street, but does not appear to address underlying parental concerns about CIM, or to expand children's home territory much beyond the immediate vicinity of the home. The evidence base on School Travel Plans and walking school bus is mixed in terms of success, and again, focuses on a set of specific routes to one place (the school) rather than the entire community. A more holistic emphasis on children's participation in planning, encompassing both physical design and social change, is evident in Child Friendly Cities, but there is, at present, limited evidence that this approach works to change environments, let alone change behaviors or lead to resultant improvements in health and well-being. More holistic research is needed on how children actually travel: their needs, desires, and the built and social environment factors that may work to make children free to explore their local communities and lead healthier active lives.

Acknowledgement

The authors would like to acknowledge the financial support of the Australasian Centre for the Governance and Management of Urban Transport (GAMUT).

References

1 Hillman M, Adams J, Whitelegg J: One False Move ... A Study of Children's Independent Mobility. London: Policy Studies Institute, 1990.

2 Hillman M: Are We Developing Battery-reared or Free-range Children? Perth: Western Australia Pedestrian Advisory Council Seminar, 2002.

3 O'Brien M, Jones D, Sloan D: Children's independent spatial mobility in the urban public realm. *Childhood* 2000; **7**: 257–277.

4 Tranter PJ: Overcoming social traps: a key to creating child-friendly cities. In: Gleeson BJ, Sipe N, eds. Creating Child Friendly Cities. London: Routledge, 2006:121–135.

5 Kingham S, Ussher S: An assessment of the benefits of the walking school bus in Christchurch, New Zealand. *Transp Res Part A* 2007; **41**:502–510.

6 Salmon J, Timperio A, Cleland V, Venn A: Trends in children's physical activity and weight status in high and low socio-economic status areas of Melbourne, Victoria, 1985–2001. *Aust N Z J Public Health* 2005; **29**:337–342.

7 Romero V: "I will be not a nerd": children's development, the built environment, and school travel. 3rd State of Australian Cities Conference, Adelaide, November 2007.

8 Sturm R: Childhood Obesity: what we can learn from existing data on societal trends. *Prev Chronic Dis* 2005; **2**:1–9.

9 Mackett R, Lucas L, Paskins J, Turbin J: Walking Buses in Hertfordshire. London: Centre for Transport Studies, University College, 2004.

10 O'Brien C: Transportation that's actually good for the soul. National Centre for Bicycling and Walking Forum, Article no. 12-03-1—December 2003.

11 Tranter P, Pawson E: Children's access to local environments. *Local Environ* 2001; **6**:27–48.

12 Mackett R, Lucas L, Paskins J, Turbin J: Understanding the car dependency impacts of children's car use. Children and Traffic Conference, Copenhagen, Denmark. 2002.

13 Thomsen TU: Children—automobility's immobilized others? *Trans Rev* 2004; **24**:515–532.

14 Malone K: The bubble-wrap generation: children growing up in walled gardens. *Environ Educ Res* 2007; **13**:513–527.

15 Curtis C, Olaru D, Scheurer J: Children travel and accessibility in conventional suburbia. Forthcoming 2009.

16 Timperio A, Crawford D, Telford A, Salmon J: Perceptions about the local neighbourhood and walking and cycling among children. *Prev Med* 2004; **38**:39–47.

17 Prezza M, Alparone F, Cristallo C, Luigi S: Parental perception of social risk and of positive potentiality of outdoor autonomy for children. *J Environ Psychol* 2005; **25**: 437–453.

18 Sanger C: Girls and the getaway: cars, culture, and the predicament of gendered space. *Univ PA Law Rev* 1995; **144**: 705–756.

19 Dowling R: Cultures of mothering and car use in suburban Sydney. *Geoforum* 2000; **31**:345–353.

20 Rissotto A, Giuliani MV: Learning neighbourhood environments. In: Spencer C, Blades M, eds. Children and their Environments. Cambridge: Cambridge University Press, 2006:75–90.

21 Valentine G: "Oh Yes I Can" "Oh No You Can't": children and parents' understandings of kids' competence to negotiate public space safely. *Antipode* 1997; **29**:6589.

22 Valentine G, McKendrick JH: Children's outdoor play: exploring parental concerns about children's safety and the changing nature of childhood. *Geoforum* 1997; **28**:219–235.

23 Collins D, Kearns RA: The safe journeys of an enterprising school. *Health Place* 2001; **7**:293–306.

24 Wen ML, Fry D, Rissel C, Dirkis H, Balafas A, Merom D: Factors associated with children being driven to school. *Health Educ Res* 2008; **23**:325–334.

25 Pooley C, Turnball J, Adams M: The journey to school in Britain since the 1940s. *Area* 2005; **37**:43–53.

26 Timperio A, Salmon J, Ball K: Evidence-based strategies to promote physical activity among children, adolescents, and young adults. *J Sci Med Sport* 2004; **7**(1 Suppl.) 20–29.

27 Veitch J, Salmon J, Ball K: Children's active free play in local neighbourhoods. *Health Educ Res* 2007; **23**:870–879.

28 Mackett R: Are We Making Our Children Car Dependent? Dublin: Trinity College Dublin, 2001.

29 VicHealth [Victorian Health Promotion Foundation]. The Walking School Bus 2001 2002. Melbourne: VicHealth, 2002.

30 Engwicht D: Towards an Eco-City. Sydney: Envirobook, 1992.

31 Bartlett S, Hart R, Satterthwaite D, de la Barra X, Missair A. Cities for Children. London: Earthscan, 1999.

32 Hewson P: Child pedestrian accidents in the UK. *Radic Statistics* 2002; **79/80**:1–27.

33 Gill T. Can I Play Out …? Lessons from London Play's Home Zones Project. London: London Play, 2007.

34 Gill T. No Fear: Growing Up in a Risk-Averse Society. London: Calouste Gulbenkian Foundation, 2007.

35 Clayden A, McKoy K, Wild A: Improving residential liveability in the UK: home zones and alternative approaches. *J Urban Design* 2006; **11**:55–71.

36 Tranter PJ: Children's Mobility in Canberra. Monograph Series No 7. Department of Geography and Oceanography, University College, UNSW, 1993.

37 Hume C, Salmon J, Ball K: Children's perceptions of their home and neighbourhood environments and their association with objectively measured physical activity. *Health Educ Res* 2005; **20**:1–13.

38 Babey SH, Hastert TA, Yu H, Brown ER: Physical activity among adolescents. When do parks matter? *Am J Prev Med* 2008; **34**:345–348.

39 Frank L, Kerr J, Chapman J, Sallis J: Urban form relationships with walk trip frequency and distance among youth. *Am J Health Promot* 2007; **21**(Suppl. 4):305–311.

40 Norman G, Nutter S, Ryan S, Sallis J, Calfas K, Patrick K: Community design and access to recreational facilities as correlates of adolescent physical activity and body-mass index. *J Phys Act Health* 2006; **3**(Supp. 1)S118–S128.

41 Engwicht D: Mental Speed Bumps: The Smarter Way to Tame Traffic. Annandale, NSW: Envirobook, 2005.

42 McMillan T: Urban form and a child's trip to school. *J Plann Lit* 2005; **19**:440–456.

43 Mackett R, Lucas L, Paskins J, Turbin J: A methodology for evaluating walking buses as an instrument of urban transport policy. *Trans Policy* 2003; **10**:179–186.

44 Taylor M, Ampt E: Travelling smarter Down Under. *Trans Policy* 2003; **10**:165–177.

45 Staunton C, Hubsmith D, Kallins W: Promoting safe walking and biking to school. *Am J Public Health* 2003; **93**: 1431–1434.

46 Kearns R, Collins D, Neuwelt P: The Walking School Bus: extending children's geographies? *Area* 2003; **35**:285–292.

47 Engwicht D: Is the Walking School Bus Stalled in an Evolutionary cul de sac? Brisbane: Creative Communities International, 2003.

48 Mackett R, Lucas L, Paskins J, Turbin J: The effectiveness of initiatives to reduce children's car use. European Transport Conference. Strasbourg, France. 2003.

49 Collins D, Kearns RA: Geographies of inequality: child pedestrian injury and walking school buses in Auckland, New Zealand. *Soc Sci Med* 2005; **60**:61–69.

50 Malone K: Children, youth and sustainable cities. *Local Environ* 2001; **6**:5–12.

51 Gleeson B, Sipe N, eds. Creating Child Friendly Cities. London: Routledge, 2006.

52 Child-Friendly Cities. UNICEF (United Nations Children's Foundation); Child-Friendly Cities Partnerships and Networking-Italy. ••. www.childfriendlycities.org/networking/italy.html (accessed 28 June 2008).

53 Bartlett S: Review of Child Friendly Cities Database. Stockholm: Save the Children, 2006.

54 European Commission: Kids on the Move. Luxembourg: European Commission, 2002.

55 O'Brien C: Child-Friendly Transport Planning. Winnipeg: Centre for Sustainable Transportation; 2004.

CHAPTER 14

Evidence on the food environment and obesity

Deborah A. Cohen
The RAND Corporation, Santa Monica, CA, USA

Summary and recommendations for practice

Although weight is a function of the balance between what we eat and how much we exercise, a growing consensus points to food intake as the primary cause of the obesity epidemic.[1–3] The dominant thinking about the obesity epidemic is that it could be solved if people would exercise more self-control; thus, multiple interventions have been designed to increase self-efficacy, knowledge and skills with respect to nutrition and dieting.[4–6] However, most people know that if they eat too much and exercise too little, they will gain weight, and they also know that if they would just eat less and exercise more, they will lose weight. Furthermore, most people know that certain foods increase the odds of gaining weight, like chips, sodas, donuts, ice cream, candies and big portions of foods such as French fries and meat, yet these products continue to be among the best-selling items in America and other parts of the developed world. Knowledge appears to be less a problem than willpower.

Yet lack of willpower appears to be an implausible explanation as well. Given that people tend to gain weight when they move to a society where more people are overweight,[7,8] it would mean that an individual's character changes just by emigrating. If loss of willpower was the source of the problem, it would suggest that there would be significant differences in willpower by race, gender, ethnicity and age and, more importantly, by country of residence or historical

Preventing Childhood Obesity. Edited by
E. Waters, B.A. Swinburn, J.C. Seidell and R. Uauy.
© 2010 Blackwell Publishing.

cohort. Is it conceivable that 30 years ago when fewer were overweight and obese, people had more willpower than they do now?

This paper is the result of searching the literature for counterfactual evidence that would indicate that the dominant conceptualization that people eat too much because they lack self-control or have insufficient knowledge is plain wrong. Rather, the problem of obesity can be traced to the dramatic changes in our food environments and their interaction with human neurophysiology. This chapter describes how environments affect people in manners that defy personal insight or are below individual awareness. If people are unaware of the environmental forces and cues that are artificially making them feel hungry and leading them to eat too much, they cannot possibly control how much they eat.

Introduction

Eating is not a rational behavior. Eating is not like studying for a test, memorizing facts, understanding and manipulating sophisticated mathematical equations, painting a portrait or writing a book. It is not an advanced behavior, but a primitive one—one that is instinctual, hard-wired and in many ways uncontrollable. Humans are endowed with a metabolic pathway that allows them to store extra energy as fat. One might argue the existence of a pathway to create and store energy means that people were actually designed to eat too much. Given that more food is available in today's world compared to the past, individuals are functioning normally and responding in the manner in which they were designed. Nothing is wrong with us. The problem is the environment in which we now live.

Changes in the food environment—the nutrition transition

Beginning in the 1960s, the green revolution increased the production of cereals, rice, wheat and maize—staples for much of the world. As a consequence, three major changes have occurred:

1. the relative price of food has declined, especially for high calorie foods filled with fat and sugar;
2. food is increasingly easily accessible; and
3. multi-national corporations have invested heavily in advertising and marketing to sell more of their products, making cues to eat more salient.

Together, these three changes have made it possible for people to eat as much as they can whenever they want, as well as making people eat too much, and artificially stimulating people to feel hungry when they do not need to eat.

Food prices

The increasing yields and production of all staples have led to lower food prices overall in relation to income,[9] and in the United States, in 2006, the average family spent only 9.9% of their income on food compared to 14.8% 40 years earlier and nearly 25% in the 1920s.[10] Interventions that have manipulated the price of food have shown that when healthier foods are less expensive people are more likely to buy them.[11–13] Another study, examining the incidence of obesity in elementary school children, showed that in communities where the cost of meat was high and vegetables were low, children were less likely to become overweight than in communities where meat prices were low and fruits and vegetables were high.[14] People are sensitive to price, and when food is cheap, they are able to purchase more. When high-calorie foods are cheaper than lower-calorie foods, more people purchase and eat too many calories.[15]

Food accessibility and portion sizes

Another dramatic change in the food environment has been the increase in portion sizes. Portions for beverages in 6 oz and 8 oz sizes, for example, are no longer sold in the US, in favor of 12 oz, 16 oz, 20 oz and larger sizes. The typical American restaurant now serves portions that are 2–5 times in excess of what individuals typically require to stay in energy balance.[16–18] Beyond portion sizes, the number of places that now sell food has also increased dramatically. While the number of convenience stores and restaurants has increased dramatically, especially fast-food restaurants, a large proportion of non-restaurant outlets such as supermarkets and businesses that previously did not sell prepared food now do. Food that you can eat right away ("convenience food"—especially candy, cookies, chips and sodas) can be purchased in book stores, car washes, hardware stores and even building supply warehouses. One survey of multiple cities estimated that about 40% of non-food outlets in the United States now sell food (personal communication, Tom Farley, February 2008). Furthermore, the availability of vending machines has multiplied several times over the last couple decades,[19] and these machines now sell food in office buildings, public buildings, parks, petrol stations—practically anywhere. And the types of food items sold are predominantly high-calorie salty snacks (e.g., chips), cookies, candy and sugar-sweetened beverages.

Food advertising—cues

Along with increased food availability is the massive increase in advertising and marketing for food products. The amount of funds spent on commercial advertising and marketing research exceeds funds available for nutrition education more than 10-fold.[20–22] Further, the sophistication of advertising and the ability to target subgroups has advanced substantially. Some studies investigating the differential exposure to age, race and ethnic groups indicate that children and racial ethnic minorities are differentially targeted to receive a high proportion of food advertising not only in television, but in magazines as well.[23] Tirodkar and Jain compared the number of commercials shown on prime-time shows with African American characters to prime-time shows with predominantly white characters.[24] Not only did the shows targeting African Americans air 66% more commercials about food (4.8 spots for a 30-minute show vs 2.9 advertisements for white audiences), but the advertisements shown to the African-American audiences were more likely to promote unhealthy items. For example, 30% of the food commercials for African American audiences were about candy and chocolate whereas there were only 14 % for white audiences; 13% advertised soda during Black prime time as opposed to only 2% for white audiences.[24] Given that studies indicate that exposure to food advertisements influence food preferences, this level of exposure could explain, in part, the health disparities seen among racial and ethnic minorities.[25]

Automatic responses to the food environment

Understanding the way in which humans respond to environmental stimuli is critical to identifying how the dramatic changes in the food environment have been able to transform the eating behavior of Americans, and is now quickly influencing people across the entire globe. People are hardwired to respond automatically to food and images of food. These responses are immediate and the physiological reflexive responses are largely uncontrollable. For example, when people are exposed to images of appetizing food, their brains automatically and reflexively secrete dopamine, activating at least five separate reward centers in the brain.[26] This activation leads to food cravings. The physiological pathway involving dopamine excretion in response to food images involves the same neural pathways that are associated with drug addictions.[27] The magnitude of the arousal of the reward centers varies considerably across individuals and is believed to explain the variability of drives for food, hyperphagia and obesity.[26] Given that food advertising and food availability have mushroomed, people are being artificially stimulated throughout the day to feel hungry and crave food.

Limited ability to exercise control

Not only are people unable to prevent the automatic, reflexive responses to food images and foods (including salivation), but it may be difficult for many people to distinguish between artificially induced hunger and desire for food and true hunger that comes from a low blood sugar. Moreover, people may be unable to recognize that they are being artificially stimulated to feel hungry, since many of the cues are imperceptible.[28] Humans have the ability to perceive images through visual systems that are not perceived by the part of the brain that provides conscious awareness.[29,30] Although this type of stimulation may occur during a small proportion of the time, it does not require much for individuals to be out

of energy balance. Large amounts of calories are available in small volumes of food; a small candy bar has over 200 calories. Relatively small amounts of calorie excess are believed to be fueling the obesity epidemic.[31]

Evidence that people can be stimulated to eat too much without their awareness or insight comes from a variety of studies. In one study, subjects exposed to subliminal images that were unrelated to food, were influenced to drink a greater quantity of an energy drink, and rate it more favorably. They had no subjective awareness that their behavior was affected in the least.[29]

Another study that showed people lacking insight into the quantity of food consumed was demonstrated when subjects were provided with soup in self-refilling bowls. Without cues that let people judge quantity, subjects ate 73% more than the participants given soup in normal bowls, yet did not feel more satiated.[32] People also have a limited capacity to judge volume and portion sizes. In several studies, individuals were unable to correctly judge the volume held by two glasses of different shapes and incorrectly thought that a tall narrow glass held more liquid than a short wide glass.[33,34] Since people do not have any internal signals that allow then to regulate the quantity of food to eat,[3,35] they rely on external cues, such as portion sizes, to determine how much to consume.

People usually consume more calories than they need to when offered too many, and they do not compensate for the excess by eating less at subsequent meals.[36–39] Instead, excess calorie consumption initiates the pathway to store excess energy as fat. People cannot easily judge when this happens.

Studies in the field of behavioral economics indicate that individual choices are strongly influenced by the means through which the choices are presented.[40] People exercise a limited amount of cognitive decision making, and typically rely on specific heuristics to make decisions, particularly when they are overwhelmed by too much information or are under stress. In these cases, people rely on default, impulsive reactions, rather than considered cognitive decision making.[41,42] Heuristics governing food choices have more to do with factors such as price, convenience and emotional associations rather than concerns about health.

115

Promising interventions—regulating the food environment

A wide variety of interventions are likely to be successful if they address our natural proclivity to be attracted to food, to be stimulated to feel hungry when confronted with food cues (regardless of how full we are), and to maximize the quantity and variety of food we eat. The following are be discussed:

- price incentives
- regulating portion sizes and labeling calorie information
- counter-advertising campaigns
- controlling food cues
- regulating food accessibility.

There is limited evidence for the effectiveness of these interventions, since they have never been tried on the scale needed to have an impact. Given that these would address pathways shown to be causally related to overconsumption, they are, nevertheless, the most promising.

While regulating the food environment may seem heavy handed, what people fail to appreciate is how much it is currently being engineered so that people will automatically eat more than they need, eat more unhealthy foods than they should, and, as a consequence, develop chronic diseases that shorten their lifespan. The limitations of human cognition make it very difficult for people to have insight into the process. People cannot naturally identify which nutrients and calorie amounts are present in specific foods, particularly those that are processed and transformed from raw ingredients, nor can they prevent being artificially stimulated to desire foods that are high in sugar and fat. Thus, there is a role for government to regulate the food environment so that people will automatically have the optimal quality and quantity of food available for them to choose.

Regulating prices

Currently, unhealthy foods like salty snacks, cookies and candy and sugar-sweetened beverages are less expensive per calorie than healthier foods such as fruits and vegetables.[43,44] Taxing the unhealthy foods and subsidizing the healthy ones has been proposed, and has been implemented in a very minimal way in several states in the USA.[45] However, the fact that people are very price sensitive when it comes to food purchases, suggests that this is a promising approach. There is enormous scope for adding taxes to unhealthy foods, which could be used to subsidize healthy ones.

Labeling and regulating portion sizes

Labeling of calories in food items is beginning to have some traction in the United States. Although New York City has implemented a rule that requires certain restaurants and food outlets to label food items, it has been held up by litigation at the time of writing.[46] Point-of-purchase labeling and signage do appear to have a significant impact on behaviors.[11,47] However, given people's limited cognitive capacity, it may be difficult for many to keep track of all the calories they consume over the course of a day. Another solution that might be helpful to individuals would be to regulate the portion sizes, so that when a person is served, they are given a default amount that is appropriate to their needs. For example, a person would be given an entire cup of vegetables, rather than half a cup, but only 3–5 oz of meat in any given meal, or only 150 calories worth of French fries, and a small beverage or a no-calorie beverage. (The McDonalds small portion of French fries is now 2.6 oz and 250 calories and the small fountain soda is 16 oz for an adult at 150 calories. www.mcdonalds.com/app_controller.nutrition.index1.html). Currently, the smallest sizes of many items may be too large for most people. Requiring food outlets to make smaller portions available would help people obtain more appropriate quantities of food.

Counter advertising/restricting cues

Currently, there are minimal, if any, counter-advertisements that can help people resist the ubiquitous cues that stimulate hunger and the desire for food. In the anti-tobacco campaigns it was documented that even having only one counter-advertisement for every 12 pro-tobacco advertisements was effective in helping to reduce tobacco consumption.[48,49] If people are reminded of the appropriate and preferred behaviors, automatic responses to food cues can be interrupted, and it may be easier for people to resist foods. A barrier to negative advertising is the perception that negative messages may increase food problems such as anorexia and bulimia, although there are no scientific data to support these concerns. In fact, studies indicate the opposite: that negative messages are better attended and more memorable than positive ones.[50,51]

Regulate food accessibility (schools, worksites, public settings)

Food accessibility can be controlled in settings where managers and administrators have a vested interest in controlling the health of those who use the facilities. For example, schools are increasingly becoming sensitive to the problem of obesity and are replacing unhealthy cafeteria foods with healthier choices; they are eliminating some vending machines or the unhealthy choices in them. Control of food accessibility can occur at worksites as well, where employers have an interest in reducing the medical problems of their employees. They too could remove vending machines and regulate what foods are available in company cafeterias. They can offer calorie-appropriate portions and develop policies that restrict locations where food can be eaten and the types of snacks that can be served at company meeting and events. Government agencies can also regulate the food available in public buildings and settings, as well as prohibit the consumption of food in specific areas. Another possibility is to restrict the number and type of outlets that may sell foods. Just as alcohol licences are typically limited, food sales in businesses that do not sell food as their major mission (book stores, hardware stores, car washes) could be restricted. Reducing food availability would reduce the cues that artificially stimulate feelings of cravings and hunger as well limit opportunities for excessive caloric intake.

Conclusion

We will be able to control our weight when the food environment is one that does not artificially make us hungry, that automatically provides the variety of foods that we need, and that limits the accessibility of the foods that make us sick. Needless to say, the changes required would precipitate a multitude of barriers and opposition, because many companies would stand to lose profits from the sales of food that are making people sick. Making the necessary changes would require political genius and indefatigable will-power and conviction.

Since eating is largely an automatic behavior, the current situation that requires each and every person to think very carefully and control what they eat in order not to gain weight constitutes an undue burden and is likely to interfere with our abilities to do other things. Given that the majority of people are overweight, this burden is too much for most of us. In fact, many people on diets suffer from a loss of executive functioning and impaired decision making.[52] Our thinking power is best devoted to solving everyday problems with our jobs, our friends, our homes, our families and our plans for the future. Most people do not have the spare cognitive capacity to count every last calorie, vitamin and mineral. If we want a diet that promotes optimal health, people will need a lot of help. Just as we make sure the water that is available is safe to drink, the food that is available should also be safe, provided in the appropriate quantities for every person, neither too much nor too little. We just have to accept the fact that it is too hard for most individuals to do this on their own.

References

1 Cutler DM, Glaeser EL, Shapiro JM: Why Have Americans Become More Obese? Cambridge: National Bureau of Economic Research, 2003.
2 Davey RC: The obesity epidemic: too much food for thought? *Br J Sports Med* 2004; **38**(3):360–363.
3 Levitsky DA: The non-regulation of food intake in humans: hope for reversing the epidemic of obesity. *Physiol Behav* 2005; **86**(5):623–632.
4 Zhang L, Rashad I: Obesity and time preference: the health consequences of discounting the future. *J Biosoc Sci* 2008; **40**(1):97–113.
5 van den Bos R, de Ridder D: Evolved to satisfy our immediate needs: self-control and the rewarding properties of food. *Appetite* 2006; **47**(1):24–29.
6 Sharma M, Wagner DI, Wilkerson J: Predicting childhood obesity prevention behaviors using social cognitive theory. *Int Q Community Health Educ* 2005; **24**(3):191–203.
7 Fuentes-Afflick E, Hessol NA: Acculturation and Body Mass among Latina Women. *J Womens Health (Larchmt)* 2008; **17**(1):67–73.
8 Koya DL, Egede LE: Association between length of residence and cardiovascular disease risk factors among an ethnically diverse group of United States immigrants. *J Gen Intern Med* 2007; **22**(6):841–846.
9 Khush G: Productivity improvements in rice. *Nutr Rev* 2003; **61**(6 Pt 2):S114–S116.

10 USDA-ERS: Food CPI, Prices and Expenditures: Food Expenditures by Families and Individuals as a Share of Disposable Personal Income. 2007. www.ers.usda.gov/Briefing/CPIFoodAndExpenditures/Data/table7.htm.

11 French SA: Pricing effects on food choices. *J Nutr* 2003; **133**(3):841S–843S.

12 French SA, Jeffery RW, Story M et al: Pricing and promotion effects on low-fat vending snack purchases: the CHIPS Study. *Am J Public Health* 2001; **91**(1):112–117.

13 French SA et al: A pricing strategy to promote low-fat snack choices through vending machines. *Am J Public Health* 1997; **87**(5):849–851.

14 Sturm R, Datar A: Body mass index in elementary school children, metropolitan area food prices and food outlet density. *Public Health* 2005; **119**(12):1059–1068.

15 Drewnowski A, Specter SE: Poverty and obesity: the role of energy density and energy costs. *Am J Clin Nutr* 2004; **79**(1): 6–16.

16 Nestle M: Increasing portion sizes in American diets: more calories, more obesity. *J Am Diet Assoc* 2003; **103**(1):39–40.

17 Young LR, Nestle M: The contribution of expanding portion sizes to the US obesity epidemic. *Am J Public Health* 2002; **92**(2):246–249.

18 Nielsen SJ, Popkin BM: Patterns and trends in food portion sizes, *1977*–1998. *JAMA* 2003; **289**(4):450–453.

19 USCensus: Manufacturing—Industries Ranked by Growth in Value of Shipments 1992 to 1997. 1997. www.census.gov/epcd/ec97sic/RANKUSD8.HTM (accessed 8 November 2004).

20 Nestle M: Food marketing and childhood obesity—a matter of policy. *N Engl J Med* 2006; **354**(24):2527–2529.

21 Rivkees SA: Advertised calories per hour … 2000+: anti-obesity announcements per hour … 0. *J Pediatr Endocrinol Metab* 2007; **20**(5):557–558.

22 Gallo A: Food Advertising in the United States. 1999. www.ers.usda.gov/publications/aib750/aib750i.pdf, in Food Advertising. USDA/ERS.

23 Kumanyika S, Grier S: Targeting interventions for ethnic minority and low-income populations. *Future Child* 2006; **16**(1):187–207.

24 Tirodkar MA, Jain A: Food messages on African American television shows. *Am J Public Health* 2003; **93**(3):439–441.

25 Coon KA, Tucker KL: Television and children's consumption patterns. A review of the literature. *Minerva Pediatr* 2002; **54**(5):423–436.

26 Beaver JD et al: Individual differences in reward drive predict neural responses to images of food. *J Neurosci* 2006; **26**(19): 5160–5166.

27 Volkow ND, Wise RA: How can drug addiction help us understand obesity? *Nat Neurosci* 2005; **8**(5):555–560.

28 Bargh JA: Losing consciousness: Automatic influences on consumer judgment, behavior, and motivation. *Journal of Consumer Research* 2002; **29**(2):280–285.

29 Berridge KC, Winkielman P: What is an unconscious emotion? (The case for unconscious "liking"). *Cogn Emot* 2003; **17**(2):181–211.

30 Dijksterhuis A, Aarts H: On wildebeests and humans: The preferential detection of negative stimuli. *Psychol Sci* 2003; **14**(1):14–18.

31 Hill JO et al: Obesity and the environment: where do we go from here? *Science* 2003; **299**(5608):853–855.

32 Wansink B, Painter JE, North J: Bottomless bowls: why visual cues of portion size may influence intake. *Obes Res* 2005; **13**(1):93–100.

33 Wansink B, Van Ittersum K: Bottoms up! The influence of elongation on pouring and consumption volume. *J Consum Res* 2003; **30**(3):455–463.

34 Wansink B, van Ittersum K: Shape of glass and amount of alcohol poured: comparative study of effect of practice and concentration. *BMJ* 2005; **331**(7531): 1512–1514.

35 Levitsky DA et al: Imprecise control of energy intake: absence of a reduction in food intake following overfeeding in young adults. *Physiol Behav* 2005; **84**(5):669–675.

36 Orlet Fisher J, Rolls BJ, Birch LL: Children's bite size and intake of an entree are greater with large portions than with age-appropriate or self-selected portions. *Am J Clin Nutr* 2003; **77**(5):1164–1170.

37 Rolls BJ, Morris EL, Roe LS: Portion size of food affects energy intake in normal-weight and overweight men and women. *Am J Clin Nutr* 2002; **76**(6):1207–1213.

38 Rolls BJ et al: Increasing the portion size of a packaged snack increases energy intake in men and women. *Appetite* 2004; **42**(1):63–69.

39 Rolls BJ, Roe LS, Meengs JS: Larger portion sizes lead to a sustained increase in energy intake over 2 days. *J Am Diet Assoc* 2006; **106**(4):543–549.

40 Kahneman D: A perspective on judgment and choice: mapping bounded rationality. *Am Psychol* 2003; **58**(9): 697–720.

41 Schwartz B: The Paradox of Choice: Why More is Less. NY: Ecco, HarperCollins, 2003.

42 Shiv B, Fedorikhin A: Heart and mind in conflict: The interplay of affect and cognition in consumer decision making. *J Consum Res* 1999; **26**(3):278–292.

43 Drewnowski A, Darmon N: The economics of obesity: dietary energy density and energy cost. *Am J Clin Nutr* 2005; **82**(1 Suppl.):265S–273S.

44 Drewnowski A, Darmon N: Food choices and diet costs: an economic analysis. *J Nutr* 2005; **135**(4):900–904.

45 Jacobson MF, Brownell KD: Small taxes on soft drinks and snack foods to promote health. *Am J Public Health* 2000; **90**(6):854–857.

46 AssociatedPress, Enforcement of calorie listings on NYC menus is blocked. 2008. www.chron.com/disp/story.mpl/ap/fn/5727634.html.

47 Jeffery RW et al: An environmental intervention to increase fruit and salad purchases in a cafeteria. *Prev Med* 1994; **23**(6):788–792.

48 Tye JB, Warner KE, Glantz SA: Tobacco advertising and consumption: evidence of a causal relationship. *J Public Health Policy* 1987; **8**(4):492–508.

49 Warner KE: The effects of the anti-smoking campaign on cigarette consumption. *Am J Public Health* 1977; **67**(7): 645–650.

50 Dijksterhuis A et al: Yes, there is a preferential detection of negative stimuli: a response to labiouse. *Psychol Sci* 2004; **15**(8):571–572.

51 Shiv B, Britton J, Payne J: Does elaboration increase or decrease the effectiveness of negatively versus positively framed messages? *J Consum Res* 2004; **31**(1):199–208.

52 Kemps E, Tiggemann M: Working memory performance and preoccupying thoughts in female dieters: evidence for a selective central executive impairment. *Br J Clin Psychol* 2005; **44**(3):357–366.

CHAPTER 15

Food and beverage marketing to children

Gerard Hastings and *Georgina Cairns*
Institute for Social Marketing, University of Stirling and the Open University, Stirling, UK

Summary and recommendations for practice

- Marketing has a powerful influence on all our behaviors.

    It comprises consumer orientation, multi-faceted working and strategic planning.

    When harnessed to energy dense foods it has contributed to the obesity pandemic.

    It can also be a force for good in the form of social marketing.

- Experience from tobacco control suggests how this potential can be realized.

- The ultimate need is to significantly reduce the commercial marketing for food and beverages to children and to strategically increase the social marketing approaches to tackle childhood obesity.

Introduction

Marketing is based on a very simple idea: putting the consumer—rather than production—at the heart of the business process. This simple but powerful concept underpins the effects marketing has had in encouraging childhood obesity; this chapter argues that, not only does this obesogenic marketing need to be reduced, but that the concepts as applied through social marketing can also guide efforts to combat childhood obesity.

Consumer focus is only part of the marketing story. Successful marketing begins with a critical analysis of

Preventing Childhood Obesity. Edited by
E. Waters, B.A. Swinburn, J.C. Seidell and R. Uauy.
© 2010 Blackwell Publishing.

the broad environmental factors that encourage individualized choices. The resulting insights guide the development of micro-level offers. Applying a marketing approach to the challenge of childhood obesity generates opportunities to make health-reinforcing behaviors desirable and accessible, and inform multi-sectoral, multi-disciplinary policy progress. To harness the power of marketing, however, its potential scope and force must first be recognized by the broad stakeholder community, and a marketing mindset applied from the beginning of the planning process.

This chapter begins by explaining the need for marketing thinking. It examines the evidence base on food promotion to children, which has not only established that there is an effect, but has also informed UK policy-makers in their decision to impose restrictions on unhealthy food marketing to children. This path has been well trodden by tobacco control, and the chapter goes on to identify significant learning points that emerge from this experience. Finally, drawing on tobacco control, commercial marketing and social marketing experiences, the chapter concludes with calls to reduce obesogenic marketing to children and to take social marketing-oriented strategic action. The necessary behavior changes to reverse the rising rates of childhood overweight and obesity will not be achieved by ad hoc, isolated interventions driven by the supply side (be that public policy or commercial interests). Comprehensive, large-scale interventions require strategic planning. Effective planning needs to be informed and shaped by the recognition that we are caught in both the firm grip of an obesogenic environment and a somewhat passive acceptance of the trend towards overweight and obesity as the norm, rather than the exception, by many lay persons, and indeed professionals. In this way marketing can indeed promote healthy weight.

The nature of marketing

Familiarity with customer desires and needs requires consistent and multi-method research. Marketers attempt to get inside our heads, see the world as we see it and adjust their offerings accordingly. Because people differ, this often means that a degree of customization is needed, so markets are segmented into homogenous subsets and target groups selected for bespoke attention. Customization also includes the choice of communication channels—and with the growing sophistication of electronic communication technologies the opportunities for segmentation even to individual level, becomes a reality. The only limits to innovation and the responsiveness of the commercial marketing mix are that shareholder value has to be enhanced. The key lesson is that meeting customer needs more accurately is good for business.

The need for this degree of sensitivity to the customer is quite simply because their behavior is voluntary. Marketers cannot force people to buy, so they have to engage, entice, persuade and seduce: the aim is to create motivational exchanges in which people will freely, indeed gladly, engage.

For marketers, children represent an important target group: their independent purchasing power makes them a valuable market in their own right; they also influence household purchase decisions and ultimately they represent tomorrow's brand-loyal adult market.

It is challenging to put precise figures on these phenomena, but as a rough guide, the US Institute of Medicine Report on Food Marketing to Children and Youth[1] suggested that one third of children's annual $30 billion direct purchases were on food and beverages. In addition, the US Market for Kids' Foods and Beverages, 2003 report estimated that children and adolescents influence $500 billion of purchase decisions at the household level.[2] This represents more than half of the total US annual spending on food and beverages (estimated at $895.4 billion in the 2004 US Department of Agriculture Economic Research Service Food Expenditure Series).[1]

The public health community also has strong social and economic motivations to invest in influencing children's purchase and consumption behaviors. The Foresight report projected a seven-fold increase in total societal costs for obesity in England to just under £50 billion by 2050.[3] Many intervention campaigns want to ameliorate these projected trends by encouraging children and adults to accept added-value offerings—whether these are to eat more fruit and vegetables, cook or take exercise. And just as with breakfast cereals or soft drinks, individuals are free to accept or reject these offerings. The effectiveness of such public health initiatives is dependent on the voluntary action of the target audience. Public health therefore has to learn to be engaging, enticing, persuasive and seductive.

Sensitive research, customization and partnership working have to become second nature. The opportunities to intervene and encourage healthy diet and lifestyle choices using marketing theory and practice are only just beginning to be recognized and, therefore, the evidence on what works and what does not is still being amassed. There is however, much transferable experience and learning from other sectors that can be interpreted, adapted and applied in childhood obesity prevention. Two of the most valuable are current commercial marketing theory and practice, and retrospective analysis of tobacco control.

The power of marketing: the food business

In 2003, a systematic review of the literature on the extent, nature and effects of food promotion to children was commissioned by the Food Standards Agency.[4] It concluded (see Box 15.1) that food was promoted to children more than any other product group, and that the types of food being advertised were consistently contrary to recommended dietary guidelines. Television was the dominant medium for this advertising, but the review noted the increasing importance other channels, including sponsorship, in-school marketing, point-of-sale materials and incentives, free gifts and samples, loyalty schemes, and new media in the communications mix.

The review also showed that this promotional activity does influence children's food knowledge, preferences, behaviors and diet-related health status. It impacts on food categories (e.g., breakfast cereals) as well as specific branded items (e.g., particular

Box 15.1 The findings of reviews in relation to the extent and nature of food promotion

- Food dominates advertising to children.
- Five product categories dominate this advertising (soft drinks, pre-sugared cereals, confectionery, snacks and fast-food restaurants).
- The advertised diet contrasts dramatically with the recommended diet.
- Children engage with and enjoy this "unhealthy" advertising.

The findings in relation to the effects were that:

- Food promotion influences children's nutritional knowledge, food preferences, purchasing and purchase-related behavior, consumption, and diet and health status.
- The extent of the influence is difficult to determine (though advertising is independent of other factors).
- Food promotion affects both total category sales and brand switching.

Source: Food Standards Agency, 2003[4]

pre-sweetened breakfast cereals). Furthermore, the influence is independent of other influencing variables such as parental behavior or pricing.

The review was updated for WHO in 2006[5] and 2009,[6] taking in a global perspective. The updates showed that, while the more complex studies have all been undertaken in developed countries, children respond to advertising in much the same way across the globe. In fact, there is reason to believe that young people in poorer countries may be even more vulnerable to food promotion than their wealthier peers, because they are less advertising literate and associate developed countries' brands with desirable attributes of life. They also provide a key entry point for multinationals because they are more flexible and responsive than their parents.

Following on from the first systematic review, research by the UK's regulatory body for the communications industries, which includes broadcast advertising (Ofcom), also concluded that TV advertising influences children's food behaviors and that restrictions on TV advertising were, therefore, warranted.[7] These were phased in during 2007–8 and limited the advertising of high fat, salt, sugar (HFSS) foods (as defined by using the UK's nutrient profiling system) on children's TV programming and dedicated children's channels.

Concerns were raised that the restrictions would accelerate the trend for marketing spend to shift from broadcast advertising to alternative (unregulated) marketing channels. There is evidence to support this in the initial Department of Health evaluation[8] of the regulations, which show that a 41% decrease in HFSS television advertising to children is offset by a 42% increase in press advertising, and 11% increase in radio, cinema and internet advertising. In addition, a number of recent studies in the UK and internationally have analysed the content of food and beverage marketing in these other media, including children's websites,[9–11] children's magazines,[12] in-store promotions[13] and direct mailings[14] and found that HFSS foods continue to predominate.

There has also been substantial research on parental responses to the influence of marketing on their children. There is a growing and consistent body of evidence that parents perceive food marketing as a driver of children's food requests, and that it acts both as a barrier to their efforts to encourage healthy food choices and a source of parent–child conflict.[15,16]

In summary then, the power of marketing to encourage unhealthy behavior is well established. It is becoming clear, however, that it can also push in the opposite direction. Tobacco control provides some interesting insights into how restrictions on commercial marketing can be combined with proactive social marketing.

Tobacco control: ten marketing lessons

In 1954, when Richard Doll first published his research on British GPs showing the lethal qualities of tobacco, some 80% of UK men smoked and women were enthusiastically catching them up.[17] Today cigarettes are used by fewer than a quarter of the UK population, and in other countries this proportion is well under a fifth.

Dietary behaviors and stakeholder responses are still in 1954. The full enormities of the pandemic of diet and inactivity-related non-communicable chronic diseases are just now being appreciated. Two things are already certain, however: the toll will continue to rise to at least match that from tobacco,[18,19] and public health cannot afford to take fifty years to find an effective response. The purpose of learning lessons from tobacco is, therefore, to find short cuts to effective solutions.

Smoking, diet and physical activity are strongly influenced by a range of social, cultural and economic risk factors. In the case of less healthy eating patterns, such as excess consumption of fat, refined sugars and salt, there are also strong biological drivers. These biological drivers, although strongly embedded in our physiological "hard-wiring", are nevertheless potentially responsive to interventions. Establishing the relative influences and how these interact is vital to our understanding of how to respond. However, we are unlikely ever to understand this perfectly, and, as Yach et al[20] emphasize, we cannot delay taking action until we do. Good science can reduce uncertainty, it cannot produce certainty—nor can it make decisions for us. Rigorous, transparent reviews of the evidence and expert interpretation of the evidence base overall, however, does provide a substantial foundation from which to build well-informed policy response.

Restricting marketing, not just advertising

Several decades of research have shown beyond reasonable doubt that tobacco marketing is a significant causal factor in both the onset and continuance of young people's smoking. Inevitably, this research focused initially on advertising and the other forms of marketing communications discussed above, but it has also looked at marketing more widely. This has resulted in controls on advertising being matched by controls on product design (through an EU Directive in tar levels), pricing (through taxation) and packaging (through mandated and increasingly prominent health warnings). There are also currently active debates about restricting the number of outlets and introducing generic packaging.[21]

Furthermore, this broader perspective shows that it is not just the impact of individual marketing tools that matters, but their cumulative effect. This is not surprising; marketing strategies are deliberately designed to be internally consistent and self-reinforcing. Typically, this effort is focused on developing and honing evocative brands, and recent research in the UK shows that these continue to drive youth smoking even after a complete ban on tobacco advertising.[22]

Lesson One: The power of marketing extends well beyond its most visible manifestations such as advertising. Controls on advertising in isolation will most likely move investment into the myriad of other marketing channels; regulatory controls and voluntary codes of conduct must take these realities into account.

Prevention and direct interventions

In recent years, tobacco control strategies have diverged. Australasia, North America and those parts of the developing world that are active in tobacco control have opted for population level strategies. The aim is to get the message out as widely as possible that smoking is a bad idea, that you should not take it up, and that if you have done, you should stop. In this way it harnesses social norms and Robert Cialdini's notion that "most people will do the right thing if they believe it is the norm."[23]

The UK has opted for a more intensive, clinically based approach of offering high quality smoking cessation services. However, they are labor intensive, so cannot reach large numbers of the population or have any significant impact on prevalence levels. They also soak up budgets: as Chapman points out, in the UK over recent years "five times more has been spent on assisting cessation than on trying to encourage more smokers to make quit attempts, and instil in them the confidence to do so" (Chapman, p. 141).[24] He goes on to argue that this distortion of priorities has had a detrimental effect on outcomes: "in Australia and Canada two decades of quit campaigns see smoking prevalence today about 10 years ahead of where the UK is today".

Lesson Two: Population level strategies are essential in the fight against obesity; they should never have to compete with clinical interventions for resources.

Working with industry

The potential for cooperation with the tobacco industry is extremely limited because there is so little common interest with public health. The tobacco control endgame is the elimination of tobacco use; no tobacco company is going to share this vision. Clive Bates, former CEO of the Action on Smoking and Health, took this thinking a step further advocating a "scream test" to check out any new policy option: if it makes the tobacco industry scream, it is probably worth doing.

123

Food, however, is not tobacco. It does not harm when used as intended, nor does anyone want to eliminate its consumption, so collaboration is, therefore, at least a theoretical possibility.

For joint working to succeed, public health needs to have clearly thought through its aims. What is the endgame? What should the food market to look like in 5, 25 and 50 years' time? We also need to approach the task with our eyes open. The legally binding fiduciary responsibilities of corporations mean that they will only cooperate as long as it is in their shareholders' interests. They cannot do otherwise. It is up to others to ensure that their actions genuinely benefit public health.

Therefore, unless we in obesity prevention and control have a clear set of aims to guide our thinking, collaboration with even well-intentioned partners in the corporate sector will, like a lump of metal too close to a compass, inadvertently drag us off course.

Lesson Three: Cooperation with industry is only productive if public health has clearly stated goals and monitors the public health impact of industry partners' actions. Win-wins are possible but elusive.

A global response to a global problem

Those involved with tobacco control have long recognized the international dimensions of its task; global brands like Marlboro and Lucky Strike make it all too apparent. This has resulted in an established history of international working. Under the leadership of WHO this work has culminated in the Framework Convention on Tobacco Control (FCTC), the world's first public health treaty, which is in the process of laying down standards for effective tobacco control. The FCTC is also the world's most successful treaty—with more signatories than any other.

Apart from its great geographical reach, the FCTC has the enormous advantage of bringing together experts from across the world to engage in a unified effort to tackle the tobacco pandemic. This ensures both collective learning and the capacity to assess and meet the varying needs of different parts of the world, especially those of low and middle income countries.

Obesity is equally insensitive to national boundaries, and Coca-Cola has the reach of Philip Morris International—so global solutions are also needed. The WHO review of the global impact of energy-dense food promotion[5] shows that young people in

low and middle income countries are also affected by it—and may indeed be particularly vulnerable. As countries develop and industrialize this problem is likely to get worse.

Lesson Four: there needs to be a "Framework Convention on Obesity Control" (or at least an International Code on Marketing to Children) to match the FCTC.

Know your customer

The success of the fast-food industry in purveying its products may be a cause for concern. However, it also presents a great opportunity. Public health can and should be analysing the success of Coke and taking lessons for their own campaigns and interventions. At base they are good at getting us to do things—influencing our voluntary consumer behavior; and public health is also in the voluntary behavior change business.

Unhealthy commercial marketing needs to be reduced, as noted above, but can also be counteracted by healthy social marketing.[25]

Lesson Five: the first step in successful social marketing is to listen to our customers and then devise offerings that genuinely meet their needs. If our efforts do not produce results, reach for the ear trumpet not the megaphone.

Emotion, branding and relationships

The power of branding is built on the recognition that human decision making is not just driven by rational logico-deductive reasoning. Emotions and heuristics (or short cuts) also play a big part: consuming chocolate is as much about sex as it is eating, and trips to the supermarket would be impossible if shoppers rationally weighed up the pros and cons of every choice.

Brands, which were initially devised to make the early corporations seem more human,[26] provide a perfect vehicle for meeting these more subtle needs. They can make us feel happy as well as full, and cool as well as warmly clad. Public health can also use branding.[27] The anti-tobacco Truth campaign offers a good example: it built up a degree of trust with young people in the USA and drove down smoking prevalence.[28]

Building brands takes time. Indeed as business has recognized for some decades, behavior change takes time and benefits greatly from continuity. There is much more money to be made if customers come back again and again. That is why supermarkets and airlines reward regulars with loyalty cards, special deals and chatty magazines. They have moved beyond mere exchanges and want to start building relationships with us. And all the evidence is that, despite their obvious mercenary motivations, it works. We do respond with brand loyalty and regular visits. This relational thinking can be applied equally well—if not better—in social marketing.[29]

Lesson Six: behavior change takes time—we should build brands and relationships.

The whole marketing mix

Behavior change takes more than communication. The importance of distinguishing between advertising and marketing when considering regulation has already been noted; it is equally important here. Eating and exercise behavior can be influenced by media campaigns—the evidence from tobacco control puts this beyond dispute[30-35]—but it is equally clear that multi-faceted interventions are more powerful. A switch from burgers to carrots is more likely if the communications that boost the attractiveness of carrots are backed by pricing that reinforces this attraction and makes them affordable, distribution and packaging that makes them accessible, and a product that delivers satisfaction. Branding can then be used to confirm and enhance this satisfaction.

Lesson Seven: communications are only a small part of the game. Glossy advertising campaigns—especially isolated ones—are not the answer.

Context matters

The individual's power to make decisions is limited by their social and environmental context. Visiting a fast-food outlet will partly reflect personal choice, but also the availability of alternatives, income, family circumstances and, harking back to social norms, the behavior of those around us. Marketers take careful note of this context and do their best to influence or adapt to it.

The tobacco industry, for instance, puts a great deal of effort and resource into liaising with policy-makers, and has had considerable success across Europe in ensuring that they make decisions that favor the industry.[36] Similarly, the tobacco companies focus their efforts on retailers, stakeholders and potential allies (e.g., in the fight to fend off smoke-free laws) as well as final customers, to make sure the circumstances are as supportive as possible of their interests.

The importance of this debate for weight control is highlighted by the concept of the obesogenic environment. This is created by many actors—planners, the food industry, governments, other commercial operators—and all have to change their behaviors to deliver improvement in public health. The principles of bringing about these changes are the same as for ordinary citizens—listen to their needs and deliver.

Tobacco control has also managed to gain an extra degree of traction with policy-makers because of the collateral damage caused by second-hand smoke. Perhaps the nearest equivalent for obesity is the economic cost to everyone, which has begun to emerge as the external environment (from health service weighing scales to impact on post-operative complications) adapts to increases in size and excess weight among a section of the population.

Lesson Eight: good health is the product of many complex factors—including government policy, commercial marketing, education and wealth—as well as individual lifestyle choices, and progress will depend on action on all these fronts. Stakeholders are a key target group in social marketing.

Competitive analysis

In some instances, commercial stakeholders will not cooperate with public health, however seductive the approach. The tobacco industry has long resisted almost all attempts to control its marketing. The only solution in this case has been to legislate and, indeed, through the FCTC, to do so on a global basis. It remains to be seen whether obesity control will ultimately have to follow the same route as tobacco control, but nevertheless, studying the competition is a great way of learning how better to influence behavior.

Lesson Nine: competitive analysis is an invaluable tool. One of the principal reasons we have so many smokers and unhealthy eaters is that the commercial sector has been better at marketing than we have.

Research

Marketing depends on research: customer orientation; relationship building; stakeholder marketing and competitive analysis each needs to be informed by up-to-date intelligence about the people with whom we want to do business—or at least deal with—and the world that they and we inhabit. Research can also guide progress and help map the route to the final goal.

Thus marketing research acts as a navigational aid, to guide progress and aid decision making. It can and should transcend ad hoc interventions. Coca-Cola did not build its brand by conducting a randomized control trial, but gradually honed it by consistently delivering consumer satisfaction and developing its understanding of its customers and stakeholders. Public health should adopt a similarly long-term and flexible approach to research.

Lesson Ten: research is a navigational aid that will help us to understand our customers and stakeholder.

Translation into practice

Marketing has a great deal to offer the fight against childhood obesity, and the lessons learned from tobacco control need to be applied to obesity. The first priority is to reduce the pressure of commercial marketing of HFSS foods and beverages on children. This should be matched with well-informed social marketing interventions at all levels of the interlocking obesogenic system to encourage healthy behaviors. These activities should be coherent, research led and strategic; Box 15.2 presents a planning tool for ensuring that they are.

The diagram illustrates three key characteristics of marketing planning. The first reflects what might be called its gestalt. Seen as a whole, the plan becomes more than the sum of its parts. It provides a progressive process of learning about the market and its particular exchanges. This learning takes place *within* particular initiatives. For example, a systematically produced and carefully researched healthy eating initiative for school children will enable social marketers to improve their understanding of school children and their desires, and thereby to enhance the initiative. There are parallels here with building brand equity in a commercial context. Continuously refining and improving the product offered in response to target audience feedback can establish and deepen the relationship between parties. Deeper understanding enables marketers to reflect more closely the values and aspirations of their target population.

Box 15.2 A social marketing plan

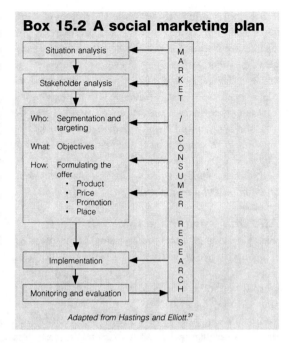

Adapted from Hastings and Elliott.[37]

Second, the learning process also takes place *between* initiatives. The social marketer will be able to use the lessons learned from one initiative as a basis for future projects. For example, consumer insights on children's responses to a school-based intervention can inform family-focused in-store campaigns and may contribute to policy research on children's unique vulnerabilities and motivations. Internally, consistent objectives and messaging of multiple interlocking initiatives have the potential to greatly strengthen policy impact. Thus the process is not just progressive but cyclical; hence the return arrows in Box 15.2.

Third, the situation and stakeholder analyses at the outset of the planning process ensure that the full extent of the task is realized. Voluntary behavior change requires resolve and motivation, not just at an individual level, but also at community and political level. The Wanless Report noted that substantial population level change required healthy choices to be easy, convenient, "low cost" choices.[38] To achieve this, a multi-agency, trans-disciplinary analysis of major population-level barriers and drivers can be used to map critical factors. Chapter 28 provides a detailed account of the application of social marketing to childhood obesity.

Conclusion

Marketing encompasses the development, distribution, pricing and promotion of food and is extremely pervasive. When harnessed to energy-dense foods it is contributing to the obesity epidemic and, therefore, needs to be restrained and—if voluntary steps do not produce results—regulated.

However, marketing can also be part of the solution. In the case of industry it underpins not just the success of burgers but fruit juices, and even in the hands of the fast-food sector can be harnessed to good effect if the right incentives are in place. In the hands of public health, it can also even the balance in favor of healthier foods.

To achieve these benefits there is a need for some systematic social marketing planning that will define long-term aims, identify the key drivers and players and set clear and measurable objectives for each. The strategy should then combine regulation, cooperation and coherent mechanisms for building relationships with all the key players. Research should act as a compass guiding all these processes as well as overall progress.

Thus that bête noire of public health, the Marlboro cowboy, can help enhance our efforts. Or as Nietzsche put it: What does not kill us, makes us stronger.

References

1 Mcginnis JM, Appleton Gootman J, Kraak VI: Institute of Medicine. Food Marketing to Children and Youth: Threat or Opportunity? Washington, DC: National Academies Press, 2006.

2 Barbour J: The U.S. Market for Kids Foods and Beverages, 5th edn [abstract]. Rockville, MD: Packaged Facts. 2003. www.packagedfacts.com/Kids-Foods-Beverages-849192/ (accessed 9 June 2009).

3 Butland B, Jebb S, Kopelman P et al: Foresight Tackling Obesities: Future Choices—Project Report, 2nd edn. UK Government Foresight Programme, Government Office for Science 2007.

4 Hastings GB, Stead M, McDermott L et al: Review of Research on the Effects of Food Promotion to Children—Final Report and Appendices. London: Food Standards Agency, 2003.

5 Hastings G, McDermott L, Angus K, Stead M, Thompson S: The Extent, Nature and Effects of Food Promotion to Children: A Review of the Evidence. Technical paper prepared for the World Health Organization by the Institute for Social Marketing, Stirling. Geneva: World Health Organization, 2007.

6 Cairns G, Angus K, Hastings G: The Extent, Nature and Effects of Food Promotion to Children: A Review of the Evidence to December 2008. Prepared for the World Health Organization. Stirling: Institute for Social Marketing, 2009.

7 Ofcom: Ofcom Final Statement on the Television Advertising of Food and Drink Products to Children (webpages). London: Office of Communications. www.ofcom.org.uk/media/mofaq/bdc/foodfadsfaq (accessed 2008 March 28).

8 Department of Health: Changes in Food and Drink Advertising and Promotion to Children: A Report Outlining the Changes in the Nature and Balance of Food and Drink Advertising and Promotion to Children, from January 2003 to December 2007. London: Department of Health, 2008.

9 Alvy LM, Calvert SL: Food marketing on popular children's web sites: a content analysis. J Am Diet Assoc 2008; 108(4): 710–713.

10 Moore ES, Rideout VJ: The online marketing of food to children: is it just fun and games? J Public Policy Mark 2007; 25:202–220.

11 Weber K, Story M, Harnack L: Internet food marketing strategies aimed at children and adolescents; a content analysis of food and beverage brand web sites. J Am Diet Assoc 2006; 106(9):1463–1466.

12 Cowburn G, Baxter A: Magazines for children and young people and the links to the Internet food marketing: a review of the extent and type of food advertising. Pub Health Nut 2007; 10(10):1024–1031.

13 Chapman K, Nicholas P, Banovic D, Supramaniam R: The extent and nature of food promotion to directed to children in Australian supermarkets. Health Prom Int 2006; 21(4): 331–339.

14 Eagle L, Brennan R: Beyond advertising: in-home promotion of "fast food". Young Consumers 2007; 8(4):278–288.

15 Noble G, Stead M, Jones S, McDermott L, McVie D: The paradoxical food buying behaviour of parents: insights from the UK and Australia. Br Food J 2007; 109(5):387–398.

16 McDermott L, O'Sullivan T, Stead M, Hastings G: International food advertising, pester power and its effects. J Adv 2006; 25(4):513–540.

17 Doll R, Hill AB: The mortality of doctors in relation to their smoking habits; a preliminary report. Br Med J 1954; 1(4877):1451–1455.

18 Olshansky SJ, Passaro DJ, Hershow RC et al: A potential decline in life expectancy in the United States in the 21st century. N Engl J Med 2005; 352(11):1138–1145.

19 Wyatt SB, Winters KP, Dubbert PM: Overweight and obesity: prevalence, consequences, and causes of a growing public health problem. Am J Med Sci 2006; 331(4): 166–174.

20 Yach D, McKee M, Lopez AD, Novotny T: Improving diet and physical activity: 12 lessons from controlling tobacco smoking. BMJ 2005; 330(7496):898–900.

21 Hastings G, Angus K: Forever Cool: The Influence of Smoking Imagery on Young People. London: British Medical Association Board of Science, 2008.

22 Grant IC, Hassan L, Hastings G, MacKintosh AM, Eadie D: The influence of branding on adolescent smoking

behaviour: exploring the mediating role of image and attitudes. *Int J Nonprofit Volunt Sector Mark* 2007, online early view. doi: 10.1002/nvsm.329

23 Kettle M: Our Ministers should Forget America and Study the Mail. *Guardian.* 2008:35.

24 Chapman S: Public Health Advocacy and Tobacco Control: Making Smoking History, 1st edn. Oxford: Blackwell Publishing, 2007.

25 Hastings G. Social Marketing: Why should the Devil have all the Best Tunes? Oxford: Butterworth: Heinemann, 2007.

26 Bakan J: The Corporation: The Pathological Pursuit of Profit and Power. London: Constable, 2004.

27 Evans WD, Hastings G: Public Health Branding: Applying Marketing for Social Change. Oxford: Oxford University Press, 2008.

28 Niederdeppe J, Farrelly MC, Haviland ML: Confirming "truth": more evidence of a successful tobacco countermarketing campaign in Florida. *Am J Public Health* 2004; **94**(2): 255–257.

29 Hastings GB: Relational paradigms in social marketing. *J Macromarketing* 2003; **23**(1):6–15.Jun

30 Farrelly MC, Niederdeppe J, Yarsevich J: Youth tobacco prevention mass media campaigns: past, present, and future directions. *Tob Control* 2003; **12**(Suppl. 1):i35–i47.

31 Friend K, Levy DT: Reductions in smoking prevalence and cigarette consumption associated with mass-media campaigns. *Health Educ Res* 2002; **17**(1):85–98.

32 Jepson R, Harris F, Rowa-Dewar N et al: A Review of the Effectiveness of Mass Media Interventions Which Both Encourage Quit Attempts and Reinforce Current and Recent Attempts to Quit Smoking. London: National Institute for Health and Clinical Excellence (NICE), 2006.

33 Richardson L, Allen P, McCullough L et al: NICE RAPID REVIEW Interventions to Prevent the Uptake of Smoking in Children and Young People Full Report. London: National Institute for Health and Clinical Excellence (NICE), 2007.

34 Sowden AJ, Arblaster L: Mass media interventions for preventing smoking in young people. *Cochrane Database Syst Rev* 2000;2 (Art. No.: CD001006). Doi: 10.1002/14651858. CD001006

35 Wakefield M, Flay B, Nichter M, Giovino G: Effects of anti-smoking advertising on youth smoking: a review. *J Health Commun* 2003; **8**(3):229–247.

36 Hastings G, Angus K: The influence of the tobacco industry on European tobacco-control policy. In: The ASPECT Consortium, ed. Tobacco or Health in the European Union Past, Present and Future. Luxembourg: Office for Official Publications of the European Communities, 2004:195–225.

37 Hastings GB, Elliott B: Social marketing practice in traffic safety. In: Organisation for Economic Co-operation and Development (OECD), ed. Marketing of Traffic Safety. Paris: OECD, 1993; :35–53.

38 Wanless D: Securing Good Health for the Whole Population. London: The Stationery Office, 2004.

CHAPTER 16

Poverty, household food insecurity and obesity in children

Cate Burns,[1] *Sonya J. Jones*[2] and *Edward A. Frongillo*[3]
[1] WHO Collaborating Centre for Obesity Prevention, Deakin University, Melbourne, Australia
[2] Centre for Research in Nutrition and Health Disparities, University of South Carolina, Columbia, SC, USA
[3] Department of Health Promotion, Education, and Behavior, University of South Carolina, Columbia, SC, USA

Summary

In this chapter we discuss the:
- definition of poverty and financial stress;
- definition of household food insecurity;
- prevalence of food insecurity in children in countries with developed and developing economies;
- impact of household food insecurity on well-being in children (health, mental, social well-being);
- relationship between socio-economic disadvantage, poverty and food insecurity and the prevalence of obesity in children;
- possible explanations for the overlap between poverty, household food insecurity and obesity in children;
- social, economic and public health policies to address childhood poverty and household food insecurity—can they have an impact on obesity in children?

Introduction

What is poverty?

Absolute poverty, as generally experienced in countries with developing economies, is a condition characterized by severe deprivation of basic human needs, including food, safe drinking water, sanitation facilities, health, shelter, education and information. For example, the WHO estimates that more than 45% of the population of the African region fall under the poverty-line definition, which characterizes as "poor" anyone who cannot afford a daily consumption rate of US$1.[1]

The poverty experienced in the developed world is considered relative. In these countries, people are considered poor if their living standards fall below an overall accepted community standard, and they are unable to participate fully in ordinary activities of society. This relative poverty can also be measured in terms of household income and a poverty line which is a defined income that families of different sizes need to cover essential needs. OECD countries use 50% of average disposable income to define a poverty line.[2]

What is financial stress?

Household income reflects economic resources. Measurement of financial stress concentrates on what people spend their money. It considers the extent to which households may have been constrained in their spending activities because of a shortage of money.[3] In developed countries financial stress may mean being unable to pay bills on time or needing to borrow money from friends or family or, at the extreme, being unable to afford heating and meals, or having had to

Preventing Childhood Obesity. Edited by
E. Waters, B.A. Swinburn, J.C. Seidell and R. Uauy.
© 2010 Blackwell Publishing.

pawn or sell possessions, or needing assistance from community organizations.

Financial stress impacts on household food expenditure. In households experiencing financial stress, food can become an elastic, and sometimes discretionary, expense resulting in changes in the quality and/or quantity of food purchased and available for consumption by adults and children in the household.

What is household food security?

Food insecurity is the limited or uncertain availability of nutritionally adequate and safe foods, or the limited ability to acquire foods in socially acceptable ways.

> Food insecurity ... refers to the social and economic problem of lack of food due to resource or other constraints, not voluntary fasting or dieting, or because of illness, or for other reasons. This definition, supported by ... ethnographic research ... means that food insecurity is experienced when there is (1) uncertainty about future food availability and access, (2) insufficiency in the amount and kind of food required for a healthy lifestyle, or (3) the need to use socially unacceptable ways to acquire food. Although lack of economic resources is the most common constraint, food insecurity can also be experienced when food is available and accessible but cannot be used because of physical or other constraints, such as limited physical functioning by elderly people or those with disabilities. Some closely linked consequences of uncertainty, insufficiency, and social unacceptability are assumed to be part of the experience of food insecurity. Worry and anxiety typically result from uncertainty. Feelings of alienation and deprivation, distress, and adverse changes in family and social interactions also occur ... Hunger and malnutrition are also potential, although not necessary, consequences of food insecurity.[4]

Measuring household food insecurity

The term food insecurity can be used in relation to individuals, households and communities.[5] Essentially, in high-income countries, household food insecurity is an economic and social condition of limited access to food. The food security status of households can be measured using validated tools. A variety of approaches have been used to measure household food insecurity.[6] The best known tool is the USDA 6 or 18 item US Household Food Security Survey Module. This measures food security on a continuum from:

- **High food security**—households have no problems, or anxiety about adequate food.
- **Low food security**—households reduce the quality, variety and desirability of their diets, but the quantity of food intake and normal eating patterns are not substantially disrupted.
- **Very low food security**—at times during the year, eating patterns of one or more household members are disrupted and food intake reduced because the household lacked money and other resources for food.

In low- and middle-income countries, interest in using similar tools has led to consensus on a generic questionnaire that, when adapted to the socio-cultural setting, will provide useful measurements of household food insecurity in many countries.[7] This consensus emerged from two international workshops organized by the Food and Nutrition Technical Assistance Project (FANTA), and is based on work carried out in Indonesia,[8] Bangladesh,[9] Brazil[10] and other countries.[11]

Other markers for food insecurity when no measurement tools exist

Before the development of survey questionnaire tools to measure household food insecurity, other proxy measures had been used, and are still used. Some of these methods are based on agricultural productivity, food storage, or children's nutritional status.[12] Others are based on coping strategies, food economy, community ranking and livelihood assessment.[6]

Prevalence of food insecurity in children

The most recent Australian data from the Victorian Population Health Survey found that in 2006 3.6% of two-parent families with dependent children and 20.6% of one-parent families with dependent children had in the last year run out of food and had no money to buy more[13] In the United States, from national survey data in 2006, 89% of households were food secure throughout the entire year, with the remaining 11% of households being food insecure at least some time during that year[14] Among households with dependent children, 16% were food insecure. The US prevalence of very low food security was 4% of households, with these households having disrupted eating patterns and reduced food intake during the year because the household lacked money and other resources for food. Some assessment has been done in low-income countries. For example, a survey in Java, Indonesia, at the height of the economic crisis that struck in 1998, saw substantial household food insecurity with 94.2% of households found to be uncertain or insecure about their food situation in the previous year, and 11% of respondents reported losing weight in the previous year because of lack of food.[8]

Impact of food insecurity on a child's well-being

A number of factors determine the food security status of a household including financial resources, local food access and cost, social support and networks, skills, values and attitudes and the mental and physical health of the primary care giver. The experience of food insecurity for a child has both the immediate impact of little or no food in the home but also the long-term consequences for both child and parent of an uncertain supply of food. Household food insecurity has been shown to relate to poor physical and mental health, social development, and academic performance, including higher prevalence of inadequate intake of key nutrients, depressive symptoms and suicide risk in adolescents, and poor learning and behavior problems in children.[4]

The relationship between poverty and food insecurity and the prevalence of obesity in children

Relationship poverty and obesity in children

How can children in families that are poor or otherwise disadvantaged be obese? Historically the image of poverty and disadvantage was one of a wasted child and/or parent. But this image has effectively been turned on its head. In countries with developed and, even developing economies, many people who are socio-economically disadvantaged, living on low income or in poverty, and are food insecure, are overweight or obese.

The results of early studies looking at the relationship between socio-economic status (SES) and childhood obesity were inconsistent. Sobal and Stunkard's review in 1989 of 34 such studies from developed countries published after 1941, found inverse associations (36%), no associations (38%), and positive associations (26%) were in similar proportions.[15] More recent data, however, indicate that the inverse gradient between SES and adiposity in adults[16] is becoming apparent in children. A systematic review of cross-sectional studies for the period 1990–2005[17] indicates that, within the past 15 years, the associations between SES and adiposity in children are predominantly inverse, and positive associations have all but disappeared. These findings are corroborated by recent analyses of nationally representative samples of children. For example in the UK, Stamatakis et al 2005, using data from the National Study of Health and Growth and the Health Survey for England, found that while obesity was increasing in all children, it was increasing more rapidly among children from low income homes.[18] In Australia, Wake et al 2006 in the Longitudinal Study of Australian Children (LSAC) found again that obesity in children was increasing across the board but that children from highly disadvantaged neighborhoods were 47% more likely to be overweight or obese compared with those from areas with more advantages.[19]

The relationship between poverty and childhood obesity is well described in a comparative study of Canada, Norway and the USA.[20] These countries were chosen because, while they are similarly affluent, they have made quite different social policy choices and have correspondingly different socio-economic outcomes for children. Canada and the USA can both be considered welfare states with relatively low levels of public spending, income transfers which are targeted to the poor rather than universally available and high rates of child poverty. In contrast, Norway has higher levels of public spending, more universal and generous spending and much lower rates of child poverty. In this study, the patterns of poverty and child obesity were lowest in Norway. In both Canada and the USA, there was a greater extent of obesity for poor than non-poor children, and this pattern was particularly marked for the USA. This study suggests that an association does exist between poverty and childhood obesity and that this may be moderated by social policies.

Studies of measures of poverty or financial stress and obesity in the USA

A number of US studies have demonstrated a modest but consistent association between food insecurity and weight status in adult women. This association and the case report published by Dietz in 1995 has stimulated a number of investigations of the association between household food insecurity and weight status in children.[21] While many of the studies cannot provide evidence of causal relationship, owing to limitations in study design and measurement, these studies generally find only limited evidence of any relationship between food insecurity and child overweight. In secondary data analysis of nationally representative US datasets, Casey[22] found no relationship between food insecurity and weight status independent of income, Alaimo[23] found that white girls aged 8–16 were slightly more likely to be overweight if they lived in a food insufficient household, and Rose[24] found that kindergarten children were less likely to be overweight if they were living in a food insecure household.

The few smaller studies published have also reported inconsistent and weak evidence of associations between food insecurity and child weight status. Matheson and colleagues[25] reported a lower BMI among children in food insecure households in a cross-sectional sample of 124 Hispanic families, but Kaiser[26] reported no association in another sample of younger Hispanic children. At the time of writing, there is only one published study that examines the longitudinal associations between food insecurity and overweight. Jyoti[27] found that girls from food insecure households had greater gains in BMI than girls from food secure households, but average BMI remained within the normal range. There are a number of plausible explanations for the lack of a clear association between food insecurity and obesity in children. It is possible that children, particularly young boys, are protected from food insecurity through their parents' coping strategies. It is also possible that programs available to protect children from the effects of household food insecurity are working, in that children are receiving adequate and healthy meals from school and child care environments.

Studies in other developed economies

Other than the USA, there are few countries with developed economies in which the relationship between food insecurity and childhood obesity has been measured. One country in which this research has been undertaken is Canada.

Canada's National Population Health Survey 1998–1999 found that 11% of children <18 years lived in households where food insecurity compromised diet. In this survey, children were five times more likely than seniors to be living in a food insecure household.[28] Using data from the Longitudinal Study of Child Development, Dubois[29] found that the presence of family food insufficiency during preschool years increased the likelihood of overweight three-fold after adjusting for income. This study reported that low birthweight children living in households that experienced food insufficiency during preschool years were at higher risk of becoming overweight at 4–5 years.

Implications for research and practice

There is evidence that an association exists between socio-economic disadvantage, poverty and obesity in children. It would appear that social policy can influence the socio-economic conditions in which children live and lessen the likelihood of a child becoming obese. Evidence for an association between food insecurity and obesity is less consistent and may be country dependent. While a very strong association has been demonstrated in Canada, the US results indicate a weaker link. Again, these differences may reflect different social policies in each of these countries that moderate either the likelihood of a household being food insecure or the impact of food insecurity on a child's health and relative body weight.

Where do we go from here? We need to improve our understanding of both how to reduce childhood poverty and disadvantage and also how to develop policies that can target solutions in the pathways between poverty and obesity in children. Research should be directed at understanding these pathways using cross-national and longitudinal comparisons. To best articulate policy regarding either childhood obesity or food insecurity, countries with developed economies need research that goes beyond examining associations of food insecurity and obesity in children. For instance, in the USA, a number of policies have been developed and programs implemented to address food insecurity in children (e.g., the School Meals Programs, The Supplemental Nutrition Program for Women, Infants and Children and The Food Stamp Program). For almost as long as the programs have been in existence, there have been concerns that they may contribute to obesity.[30] Even though most studies have demonstrated that program participation leads to better diet quality, some have also shown that children may consume more sweetened beverages and consume more fat when participating in the program. Future research regarding food insecurity and obesity in children needs to use new and innovative methods to examine the best policy options for protecting children from the negative effects of household food insecurity without exacerbating risk factors for obesity.

Why would children from poor or food insecure households be more likely to be obese?

As described elsewhere in this book, obesity is the product of an imbalance between energy intake (food intake) and energy output (physical activity). The literature consistently shows that children living in households with fewer socio-economic resources are less likely to have a healthy diet or engage in physical activity and are more likely to be unhealthy and obese.[31] It is not fully understood why this socio-economic gradient in health and lifestyle behaviors exists in adults and children.[32] It is likely that an explanation lies both within the environment, that is, our cities, neighborhoods and society in general and within the child's immediate environment, that is, their home. A good representation of the macro factors which operate at a societal and environmental level is the ecological model of health and development across the lifespan.[33] However, described in the ecological model, there are the micro factors operating at household and individual parent and child level that are also determinants of a child's health and development. The link between these factors operating within the caregiving environment (the home) and child health and development are described by the UNICEF conceptual framework.[34] The pathway between poverty, financial stress and food insecurity and childhood obesity is likely to be explained by *both* environmental factors *and* differences in caregiving and resources for caring within the home.

Macro environmental factors that may impact on the prevalence of obesity in food insecure or poor households

The effect of the economic and social environment on the development of obesity may be moderated by policies or structures that determine household economic resources. We know that those with fewer economic resources are more like to be obese.[16] Ecological studies indicate that larger increases in energy intake, obesity and diabetes, particularly among women, can be observed in developed countries where greater income disparities are also observed.[35] As described previously, studies also indicate that levels of inequity and wealth distribution influence the prevalence of childhood obesity.[20]

There is evidence that the food environment, the availability and cost of food, may increase the likelihood of those on low income or living in poverty becoming obese. Studies of the food environment indicate that the idea of poor neighborhoods having too little and too expensive healthy foods holds true only in the USA.[36] Studies in the UK[37] and in Australia[38] indicate that low income areas have good access to affordable healthy food. However, what has been consistently shown in the developed world is a strong relationship between area level disadvantage and the density of fast-food outlets. The cost of food may also accelerate obesity among the socio-economically disadvantaged.[39] Evidence is emerging that the global price of food is increasing. Data from Australia reveal that the cost of healthy staples has increased 20% above inflation while, in comparison, the price of unhealthy foods, such as soft drinks and cakes and biscuits, has steadily dropped.[40]

Studies also indicate socio-economic disparities in the built environment in terms of access to resources including playgrounds, equipment and neighborhood safety that would encourage physical activity. It is believed that these in part explain socio-economic differences observed in participation in physical activity and engagement in sedentary behaviors.

Household factors determining obesity in poor or low income households at risk of food insecurity

In addition to environmental factors, we propose that the development of obesity among children in poor and food insecure households is a product of the impact of this deprivation on parental care giving. It is well recognized that care giving practices and resources for caring have a powerful influence on children's development.[41] The significance of care has been best articulated in the extended UNICEF (1996) model of care.[34] This model has been used extensively in countries with developing economies to explore the link between food insecurity and malnutrition. We propose that the model can be adapted to explain the relationship between food insecurity and obesity, which is largely an issue in developed countries or those in economic transition. It is ironic that a model essentially used to explain malnutrition in developing countries could be applied to explain obesity in developed countries. However, obesity and malnutrition can coexist in households in developed countries and countries with developing economies and food insecurity is prevalent in these countries though not as visible as in developing countries.

Using the UNICEF model, Begin demonstrated[42] that care givers' influence on child feeding decisions, their satisfaction with life, and the help available to them, were more closely related to child development than household variables including income and the care givers' time allocation for different activities of living. We have built on this model and propose (see Figure 16.1) that, while financial resources (or lack thereof) maybe important in the development of obesity, financial hardship and food insecurity has an additional effect, which is mediated by stress on carers' resources and parental caring behaviors.

Care is the provision in the household and community of time, attention and support to meet the physical, mental and social needs of the growing child and other household members.[34]

In the current model we conceptualized resources for care as economic and organizational resources (time, money and help with children) and the human resources for care (mental and physical well-being of the care giver). We hypothesize that these resources have different mediating roles. The notion of differential mediating roles for different resources is supported by Gershoff (2007).[43] These researchers demonstrated that income mediates an effect on cognitive skills through parental investment of time, energy and support while the link between income and social and emotional competence is mediated

through material hardship and, in turn, parental stress and behaviours.[43]

There is some evidence to substantiate this explanatory model for a relationship between poverty, food insecurity and obesity. Qualitative studies describe the stress experienced by those on low and insufficient income trying to make ends meet.[44] These experiences may increase parental stress and depression which, in turn, may impact on both the eating habits of both parent and child to encourage the overconsumption of energy-dense but "valued" foods. These behaviors may be modeled in the children in these households. Stress may also modify parental feeding styles.[45] A qualitative study in USA indicated a poor food environment but also parental guilt, and that poor parenting skills and discipline result in poor feeding habits in children in disadvantaged households.[46] Mothers who report stress, depression or anxiety symptoms are at risk for non-responsive feeding styles (e.g., more controlling, indulgent and uninvolved).[45]

There is a strong literature showing that those living in poverty and on a low income, (in other words, populations at risk of food insecurity), tend to have poor food and exercise habits. The current model offers an explanation of how material hardship and food insecurity—perhaps the most extreme of hardships—can cause changes in eating habits and patterns of physical activity that are conducive to the development of obesity in children experiencing these hardships.

Public policy and practice to address obesity in financially stressed or food insecure families

Public health interventions in response to the epidemic of childhood obesity should be both universal (relating to the high prevalence across all sectors) and targeted (to those experiencing socio-economic disadvantage). Universal food and nutrition interventions are described elsewhere in this book. They include: changing the food supply, regulation of the marketing of food to children, educational policies to ensure universal health, including food skills. Vulnerable children in vulnerable households require further support: social and economic policies to ensure adequate financial resources for a modest but nutritionally adequate and socially appropriate diet; subsidizing the

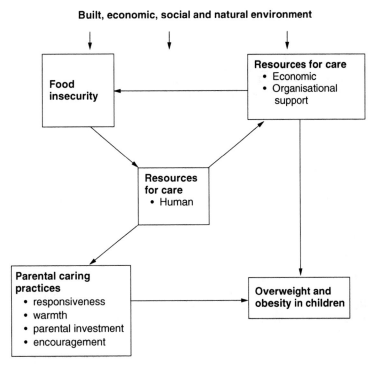

Built, economic, social and natural environment

Figure 16.1 Model of the relationship linking food insecurity, resources for care and parental caring practices to overweight and obesity in children within the context of the built, economic, social and natural environments.

cost of healthy food; social policies that ensure social inclusion and support; education programs for positive parenting; housing policies that ensure adequate and appropriate housing for children and the preparation of healthy food; and training of community workers to detect, assess and assist food insecure households. Further research is required to confirm the model we propose here. Ideally, this research would use panel datasets including all the predictive variables identified. This will help policy makers to decide on the best strategies and investments for improving household food security and reducing its impact on childhood obesity.

References

1 Feachem RG: Poverty and inequity: a proper focus for the new century. *Bull World Health Organ* 2000; **78**(1):1–2.

2 Senate Community Affairs References Committee Secretariat: A Hand Up Not a Hand Out: Renewing the Fight Against Poverty. Report on Poverty and Financial Hardship. Canberra: Commonwealth of Australia, 2004. www.aph.gov.au/Senate/committee/clac_ctte/poverty/report/index.htm (accessed 22 December 2008).

3 Bray JB. Hardship in Australia: An analysis of financial stress indicators in the 1998–1999 Australian Bureau of Statistics Household Expenditure Survey. Canberra: Department of Family and Community Services, 2001. www.aph.gov.au/Senate/Committee/clac_ctte/completed_inquiries/2002-04/poverty/submissions/sub165a.pdf (accessed 22 December 2008).

4 Panel to Review US: Department of agriculture's measurement of food insecurity and hunger. In Wunderlich G, Norwood J, eds. Food Insecurity and Hunger in the US: An assessment of the measure. Washington: National Academies Press, 2006:4.

5 Pelletier D, Olson C, Frongillo E: Food insecurity, hunger and undernutrition. In: Bowman B, Russell R, eds. Present Knowledge in Nutrition, Ninth edn. Washington DC: International Life Sciences Institute Press, 2006:906–922.

6 Wolfe W, Frongillo EA: Building household food security measurement tools from the ground up. *Food Nutr Bull* 2001; **22**:5–12.

7 Coates J, Swindale A, Bilinsky, P: Household Food Insecurity Access Scale (HIFIAS) for Measurement of Household Food Access: Indicator Guide. Washington DC: Academy for Educational Development, 2007. www.fantaproject.org/publications/hfias.shtml (accessed 22 December 2008).

8 Studdert LJ, Frongillo EA, Jr., Valois P: Household food insecurity was prevalent in Java during Indonesia's economic crisis. *J Nutr* 2001; **131**(10):2685–2691.

9 Frongillo EA, Chowdhury N, Ekstrom EC, Naved RT: Understanding the experience of household food insecurity in rural Bangladesh leads to a measure different from that used in other countries. *J Nutr* 2003; **133**(12):4158–4162.

10 Marin-Leon L, Segal-Correa AM, Panigassi G, Maranha LK, Sampaio Mde F, Perez-Escamilla R: Food insecurity perception in families with elderly in Campinas, Sao Paulo, Brazil. *Cad Saude Publica* 2005; **21**(5):1433–1440.

11 Ortiz-Hernandez L, Acosta-Gutierrez MN, Nunez-Perez AE, Peralta-Fonseca N, Ruiz-Gomez Y: Food insecurity and obesity are positively associated in Mexico City schoolchildren. *Rev Invest Clin* 2007; **59**(1):32–41.

12 Webb P, Coates J, Frongillo EA, Rogers BL, Swindale A, Bilinsky P: Measuring household food insecurity: why it's so important and yet so difficult to do. *J Nutr* 2006; **136**(5): 1404S–1408S.

13 Department of Human Services: Victorian Population Health Survey 2006: Selected findings. Melbourne: Department of Human Services, Victoria, 2007. www.health.vic.gov.au/healthstatus/vphs_current.htm#download (accessed 22 December 2008).

14 Nord M, Hopwood H: Recent advances provide improved tools for measuring children's food security. *J Nutr* 2007; **137**(3):533–536.

15 Sobal J, Stunkard AJ: Socioeconomic status and obesity: a review of the literature. *Psychol Bull* 1989; **105**(2):260–275.

16 Ball K, Crawford D: Socioeconomic status and weight change in adults: a review. *Soc Sci Med* 2005; **60**(9): 1987–2010.

17 Shrewsbury V, Wardle J: Socioeconomic status and adiposity in childhood: a systematic review of cross-sectional studies 1990–2005. *Obesity* 2008; **16**(2):275–284.

18 Stamatakis E, Primatesta P, Chinn S, Rona R, Falascheti E: Overweight and obesity trends from 1974 to 2003 in English children: what is the role of socioeconomic factors? *Arch Dis Child* 2005; **90**(10):999–1004.

19 Wake M, Hardy P, Canterford L, Sawyer M, Carlin JB: Overweight, obesity and girth of Australian preschoolers: prevalence and socio-economic correlates. *Int J Obes* 2006; **31**(7):1044–1051.

20 Phipps SA, Burton PS, Osberg LS, Lethbridge LN: Poverty and the extent of child obesity in Canada, Norway and the United States. *Obes Rev* 2006; **7**(1):5–12.

21 Dietz WH: Does hunger cause obesity? *Pediatrics* 1995; **95**(5): 766–767.

22 Casey PH, Simpson PM, Gossett JM et al: The association of child and household food insecurity with childhood overweight status. *Pediatrics* 2006; **118**(5):e1406–e1413.

23 Alaimo K, Olson CM, Frongillo EA, Jr.: Low family income and food insufficiency in relation to overweight in US children: is there a paradox? *Arch Pediatr Adolesc Med* 2001; **155**(10):1161–1167.

24 Rose D, Bodor JN: Household food insecurity and overweight status in young school children: results from the Early Childhood Longitudinal Study. *Pediatrics* 2006; **117**(2):464–473.

25 Matheson DM, Varady J, Varady A, Killen JD: Household food security and nutritional status of Hispanic children in the fifth grade. *Am J Clin Nutr* 2002; **76**(1):210–217.

26 Kaiser LL, Melgar-Quinonez HR, Lamp CL, Johns MC, Sutherlin JM, Harwood JO: Food security and nutritional outcomes of preschool-age Mexican-American children. *J Am Diet Assoc* 2002; **102**(7):924–929.

27 Jyoti DF, Frongillo EA, Jones SJ: Food insecurity affects school children's academic performance, weight gain, and social skills. *J Nutr* 2005; **135**(12):2831–2839.

28 Che J, Chen J: Food Insecurity in Canadian Households. Ontario: Health Statistics Division at Statistics Canada, 2003.

29 Dubois L, Farmer A, Girard M, Porcherie M: Family food insufficiency is related to overweight among preschoolers. *Soc Sci Med* 2006; **63**(6):1503–1516.

30 Frongillo EA: Understanding obesity and program participation in the context of poverty and food insecurity. *J Nutr* 2003; **133**(7):2117–2118.

31 Lobstein T, Baur L, Uauy R: Obesity in children and young people: a crisis in public health. *Obes Rev* 2004; **5**(Suppl. 1): 4–104.

32 Marmot M, Wilkinson RG: Psychosocial and material pathways in the relation between income and health: a response to Lynch et al. *BMJ* 2001; **322**(7296):1233–1236.

33 Lynch JW, Smith GD, Kaplan GA, House JS: Income inequality and mortality: importance to health of individual income, psychosocial environment, or material conditions. *BMJ* 2000; **320**(7243):1200–1204.

34 Engle P, Menon P, Haddad L: Care and Nutrition: Concepts and Measurment. Washington DC: International Food Policy Research Institute, 1996 August. (FCND Discussion Paper No.18). www.ifpri.org/sites/default/files/publication/pubs_divs_fcnd/dp/papers/dp18.pdf (accessed 3 December 2009).

35 Pickett KE, Kelly S, Brunner E, Lobstein T, Wilkinson RG: Wider income gaps, wider waistbands? An ecological study of obesity and income inequality. *J Epidemiol Community Health* 2005; **59**(8):670–674.

36 Cummins S, Macintyre S: Food environments and obesity—neighbourhood or nation? *Int J Epidemiol* 2006; **35**(1): 100–104.

37 Cummins S, Macintyre S: A systematic study of an urban foodscape: the price and availability of food in Greater Glasgow. *Urban Stud* 2002; **39**(11):2115–2130.

38 Burns CM, Inglis AD: Measuring food access in Melbourne: access to healthy and fast foods by car, bus and foot in an urban municipality in Melbourne. *Health Place* 2007; **13**(4):877–885.

39 Drewnowski A, Specter SE: Poverty and obesity: the role of energy density and energy costs. *Am J Clin Nutr* 2004; **79**(1): 6–16.

40 Burns C, Sacks G, Gold L: Longitudinal study of the Consumer Price Index (CPI) changes in core and non-core foods in Australia. *Aust N Z J Public Health* 2008; **32**(5): 449–452.

41 Conger RD, Donnellan MB: An interactionist perspective on the socioeconomic context of human development. *Annu Rev Psychol* 2007; **58**:175–199.

42 Begin F, Frongillo EA, Delisle H: Caregiver behaviours and resources influence Child Height-for-Age in Rural Chad. *J Nutr* 1999; **129**:680–686.

43 Gershoff ET, Aber JL, Raver CC, Lennon MC: Income is not enough: incorporating material hardship into models of income associations with parenting and child development. *Child Dev* 2007; **78**(1):70–95.

44 Hamelin A-M, Beaudry M, Habicht J-P: Characterization of household food insecurity in Quebec: food and feelings. *Soc Sci Med* 2002; **54**(1):119–132.

45 Hurley K, Black MM, Papas MA, Caufield LE: Maternal symptoms of stress, depression and anxiety are related to nonresponsive feeding styles in a statewide sample of WIC participants. *J Nutr* 2008; **138**:799–805.

46 Kaufman L, Karpati A: Understanding the sociocultural roots of childhood obesity: food practices among Latino families of Bushwick, Brooklyn. *Soc Sci Med* 2007; **64**(11):2177–2188.

CHAPTER 17

Socio-cultural issues and body image

Helen Mavoa,[1] *Shiriki Kumanyika*[2] *and Andre Renzaho*[3]
[1]WHO Collaborating Centre for Obesity Prevention, Melbourne, Australia
[2]Department of Biostatistics and Epidemiology, and Department of Pediatrics, University of Pennsylvania School of Medicine, Philadelphia, PA, USA
[3]WHO Collaborating Centre for Obesity Prevention, Faculty of Health, Medicine, Nursing and Behavioural Sciences, Deakin University, Burwood, Australia

Summary

The increasing prevalence of childhood obesity and overweight is disproportionate in some ethnic groups. Drawing on data from three separate countries, we focus on three populations that have high or similar levels of obesity relative to other ethnic groups in the same countries to discuss relationships between socio-cultural factors, other environmental components and childhood obesity. We refer to: (1) indigenous Fijians (Fijians), who constitute the majority of the population in Fiji; (2) African Americans, who have resided in the United States of America for generations and remain a minority ethnic group; and (3) Africans, who have recently migrated to Australia and constitute a fast-growing minority ethnic group. We focus on:

- how socio-cultural factors underpin body-size preferences and eating and physical activity (activity) patterns
- examining socio-cultural factors in a wider context, including the physical environment and historical, social, economic and political factors
- the conceptualisation and integration of socio-cultural factors into research and contextually-relevant programs that reduce childhood obesity by encouraging a healthy lifestyle.

Introduction

Contextual background

The independent Pacific nation of Fiji comprises 57% indigenous Fijians (Fijians) and 38% Indo-Fijians.[1]

Fiji has experienced a series of influences and socio-political changes, including: the arrival of indentured labourers from India (1897–1916; the gaining of independence (1971); and four coups. Since the 1960s, Fiji has been exposed to increasing international movement of people, ideas and goods, a rural–urban shift, greater access to cash, increasing consumption of high-energy imported foods[2–4] and changes in actual and ideal body size.[5,6] There is a high prevalence of obesity among Fijian adults; 42% of males[7] and >47% of females[7–9] have a BMI >25 kg/m². The higher prevalence of obesity in young Fijian adults than Indo-Fijians[7] suggests that the physical environment is not the only influence on body size, and that socio-cultural, historical and economic factors also come into play.

African Americans (also referred to as non-Hispanic black Americans) are descendants of people brought to the USA during the slave trade. Even counting the increasing numbers of immigrants from Africa or the Caribbean who may identify themselves in this census bureau category, >90% of African Americans are US-born.[10] African Americans constitute 13% of the US population[11,12] and, until recently, were the largest US "ethnic minority" group.* In the US black population overall, people of any race who identify as "Hispanic", now outnumber African

---

---

*The term "ethnic minority" refers to a sub-population that is disadvantaged in terms of language, economic status or religion and whose people have limited space to express themselves culturally and socially. "Ethnic minority" does not necessarily imply numerical disadvantage. In Australia the term "culturally and liguistically diverse communities" is used when describing ethnic minority groups.[13,14]

Americans.[12] Although African Americans are well-integrated into many aspects of US society, they remain a distinct ethno-cultural group.[15] There are numerous demographic differences between African Americans and whites,[11,15,16] with the former having higher rates of poverty and unemployment, lower educational attainment, more female-headed households, residence in racially-segregated urban areas, and greater representation in South and South-eastern regions compared to other parts of the country. Compared to whites and other minority populations, African Americans have poorer health status and a shorter life expectancy.[17] Some aspects of adverse health profiles are confined to African Americans with low social position, while others—like high rates of low birth weight—are observed in all social strata.

The prevalence of obesity among African Americans is greater than among whites, particularly among females. Data from the US National Health and Nutrition Examination Survey (NHANES) show a higher obesity prevalence in non-Hispanic black (primarily African American) and Mexican American children than non-Hispanic white children.[18] More Mexican American boys aged 2–19 years are obese (i.e., at or above the 95th percentile of the age-sex appropriate Centers for Disease Control and Prevention BMI reference) than non-Hispanic black or white boys: 22.0% vs. 16.4% and 17.8%, respectively. Non-Hispanic black girls have a higher prevalence of obesity than either Mexican American or white girls: 23.8% vs. 16.2% and 14.8%, respectively.[18] Obesity prevalence has been higher in black than white women in the USA since the 1960s,[19] but the relatively high prevalence of obesity in African American girls has emerged only in recent decades.[20] This may reflect greater impact of recent socio-cultural and environmental changes for African American girls than other children.[21]

Sub-Saharan African migrants are a culturally- and linguistically-diverse ethnic minority group comprising 43 different cultures; about half are from the Horn of Africa (Somali, Ethiopia and Eritrea), South Sudan, Sierra Leone and Liberia.[22] Each subgroup has different socio-cultural contexts and holds different value systems from mainstream Australians. The term "African migrant group" is used to refer to this heterogeneous group of migrants with a recent history of migration to Australia, the majority of whom are refugees or humanitarian entrants who immigrated directly from refugee camps or transitional countries.

Africans appear to be at increased risk of obesity and related diseases such as diabetes following migration to Australia and other Western countries.[23–25] Recent work indicated that 27% of 3–12-year-old African migrant children were obese.[26] While this obesity prevalence is similar to that reported for other Australian children, African migrants have been in Australia for only six years on average. Further, many African migrant children have come from deprived environments where undernutrition prevails (20–40% have chronic malnutrition).[27] It is highly likely that African migrant children entered Australia with lower BMIs, which have increased following arrival.[26] Obesity among African migrant children in Australia has been associated with lower household income level, fewer siblings, single-parent households and western African background.[26]

As illustrated, children in each of these ethnic "groups" have been exposed to recent changes, including greater access to fast foods, sweetened drinks and greater exposure to the media compared to previous generations. African migrant children in Australia have experienced marked dietary acculturation[28] and changes in language, religion and cultural values,[29] especially children who were born prior to arriving in Australia.

We examine some environmental factors that may explain the high prevalence of obesity among Fijian and African American children relative to other ethnic groups in their respective countries, and African migrant children in their new (Australian) environment. The Analysis Grid for Environments Linked to Obesity (ANGELO) framework is used as part of the priority-setting process for obesity prevention action in communities. The ANGELO framework conceptualizes four environments (socio-cultural, physical, political, economic),[30] and is premised on individuals or groups interacting with environments in multiple settings, including homes, schools and neighborhoods. The family is the most fundamental influence on children's behaviors.[31,32] Next, we consider ways that the socio-cultural environment influences actual and ideal body size, as well as eating and activity patterns.

The socio-cultural environment

The socio-cultural environment influences body-size preferences, as well as eating and activity patterns.[21,32] This environment comprises structural characteristics and the dominant ethos, as well as culturally-shaped values, beliefs, attitudes and expectations.[31–33] The structure of a cultural group impacts on food-related practices in families, households and wider communities, thus impacting on the body size of group members.[32] The hierarchical structure of a group is defined by the relative rank and status of individuals and/or families. Status is determined by a range of variables, including gender, seniority, life stage, education, employment and wealth. Body size, eating and activity patterns are often associated with the relative status of group members. For example, older Fijian men are given more prestigious and greater quantities of food than women and younger men.[34] A large body size characterizes social rank, status and power for sub-Saharan Africans.[35] In any group, high-status family members are likely to make key decisions about the nurturing of children and the acquisition, preparation and distribution of food. For example, grandmothers in intergenerational African American households often influence infant feeding practices.[36]

The prevailing ethos or world-view within an ethnic group also influences body-size preferences and eating and activity patterns.[32] A collective ethos is characterized by expectations of interdependence, awareness of others, a sense of duty and cooperation.[37–39] The family is the most fundamental social unit.[32] There is often greater connectedness with extended family members and elders are more directly involved in child-rearing among Fijian families,[40,41] ethnic minority groups in the USA[21,42,43] and Africans[44] compared to white families.

Values, beliefs, attitudes and expected behaviors also impact on body size and eating and activity patterns.[21,32] While socio-cultural influences on body size are universal, their expressions differ among populations, classes and ethnic groups.[21] For example, ideas about what constitutes a well-nurtured or healthy body are culturally shaped. The WHO's definition of an optimal body mass index ($18.5–25 \text{ kg/m}^2$) does not necessarily concur with the views of all ethnic groups. Fijians,[6,32] African Americans[21] and sub-Saharan

Africans[35] prefer larger body sizes than Europeans, although emerging evidence suggests that Fijian preferences are shifting toward Western ideals.[5,45]

Although attitudes may coexist among cultural groups sharing the same environment over time, the persistence of different body ideals is evident in data for African Americans vs US whites. Several qualitative studies report that African Americans tolerate large body sizes and view the meaning of large body size differently from health professionals.[21] A study of low-income mothers of preschool children, the majority of whom were African American, indicated that having a larger body size than the growth charts was acceptable, providing children were healthy, active and had good self-esteem.[46] A study of 9–10-year-old white and African American girls reported that African American girls with a "normal" weight were more likely to receive maternal messages that they were underweight than white girls.[47] Similarly, African migrant adults may have maintained their preference for a large body size after migration to Australia, continuing to view a robust body as beautiful and as an expression of a family's wealth.[35] However, it is not yet clear whether African migrants' body-size ideals will persist in Australia, given the increasing prevalence of obesity and awareness of obesity-related diseases.

Parents and/or primary caregivers have a major influence on their children's eating and activity patterns via their ideals about a healthy body, knowledge about healthy eating and exercise, food available at home, structuring of family meals, shaping of opportunities for physical activity and modeling of acceptable behaviors and body sizes.[48] Eating and activity patterns that result in a large body size may be considered acceptable, or even desirable, to achieve a "healthy looking" child. A well-nurtured body may indicate high status and good health, as well as being associated with fertility in environments where people have been undernourished, for example, in some parts of Africa.[49] These associations between a robust body, social status and health are reflected in the post-migration eating patterns of African migrants in Australia, with reduced consumption of foods that are considered less desirable and seen as survival food for poor people, for example, vegetables and fruit.[35]

Parents' and children's respective roles are culturally influenced and are likely to differ across ethnic groups. For example, many children in Western/white families have substantial control of what and how much they eat,[50] especially during adolescence.[48] This is not necessarily the case for children from all ethnic groups; many parents in Fijian[51] and African[44] families have an authoritarian parenting style, with children having little control over their eating patterns. This has also been reported for African American families.[21]

The expression of socio-cultural factors varies within ethnic groups. For example, children experience the same exposures differently from their parents, who in turn have different perceptions from older generations. These intergenerational differences have major implications for body-size preferences, as well as ideas about how to attain the optimal body size. Studies with Fijians,[52] African Americans[47] and African migrants in Australia[28,35] all report that adolescents preferred a leaner body than their parents. Thirty-one percent of Fijian adolescent females believed that that their parents wanted them to eat more than they thought was ideal.[5] In a US cohort study of pre-adolescent girls, African Americans were much more likely than white girls to report trying to gain weight.[47] Weight-gain strategies were associated with parents, especially in those with less education, telling girls that they were too thin.[47] African migrant parents reinforced traditional African body-size ideals using weight-gain strategies to achieve a culturally-desired body size, overfeeding their offspring and/or promoting energy-dense foods.[53] These strategies were often resisted by young African migrants.[53]

There are also intergenerational differences between parents and older family members in terms of body-size preferences and body-change strategies. Fijian mothers reported that their mothers/mothers-in-law shaped their ideas about appropriate infant feeding and optimal body size.[54] Co-resident grandmothers often dominated feeding decisions in African American families, especially when they were key caregivers.[21]

Children from all three ethnic groups are exposed to a wide continuum of values and expectations from parents, older generations, siblings and peers. Children in ethnic minority groups are likely to experience a wider spectrum of body-size ideals and eating and activity practices compared to Fijians, the largest ethnic group in Fiji. African American and African migrant children are not only exposed to the different values, ideals and practices within their own group, but also those of other ethnic groups with whom they live while retaining a separate cultural identity. Both realities may be influential. When competing cultural perspectives are incongruent, the context, for example, the types and amounts of interactions with the mainstream groups, will determine which perspectives are most influential and the types of intrapersonal conflicts that arise from trying to be bicultural.[33]

Cultural influences are also derived from various media sources and marketing strategies that interact with culturally-shaped preferences and practices—reflecting the larger culture in the case of ethnic minority groups—thus influencing body-size preferences and eating and activity patterns. For example, within three years of television exposure in Fiji, Fijian female adolescents[5] and adults[6] changed their body-size ideals; compared to a pre-television cohort. More adult females: were dissatisfied with their bodies; believed that body size could be changed; and made an effort to do so.[6] Marketing practices also contribute to an obesogenic environment for African American children.[55,56] Studies examining the frequency and content of food advertisements in television markets with a high viewership of African American children have documented the higher than average occurrence of food advertisements, especially targeting high-calorie snack foods, soft drinks and candy, relative to advertisements in predominantly white markets.[21,57–59] The impact of the Australian media and marketing on African migrant children in Australia has yet to be studied.

While socio-cultural factors underpin body size, eating and activity patterns, the socio-cultural environment is shaped by historical,[21,32] physical and economic factors.[21,30,60] We now discuss interactions between the socio-cultural environment and historical and economic factors.

The socio-cultural environment in context

Historical events influence body-size ideals and strategies to achieve these ideals. The cultural acceptability of overeating may be conditioned by economic deprivation, with feasting occurring whenever food is available.[61] The most valued foods may be associated with limited access and/or survival, for example, meat, fats, and sugars.[21] These foods are often related to high social status and symbolize integration into the US mainstream society and/or upward social mobility.[62] The status of such foods may persist for generations, even when they become cheap and abundant. The persistent preference for a large body size among African migrant adults in Australia may reflect previous experiences of hunger and deprivation, as well as experiences with tuberculosis and HIV/AIDS.[35]

In terms of the economic environment, food cost and accessibility result in people with unstable or limited discretionary incomes relying on foods with high energy density[21,63] because they are the least expensive,[64] and more accessible. These two factors are directly related to the social and economic environments of the three ethnic groups considered here. For example, increased availability of high-energy imported foods in Fiji has been associated with a concomitant reduction in the consumption of traditional foods.[3,4] In the case of African Americans, there is a disproportionate prevalence of poverty and a high absolute or relative density of "fast food" outlets in black neighborhoods and impoverished areas.[65,66] African migrant children in Australia have probably been exposed to a greater range and availability of high-energy foods in Australia than in their countries of origin. Fijian, African American[67] and African migrant families often have high levels of economic stress and insecurity, including food insecurity.

Environmental contexts are in dynamic interaction with socio-cultural factors[21,32] and can either enhance cultural predispositions[21] or limit or prevent the expression of cultural preferences.[21] The ability of parents to provide healthy foods is influenced by food availability and access, other market-related variables and economic stress,[21,28] making it critical to consider the socio-cultural environment in a broader context, albeit through a socio-cultural lens.

Translation into practice

Some programs designed to promote a healthy body size during childhood have incorporated socio-cultural components. We draw on examples of three such approaches: cultural-relevance, tailoring and cultural competence.

Culturally-relevant programs

The Pacific Obesity Prevention in Communities (OPIC) project aimed to reduce weight gain in adolescents via culturally-relevant programs where local communities set goals, determined action plans and implemented culturally-specific interventions, using the ANGELO framework.[30,68] Cultural relevance was determined via interviews that yielded adolescents' perspectives on socio-cultural factors that impacted on body size, eating and activity patterns, and consultations with adolescents and adults from target communities.[68,69] The Fiji team exchanged newly-acquired skills with community leaders and stakeholders who, in turn, advised on priorities and supported program implementation. Adolescent leaders were active in school health committees, completed health-promotion courses, and/or promoted and modeled healthy eating and activity patterns.

Culturally-tailored programs

"Tailoring" is a deliberate strategy that responds to important individual and subgroup variables when designing interventions.[70] A critical component of tailoring is identifying "focal points" for interventions, such as dinner time (setting) and parents of children in day care (population) relying on fast foods (behavior). Many elements of tailoring are related to cultural variables, for example, attitudes toward breastfeeding of African American teenage mothers enrolled in supplemental nutrition programs. Two examples of culturally-tailored programs that promote a healthy weight in young African American children are the Hip-Hop to Health Junior program for 3–5-year-old African American and Latino children in Head Start programs[71] and the Memphis Girls Health Enrichment Multi-site Studies (GEMS) project for 8–10-year-old African American girls.[72] The Hip-Hop to Health Junior program comprised "developmentally, culturally and linguistically appropriate diets and physical activity".[71] The GEMS project comprised a carefully tailored, family-based intervention that aimed to improve families' eating and activity patterns.[72]

Culturally competent programs

Obesity initiatives in Australia that adopt "the one approach fits all" are more likely to increase inequalities because most ethnic minority groups experience language difficulties, live in high-rise estates, do not understand complex health messages, and experience social exclusion, discrimination and poverty.[14] Together, these factors influence the eating and activity patterns of African migrants in Australia. These barriers can be overcome by working within a "cultural competence" framework, which extends beyond awareness of cultural differences to encompass behaviors, attitudes and policies that characterize an agency and support effective work in cross-cultural situations.[73] A system or agency is culturally competent when it: i) values diversity; ii) is capable of cultural self-assessment, iii) is conscious of the dynamics that occur when cultures interact, iv) institutionalizes cultural knowledge, and v) adapts services to reflect the diversity between and within cultures.[74]

These three culturally-specific approaches (cultural relevance, cultural tailoring, cultural competence) have common threads: recognition that the socio-cultural environment shapes body-size preferences and associated behaviors; identification and integration of socio-cultural factors; consideration of socio-cultural factors in a broad context that includes historical, physical, economic and policy environments; engagement with experts and key community members during program design and implementation.

What is the evidence to suggest that these three approaches influence either intervention uptake or outcomes in terms of BMI? Data on the effectiveness of the Pacific OPIC project intervention in Fiji are not yet available. Programs that actively engage families have been more effective in reducing childhood obesity than programs that do not.[75] Data on programs designed for young African American children suggest that parents are key to developing an environment that successfully fosters healthy eating, activity and body image.[48,72] The culturally-tailored programs with African American children described earlier have produced encouraging results in their follow-up measures. Children in the intervention group of the Hip-Hop to Health Junior program had significantly smaller increases in BMI compared to the control group.[71] Girls in the intervention group of the Girls Health Enrichment Multi-site Studies showed a significant decrease in excess weight gain, television viewing hours, and dinners eaten in front of television, compared to the control group.[76]

Conclusions/summary

In summary, socio-cultural factors shape body-size preferences and eating and activity patterns. Dominant world-views, values, attitudes and behaviors vary within and between ethnic groups. Within-group variations are often defined by intergenerational differences in body size preferences and ideas about how to attain these ideals. Intergenerational differences may be amplified with recent migration experiences, for example, with African migrants in Australia. The relatively high prevalence of childhood obesity for Fijians and African Americans, and potentially for Australian African migrants compared to other subgroups in their respective countries appears to be explained not only in terms of cultural differences, but also in interaction with economic disadvantage and physical and media environments that fail to support healthy behaviors. Emerging evidence from the USA suggests that the careful and timely integration of socio-cultural factors into culturally-tailored programs to promote healthy behaviors and body size are more effective in terms of both uptake and outcomes than those that do not address socio-cultural considerations. There is a need for more studies that measure the relative impact of socio-cultural factors on the effectiveness of programs to prevent obesity in children from different ethnic groups.

The three ethnic groups considered live in very different contexts; indigenous Fijians are the dominant ethnic group in their homeland, while both African Americans and African migrants in Australia are minority groups in their respective countries. However, the many common socio-cultural factors that appear to impact on the body size of children in these groups include: adults' acceptance of a larger body size than health professionals consider to be healthy; the generous provision of food to attain this ideal body size; and the family being the most fundamental influence on children's eating and activity patterns. Importantly, there are common principles for integrating socio-cultural factors into effective interventions designed to reduce childhood obesity in these three ethnic groups and, indeed, in other ethnic groups.

What else can be done to ensure the effectiveness of programs that promote a healthy weight for children? Given the fundamental nature of socio-cultural influences and the available evidence for these three cultural groups, we recommend that programs to promote healthy eating, activity and body size during childhood should:

- integrate socio-cultural factors and culturally appropriate approaches into their design and implementation;
- evaluate the socio-cultural environment in interaction with historical factors and economic, policy and physical environments
- recognize that culturally specific factors are an asset rather than a deficit and use cultural structures and other socio-cultural factors to ensure cultural relevance
- actively engage key family and community members and local experts throughout design and implementation phases
- emphasize healthy eating and activities rather than weight per se in order to avoid an unhealthy body image and the uptake of unhealthy strategies to attain the thin ideal that is promoted by the media and other Western influences
- recognize that there may be less motivation to prevent weight gain in ethnic groups that value a robust body size, and explore culturally tailored strategies that provide relevant and sufficiently strong motivations for change in the targeted parenting behaviors
- Recognize that children are exposed to numerous competing influences, especially children from ethnic minority groups who experience strong influences from within their own group, as well as from larger ethnic groups.

References

1 Central Intelligence Agency: The World Fact Book. Fiji. Washington DC: Central Intelligence Agency, 2008. www.cia.gov/library/publications/the-world-factbook/geos/fj.html.

2 Government of Fiji T: A Situational Analysis of Children and Women in Fiji 1996: The Government of Fiji and UNICEF, 1996.

3 Hughes R, Lawrence M: Globalisation, food and health in Pacific Island countries. *Asia Pac J Clin Nutr* 2005; **14**(4): 298–306.

4 Lako JV, Nguyen VC: Dietary patterns and risk factors of diabetes mellitus among urban indigenous women in Fiji. *Asia Pac J Clin Nutr* 2001; **10**(3):188–193.

5 Becker AE, Burwell RA, Gilman SE, Herzog DB, Hamburg P: Eating behaviours and attitudes following prolonged exposure to television among ethnic Fijian adolescent girls. *Br J Psychiatry* 2002; **180**:509–514.

6 Becker AE, Gilman SE, Burwell RA: Changes in prevalence of overweight and in body image among Fijian women between 1989 and 1998. *Obes Res* 2005; **13**(1):110–117.

7 Ministry of Health: Fiji Non-communicable Disease (NCD) STEPS Survey 2002. Suva, Fiji: Ministry of Health, 2004.

8 Saito S: 1993 National Nutrition Survey. Main Report. Suva, Fiji: National Food and Nutrition Committee, 1995.

9 Tomisaka K, Lako J, Maruyama C et al: Dietary patterns and risk factors for type 2 diabetes mellitus in Fijian, Japanese and Vietnamese populations. *Asia Pac J Clin Nutr* 2002; **11**(1):8–12.

10 Frey W: Analysis of the U.S. Census Bureau data (2001 CPS and 1970 Census). Population Today, 2002. www.prb.org/Articles/2002/ForeignBornMakeUpGrowingSegmentofUSBlackPopulation.aspx.

11 McKinnon J: The Black Population in the United States, 2002. Current Population Reports, 200www.census.gov/prod/2003pubs/p20-541.pdf.

12 U.S. Census Bureau: Quick Facts. 2008. http://quickfacts.census.gov/qfd/states/00000.html.

13 Renzaho A: Addressing the Needs of Refugees and Humanitarian Entrants in Victoria: An Evaluation of Health and Community Services. Melbourne: Centre for Culture Ethnicity and Health, 2002.

14 Renzaho A: Revisioning cultural competence in community health services: Challenges of addressing the health and welfare needs of cultrually and linguistically diverse migrants in Australia. *Aust Health Rev* 2008; **1**(32(2)):223–235.

15 Smelser J, Wilson W, Mitchell F: America Becoming. Racial Trends and Their Consequences. Washington DC: National Academy Press, 2001.

16 Iceland J, Weinberg DH, Steinmet E: U.S. Censur Bureau, Series CENSR-3. Racial and ethnic residential segregation in the United States: 1980–2000. Washington DC: U.S. Government Printing Office, 2002. www.census.gov/hhes/www/housing/housing_patterns/pdftoc.html.

17 National Center for Health Statistics. Health, United States, 2007. With Chartbook on Trends in the Health of Americans. Maryland: Hyattsville, 2007. www.cdc.gov/nchs/hus.htm.

18 Ogden C, Carroll M, Curtin L, McDowell M, Tabak C, Flegal K: Prevalence of overweight and obesity in the United States, 1999–2004. *JAMA* 2006; **295**:1549–1555.

19 Kumanyika S: Obesity in black women. *Epidemiol Rev* 1987; **9**:31–50.

20 Freedman D, Khan L, Serdula M, Ogden C, Dietz W: Racial and ethnic differences in secular trends for childhood BMI, weight, and height. *Obesity (Silver Spring)* 2006; **14**(2): 301–308.

21 Kumanyika S: Environmental influences on childhood obesity: ethnic and cultural influences in context. *Physiol Behav* 2008; **94**(1):61–70.

22 Australian Bureau of Statistics: 2006 Census of Population and Housing (cat. No. 2914.0.55.002). Canberra; 2007.

23 Renzaho A: Migrants Getting Fat in Australia: Acculturation and its Effects on the Nutrition and Physical Activity of African Migrants to Developed Countries. New York: Nova Science Publishers, 2007.

24 Rozman M: Ethiopian Community Diabetes Project Report. Footscray, Victoria: Western Region Health Centre, 2001.

25 Saleh A, Amanatidis S, Samman S: The effect of migration on dietary intake, type 2 diabetes and obesity: the Ghanaian Health and Nutrition Analysis in Sydney, Australia (GHANAISA). *Ecol Food Nutr* 2002; **41**:255–270.

26 Renzaho AMN, Gibbons C, Swinburn B, Jolley D, Burns C: Obesity and undernutrition in sub-Saharan African immigrant and refugee children in Victoria, Australia. *Asia Pac J Clin Nutr* 2006; **15**(4):482–490.

27 ACC/SCN U. UN ACC/SCN: 4th report on the World Nutrition Situation: Nutrition throughout the Life Cycle. Geneva: ACC/SCN in collaboration with the International Food Policy Research Institute, 2000.

28 Renzaho AMN, Burns C: The post migration food habits of Sub-Saharan African migrants- a cross-sectional study. *Nutr Diet* 2006; **63**:91–102.

29 Renzaho AMN, Swinburn B, Burns C: Maintenance of traditional cultural orientation is associated with lower rates of obesity and sedentary behaviours among African migrant children to Australia. *Int J Obes* 2008; 2008 Feb 5 epub ahead of print PMID 18253161.

30 Swinburn B, Egger G, Raza F: Dissecting obesogenic environments: The development and application of a framework for identifying and prioritising environmental interventions for obesity. *Prev Med* 1999; **29**:563–570.

31 Daniels S, Arnett D, Eckel R et al: Overweight in children and adolescents. Pathophysiology, consequences, prevention, and treatment. *Circulation* 2005; **111**:1999–2012.

32 Mavoa H: The "C" Factor: Cultural underpinnings of food, eating and body size. Progress in Obesity Research 10: Proceedings of the 10th International Congress on Obesity; 2006; Sydney. 2006. Paper IS0048.

33 Kumanyika S, Story M, Beech B et al: Collaborative planning for formative assessment and cultural appropriateness in the Girls Health Enrichment Multi-site Studies (GEMS): a retrospection. *Ethn Dis* 2003; **13**(1 Suppl. 1):S15–S29.

34 Ravuvu A: A Fijian cultural perspective on food. In: Jansen A, Parkinson S, Robertson A, eds. Food and Nutrition in Fiji. Suva: Department of Nutrition and Dietetics, Fiji School of Medicine and University of the South Pacific, 1991: 622–635.

35 Renzaho A: Fat, rich and beautiful: changing socio-cultural paradigms associated with obesity risk, nutritional status and refugee children from sub-Saharan Africa. *Health Place* 2004; **10**:113–115.

36 Bentley ME, Caulfield LE, Gross SM et al: Sources of influence on intention to breastfeed among African-American women at entry to WIC. *J Hum Lact* 1999; **15**(1):27–34.

37 Cicirelli V: Sibling relationships in cross-cultural perspective. *J Marriage Fam* 1994; **56**(1):7–20.

38 Greenfield P: Independence and interdependence as developmental scripts: Implications for theory, research, and practice. In: Greenfield P, Cocking R, eds. Cross-Cultural Roots of Minority Child Development. Hillsdale, NJ: Lawrence Erlbaum Associates, Publishers, 1994:1–37.

39 Suaalii T, Mavoa H: Who says Yes? Collective and individual framing of Pacific children's consent to, and participation in, research in New Zealand. *Childrenz Issues* 2001; **5**(1): 39–42.

40 Becker AE: Body, Self and Society. The View from Fiji. Philadelphia: University of Pennsylvania Press, 1995.

41 Defrain J, Defrain N, Lepard J: Family strengths and challenges in the South Pacific. *Int J Sociol Fam* 1994; **24**(2): 25–47.

42 Bentley M, Gavin L, Black MM, Teti L: Infant feeding practices of low-income, African-American, adolescent mothers: an ecological, multigenerational perspective. *Soc Sci Med* 1999; **49**(8):1085–1100.

43 McLoyd V, Hill N, Dodge J: African American Family Life. New York: Guilford, 2005.

44 Dei G: Schooling and Education in Africa: the Case of Ghana. Asmara: African World Press, 2004.

45 Williams L, Ricciardelli L, McCabe M, Swinburn B, Waqa G, Bavadra K: A comparison of the sources and nature of body image messages perceived by indigenous Fijian and European Australian adolescent girls. *Sex Roles* 2006; **55**:555–566.

46 Jain A, Sherman SN, Chamberlain LA, Carter Y, Powers SW, Whitaker RC: Why don't low-income mothers worry about their preschoolers being overweight? *Pediatrics* 2001; **107**(5): 1138–1146.

47 Schreiber G, Robins M, Striegel-Moore R, Obarzanek E, Morrison J, Wright D: Weight modification efforts reported by black and white preadolescent girls: national heart, lung and blood institute growth and health study. *Pediatrics* 1996; **98**(1):63–70.

48 Lindsay A, Sussner K, Kim J, Gortmaker S: The role of parents in preventing childhood obesity. *Future Child* 2006; **16**(1):169–186.

49 Sajdl D: Women and Food—socio-cultural aspects. 2006.

50 Dietz W, Stern L: Guide to Your Children's Nutrition. New York: Villard, American Academy of Pediatrics, 1999.

51 Schultz J, Waqa G, McCabe M, Ricciardelli L, Mavoa H: Report on Interviews with Indigenous Fijian and IndoFijian Youth. Sociocultural Studies in the Healthy Youth Healthy Community Project 2006.

52 Williams L: Body image attitudes and concerns among indigenous Fijian and European Australian adolescent girls. *Body Image* 2006; **3**:257–287.

53 Renzaho A, McCabe M, Swinburn B: Socio-cultural aspect of obesity among African migrants in Australia: examining the intergenerational conflict. Second Congress on Physical Activity and Public Health, 2008; Amsterdam, 13–16 April 2008. 2008.

54 Boggs M, Phongsavan P: Formative Research in the Suva Subdivision. A Qualitative Study to Identify Caregivers' Beliefs, Attitudes and Infant/Child Feeding Practices. Suva, Fiji: UNICEF Pacific, 2001.

55 Grier S, Kumanyika S: The context of choice: Health implications of targeted food and beverage marketing to African Americans. *Am J Public Health* 2008; **98**(9):1616–1629.

56 Kumanyika S, Grier S: Targeting interventions for ethnic minority and low-income populations. *Future Child* 2006; **16**(1):187–208.

57 Henderson V, Kelly B: Food advertsing in the age of obesity: content analysis of food advertising on general market and African American television. *J Nutr Educ Behav* 2005; **37**: 191–196.

58 Outley C, Taddese A: A content analysis of health and physical activity messages marketed to African American children during after-school television programming. *Arch Pediatr Adolesc Med* 2005; **160**:432–435.

59 Tirodkar M, Jain A: Food messages in African American television shows. *Am J Public Health* 2003; **93**:439–441.

60 Evans M, Sinclair R, Fusimalohi C, Liava'a V: Globalization, diet, and health: an example from Tonga (nutritional evaluation). *Bull World Health Organ* 2001; **79**(9):856–862.

61 Mintz S: Tasting Food, Tasting Freedom. Excursions into Eating, Culture, and the Past. Boston: Beacon Press, 1997.

62 Liburd L: Food, identity and African-American women with Type 2 diabetes: an anthropological perspective. *Diabetes Spectrum* 2003; **16**:160–165.

63 Mendoza J, Drewnowski A, Cheadle A, Christiakis D: Dietary energy density is associated with selected predictors of obesity in U.S. children. *J Nutr* 2006; **136**:1318–1322.

64 Drewnowski A, Specter S: Poverty and obesity: The role of energy density and energy costs. *Am J Clin Nutr* 2004; **79**: 6–16.

65 Block J, Scribner R, De Salvo K: Fast food, race/ethnicity, and income: A geographic analysis. *Am J Prev Med* 2004; **27**(3):211–217.

66 Powell L, Chaloupka F, Bao Y: The availaibility of fast-food and full-service restaurants in the United States: associations with neighborhood characteristics. *Am J Prev Med* 2007; **33**(4 Suppl.):S240–S245.

67 McLoyd V: The impact of economic hardship on black families and children: psychological distress, parenting, and socioemotional development. *Child Dev* 1990; **61**(2): 311–346.

68 Swinburn B, Pryor J, McCabe MP et al: The Pacific OPIC Project (Obesity Prevention in Communities)—objectives and design. *Pac Health Dialog* 2007; **14**(2):139–146.

69 Schultz J, Utter J, Matthews L, Cama H, Mavoa H, Swinburn B: Action plans and interventions—the Pacific OPIC (Obesity Prevention In Communities) Project. *Pac Health Dialog* 2007; **14**(2):147–153.

70 Rakowski W: The potential variances of tailoring in health behavior interventions. *Ann Behav Med* 1999; **21**(4): 284–289.

71 Fitzgibbon M: Two-Year follow-up results for Hip-Hop to Health Jr: a randomized controlled trial for overweight prevention in preschool minority children. *J Pediatr* 2005; **146**(5):618–625.

72 Beech B, Klesges R, Kumanyika S et al: Child- and parent-targeted interventions: the Memphis GEMS Pilot Study. *Ethn Dis* 2003; **13**:S1-40–S1-53.

73 Cross T, Bazron B, Dennis K, Isaacs M. Towards a Culturally Competent System of Care. Washington, DC: National Technical Assistance Center for Children's Mental Health, Georgetown UniversityChild Development Center, 1989.

74 RACP 2008. *An Introduction to Cultural Competency*. Royal Australian Collete of Physicians. www.racp.edu.au (Accessed 14 May 2008).

75 McLean N, Griffin S, Toney K, Hardeman W: Family involvement in weight control, weight maintenance, and weight-loss interventions: a systematic review of randomized trials. *Int J Obes Relat Metab Disord* 2003; **27**(9): 987–1005.

76 Kumanyika SK, Obarzanek, E, Robinson TN, Beech BM: Phase I of the Girls Health Enrichment Multi-Site Studies (GEMS): conclusion. *Ethn Dis* 2003; **13**(1 Suppl 1): S88–91.

CHAPTER 18

Developing countries perspective on interventions to prevent overweight and obesity in children

Laura M. Irizarry and *Juan A. Rivera*
Center for Research in Nutrition and Health, National Institute of Public Health, Cuernavaca, Morelos, Mexico

Summary and recommendations for research

- Although the prevalence of childhood obesity continues to rise in developing countries, the experiences of developed countries dominate the prevention literature.
- Diverse cultural beliefs, economic contexts, and social and political systems call for a suite of timely and comprehensive interventions that can be tailored to a specific population or geographic region.
- As countries progressively undergo rapid economic growth and urbanization, they face the challenges posed by coexisting undernutrition and obesity. Interventions must be sufficiently flexible in approach to meet the needs of heterogeneous communities.
- Evidence of both the effectiveness and the efficacy of nutrition interventions in developing countries is urgently required. While successful interventions may inform future directions, failure may also provide an important opportunity for learning. Attention to resourcing and well-founded partnerships promises to strengthen sustainability when promising interventions are increased in scale.

Preventing Childhood Obesity. Edited by
E. Waters, B.A. Swinburn, J.C. Seidell and R. Uauy.
© 2010 Blackwell Publishing.

Introduction

Previous chapters have thoroughly discussed different types of strategies and interventions aimed at halting the growing obesity epidemic and its consequences. A growing body of literature confirms that effective interventions in a variety of settings, ranging from schools to primary health care centers, have the potential to slow down the progression of obesity. However, the vast majority of childhood obesity prevention and intervention efforts found in the literature have been limited to industrialized countries, predominantly in the United States and Europe. Reported successful interventions—particularly research-based—in the developing world are few and far between.

While important lessons can be drawn from the experiences of industrialized countries in implementing effective prevention efforts, interventions that have worked for developed countries may not necessarily prove effective in the developing world. A myriad of factors including cultural beliefs, social and political systems, and the diverging nutritional reality of low- and middle-income countries call for tailor-made interventions that fit the needs of the unique context of each particular country, region or community. In light of the rising incidence of childhood obesity in the developing world, countries cannot afford to wait any longer. Investing in the identification of the environmental and individual determinants of obesity in each country, and the most effective obesity prevention interventions and strategies to address them early on, can significantly increase the chances of millions of children to live longer and healthier lives.

Setting the context for interventions

Childhood obesity trends

A detailed description of international obesity trends and prevalences has been presented in earlier chapters. Nevertheless, it is necessary to give a general overview of the current situation with regards to overweight and obesity trends in the developing world in order to ascertain the need for developing appropriate childhood obesity prevention strategies and interventions.

For over a decade the increasing prevalence of overweight and obesity among all age groups in developing countries has been documented.[1,2] Today, millions of adults and children alike, in Latin America and the Caribbean, the Middle East and North Africa, Asia and Central Europe suffer from obesity.[3-5] For the most part, the rates of obesity are still much higher among the adult population. However, the information currently available on overweight and obesity trends indicates that in many countries the problem is rapidly escalating among the younger populations.

According to WHO, in 2007 nearly 22 million children under the age of 5 years were overweight worldwide; an estimated 16.5 million of them lived in developing countries. Available data from multiple countries on childhood obesity prevalences using the International Obesity Task Force (IOTF)—cut-off points also highlight alarming trends among school-aged children worldwide. For instance, in China the prevalence of childhood overweight among 2–6-year-old children rose from 14.6% to 28.6% and the prevalence of obesity increased over 700% (1.5% to 12.6%) in less than a decade.[6] In Pakistan a two-fold increase in prevalence of obesity among 5–14-year-old children has been observed in the ten-year span between 1997 and 2007.[7] Similarly, in Thailand the prevalence of obesity in children 6–12 years of age increased by 27.9% in just two years.[8] In Latin America, evidence from Chile indicates that from 1987 to 2000 the prevalence of obesity among first grade Chilean boys and girls increased by 161.5% and 138.0%, respectively.[3] While according to the Mexican National Health and Nutrition Survey 2006 (NNHS-06) the overall national prevalence of overweight and obesity among Mexican children ages 2–18 increased from 16% in 1999 to 24.3%—a 52% increase in a seven-year period.[9]

Ironically, these countries have struggled to eradicate child hunger and undernutrition for decades. While a few countries, such as Chile, have come close to totally eradicating malnutrition, stunting is still prevalent in most other countries where a growing incidence of obesity has been documented. In turn, as countries progressively undergo rapid economic growth and urbanization they are faced with implications and challenges posed by the coexistence of undernutrition and obesity.

An example of the type of challenges brought about by this phenomenon is the recent finding that children who are undernourished in the first two years of life, but who rapidly gain weight in childhood or adolescence, are at higher risk of developing nutrition-related chronic disease later in life.[10] These children will most likely face the common long-term outcomes of suffering from undernutrition during the critical development period, including shorter adult height and reduced human capital formation, as well as the multiple social, emotional and economic costs associated with obesity later in life. The long term impact of such a cycle being repeated among large numbers of children could be catastrophic. Most notably, the majority of developing countries will not have the capacity to deal with the demands that such a cycle would pose on the medical system.

In view of the multiple short- and long-term negative implications associated with the obesity epidemic facing developing countries around the globe, particularly when the condition is observed at an early age,[11] the need for timely and comprehensive interventions is evident. However, in contrast to the recognized availability of effective actions and interventions for the prevention and control of childhood undernutrition globally,[12,13] evidence is lacking on efficacious and effective intervention for the prevention and control of overweight and obesity in both the developed and developing world.

Childhood obesity prevention interventions in the developing world

Evidence of interventions

To date, innumerable interventions, programs and initiatives have been developed and implemented to counteract childhood obesity worldwide. Innovative approaches have been undertaken in order to deal with the problem. These have been led by a variety of actors, including parents, teachers, governments, research institutions, not-for-profit organizations and, in many cases, have come about through partnerships and collaborations between some of the actors previously mentioned. Regrettably, recent reviews of the scientific literature, specifically looking at research-based prevention efforts and their effectiveness, point to only two research-based interventions that have taken place in developing countries.[14,15] While a few of the studies in developed countries have dealt with culturally diverse populations, the bulk of the evidence comes from the experience of programs in the United States and the United Kingdom and therefore the implied socio-economic context bears little resemblance to that of developing countries.

It should be noted that other efforts, while not strictly evidence-based interventions, have also been undertaken in developing countries. Considering the information drawn by monitoring systems and surveys, the important role of large-scale community wellness programs and the potential impact of public policies related to nutrition and physical activity, these types of efforts should not be completely disregarded in our examination of the evidence on interventions. Evaluating their results should be considered as part of the process for the design of future interventions or efforts to improve existing efforts. A review and brief description of key efforts identified follows.

School interventions

While there are multiple advantages and disadvantages associated with working at the school level, it is usually asserted that the school environment offers a unique opportunity to reach a large number of children over an extended period of time. Therefore, many consider it to be an optimal setting in which to carry out interventions targeted at children and adolescents (see Chapters 11 and 12). Not surprisingly, the only science-based evidence on efficacy and feasibility of childhood obesity interventions in developing countries comes from research pilots carried out in primary and secondary schools.

Following a longitudinal controlled evaluation study design, an intervention by Kain and colleagues sought to have an impact on the weight status of Chilean children from the 1st grade through to the 8th.[16] The six-month nutrition and physical education intervention program included the implementation of an educational program for children, increased availability of healthier foods at the school kiosks and the implementation of an enhanced physical activity component, along with the provision of the equipment required to support it. Parents and teachers were also considered as part of the intervention efforts and specific activities were undertaken with them to raise awareness about childhood obesity issues. While the study did not show a reduction of BMI at end line, other general improvements in nutrition and physical fitness were observed.

In Thailand, Mo-suwan and colleagues conducted an enhanced physical activity intervention with kindergarten children and monitored the impact of their intervention after six months.[17] Over the course of a seven month intervention period children assigned to the intervention group took part in a structured exercise regimen three times per week in addition to the regular physical education curriculum. The additinal activities carried out included a walk prior to morning classes and dance sessions after naptime. Contrary to the results of the Chilean study period, at the end of the study period the trial came close to showing a significant reduction in BMI. Yet, the post-intervention study revealed a rebound in the participating children's BMI scores. While the scores did not return to the level of those recorded at baseline they suggest a limited long-term impact of the intervention.

In the near future additional programmatic scientific evidence on school-based interventions in developing countries will be available from two interventions being conducted in Mexico and Brazil at this time. Funded as part of the Healthy Lifestyles Healthy People Obesity Prevention Initiative sponsored by the International Life Sciences Institute (ILSI) and the Pan American Health Organization (PAHO), both projects consist of multi-year community-based interventions aimed at preventing obesity through the modification of diet and physical activity patterns. Both projects, one working with school-aged children ages 8–11 (Mexico) and the other targeting adolescents aged 15–19 years (Brazil), will yield evidence that will allow us begin to fill the existing voids in the scientific literature to informe in the design of effective strategies in the context of everyday conditions. Preliminary results from the study in Mexico[18,19] point key environmental factors at the school level that are potentially responsible for the rapid increase in childhood obesity rates among school-age children in the country. A summary of the results follows.

An initial assessment of the school environment and the physical education program was conducted in 12 public schools in Mexico City. Qualitative and quantitative tools were used to help identify barriers and opportunities in the design and implementation of potential strategies. The focus of the initial assessment was to get a measure of food availability and intake, as well as the physical activity patterns of 4th and 5th grade students during school hours. Based on the IOTF cutt-off points and classification systems the Results from this evaluation revealed that[20]—27% of the study population was overweight and 14% was obese (41% combined prevalence). The evaluation of the school environment indicated a wide availability of food high in fat and sugar and low nutritional value and a lack of policies or regulations concerning food sales in and around schools. It was also found that on average children have five opportunities to eat over the course of the 4.5 hours they spend at school every day and that only a small minority of children bring food to eat at school from the home.

Interestingly existing food distribution programs at the school were also found to contribute a significant amount of calories to children's overall intake while at school. The menu offered as part of the National School Breakfast Program—designed at a time when undernutrition was still the most pressing nutritional challenge—distributes energy-dense foods, rich in fat and sugar, including flavored sugar-sweetened whole milk, ready-to-eat sugar sweetened cereals or bread, and other products rich in fat and sugar, cookie or dessert that is also high in fat and sugar. In turn, the program offers a limited variety of fruits about once a week. The formative research assessment also revealed that children have limited drink choices. A limited or total lack of access to potable water was documented. Consequently, for those children who do not bring water from home the only beverage option at the school is the sugar-sweetened beverages available for purchase.

In order to better capture the quality of food available within the school, a system was developed to categorize food based on nutritional value. Healthy foods included fruits, vegetables, low fat dairy products and water. Unhealthy foods were classified into two groups: foods that would be acceptable if prepared or served differently—for example, baked instead of fried or served in smaller portions—and those that could not be modified and had a low nutritional value. In addition, a food inventory was developed to quantify all food and beverage portions. Based on this evaluation system, only 19% of the foods listed were considered to be healthy, while 81% were classified as unhealthy. Of these, only 31% would be acceptable if modifications were made while 50% were packaged or processed foods with no room for improvement.

Observations of children's physical activity patterns during physical education class and recess pointed to very low physical activity levels among children. Evaluations conducted using various methodologies including the System for Observing Fitness Instruction Time (SOFIT), pedometers and accelerometers confirmed that children spent most of their time standing. Overall, during PE class children engaged in moderate to vigorous physical activity (MVPA) a total of 11 minutes per week or 26% of the time, two thirds of the time walking and only about one third in vigorous physical activity. During recess, children engaged in MVPA 36.1% of the time or an average of 10.7 minutes per day. The other 77% of the time was spent walking. Overall, the total amount of time spent engaged in physical activity physical was approximately 65 minutes per week and less than 20 minutes was devoted to activities other than walking.

Based on the information collected as part of the initial assessment previously described mentioned above a science-based school intervention was developed with the input of the Secretariat of Education and the school community. Given the breadth of the formative research conducted prior to the design of the intervention it is expected that the program will have a significant impact in food and beverage intake, activity patterns and health and nutrition knowledge. If proven to be successful, it can serve as a concrete model for other countries to follow in the near future.

There are several additional examples of other school-based initiatives, programs and policies likely to have a positive impact in halting the obesity epidemic in developing countries.[21] However, no published information was found with regards to their impact. For instance, in Brazil it is mandatory for 70% of the foods provided by the school meals program to be basic or minimally processed foods. In the same way, and along with the implementation of more nutrition education and structured physical activity into the school curriculum, notable changes have been made to Chile's National School Breakfast Program in order to provide more fruits and vegetables as part of the daily offer of food options. In China, the Ministry of Education has been encouraging schools to increase the time allocated for physical activity, while in South Korea dietitians have incorporated the school meals program staff to ensure that more nutritious and well-balanced foods are offered in schools.[22]

Community-based initiatives

Communities can play an important role in preventing childhood obesity. Most school-aged children spend a significant number of their waking hours at school; the rest are usually spent in their homes and communities. Agita, a multi-level intervention in an ongoing large-scale community based program to promote physical activity in Brazil is a model intervention for countries to consider when evaluating models for community based initiatives. Many countries have already emulated it including Colombia with Muevete Bogota & Risaralda Activa, Argentina with Amoverse, and Uruguay with Muevete Uruguay.[23] The program's main objective is to promote an active lifestyle in the general population through a variety of strategies targeting children, adolescents and adults alike. Recent findings suggest that Agita has played an appreciable role in increasing the levels of physical activity and general knowledge about its importance in São Paolo.

Other initiatives with community-wide reach targeting individuals of all ages in developing countries include: the implementation of a health promotion policy with a focus on food, nutrition, physical activity and other risk factors for nutrition-related chronic diseases in Chile,[24] a yearly healthy lifestyle campaign to raise awareness about different health issues among the Malaysian population, a variety of large-scale programs on nutrition and physical activity for disease prevention in Cuba and a pilot currently being tried in 32 South Korean health centers to evaluate the impact of providing on-site nutritional services by professional dietitians.[21] While not specifically a community intervention, another recent initiative with community and nationwide reach are the Beverage Consumption Recommendations for the Mexican Population.[25] This initiative, led by the Ministry of Health, is a response to the finding that in Mexico—among the developing countries with the highest rates of obesity among all age groups—beverages contribute a fifth of all calories consumed by Mexicans. The program is in the early stages of its implementation and impact evidence is not yet available.

Monitoring systems

Nutrition monitoring and surveillance is a strategy designed to follow and better understand populations' nutritional status and consumption patterns, as well as to identify the evolution of nutrition-related conditions over time. It is also a valuable tool at the time of developing any intervention, policy or program related to food and nutrition issues.[26,27] Several countries including China, Cuba, Iran, India, South Africa, South, Brazil, Korea and Thailand, have well-established large-scale monitoring systems that, among other nutrition issues, assess the prevalence of overweight, obesity or nutrition-related chronic diseases.[21] In Egypt, Malaysia and Mexico, representative national comprehensive national nutrition surveys are conducted periodically. By collecting and generating information on a population's nutritional status over time these data offer a framework to place and assess the effectiveness of any future childhood obesity prevention interventions in developing countries.

Evaluating the evidence

Childhood obesity prevention in the developing world represents a daunting challenge. Given that the variety of barriers in developing interventions are likely to be as diverse as the millions of children that live in low- and middle-income countries and are already afflicted by obesity or risk of developing this condition, providing specific recommendations for potential actions plans is unrealistic. The different interventions and initiatives identified and previously discussed represent a step in the right direction. However, numerous challenges need to be addressed and information gaps need to be filled.

The role of science-based research

The narrow availability of science-based evidence on childhood obesity intervention studies in developing countries precludes the development of well-informed prevention strategies. As a result, most of the initiatives undertaken to date have been implemented without confirmation that they are the most effective or appropriate ones to serve the needs of the populations targeted. Children are influenced by their immediate environment and those individuals who are closest to them. The school, household, community and health care settings are among the most popular sites for conducting all types of child-centered interventions and obesity preventions strategies are not the exception. Evaluating the impact of interventions in all of these settings in developing countries is unquestionably needed. However, the basis for identifying effective long-term strategies is to fully comprehend the nature of the underlying factors accelerating the childhood obesity that is problematic in the developing world and must seek to understand the multifactorial nature of the problem.

For example, issues of safety and accessibility to adequate facilities might disallow some children to participate in physical activity. Similarly, physical and financial barriers are known to prevent families from purchasing nutritious foods such as fruit and vegetables—as well as safe drinking water in cases when potable drinking water is not available—and coerce them to rely on more convenient cheap, non-perishable, calorie-dense products for sustenance. In some societies erroneous perceptions bring about dangerous practices such as overfeeding children or mothers opting out of breastfeeding. Moreover, taking into account information on motivation, eating behaviors and food preferences can be a valuable element in the design of interventions. These types of issues, while not initially considered as research-based studies are designed, are also an essential component of conducting comprehensive solution-oriented scientific research.

Learning by doing

Evidence-based intervention projects can yield information on efficacy or on efficiency. Efficacy refers to the impact of an intervention in a controlled setting; effectiveness refers to the impact of an intervention in a real world setting. Both types of information are valuable and necessary in the process of understanding the issue at stake. However, the rate at which the obesity epidemic is evolving means that many countries cannot afford to wait for the most efficacious programs in childhood obesity prevention to be identified to then implement them. There is a need to conceptualize and implement flexible methodologies that allow for the evaluation of large-scale interventions as they are implemented. Establishing rigorous monitoring and evaluation systems, while allowing for enough flexibility in ongoing programs to make changes as necessary, is a feasible alternative in settings where there is an urgency to intervene.

Sustainability

Effectiveness is not the sole factor determining an intervention's long-term sustainability. Even when an intervention or pilot project has proved to be effective, a number of additional factors need to be in place in order to ensure long-term sustainability or potential to be scaled-up. Lack of organizational structure and insufficient funding are usually the primary factors that lead to the cessation of otherwise successful nutrition interventions. In many cases, childhood obesity prevention interventions will call for the investment of significant resources to promote and facilitate improved nutrition and physical activity. In the context of limited resources, it is necessary that intervention undertaken among those with low and middle incomes takes into account the cost of upkeeping the initiative devised beyond the initial pilot, particularly when science-based interventions evaluated exclusively for their efficacy, energy and financial resources are invested in programs that will not be sustainable long term. In the interest f serving large numbers of individuals, emphasis should be placed on the evaluation of pilot interventions that have the potential to be sustained even when scaled up at a national level.

Building partnerships is another crucial factor to developing sustainable childhood obesity interventions and prevention efforts in developing countries. Whether carried out at school, community or household level, the relevant key actors need to be involved in the decision-making process regarding the potential strategies to be implemented. Particularly when interventions are carried out at the school and community level, building partnerships among public agencies, community members, industry and other constituents is likely to bring about a supportive environment in which any program will have better odds of having a positive impact.

The double-burden challenge

One of the most complex and inevitable challenges faced by countries developing strategies to face the growing rates of childhood obesity where undernutrition prevails is working around existing nutrition programs. One of the universal goals of most nutritional assistance and supplementary feeding programs in developing countries has been to promote normal growth and development in children. Through the provision of energy-rich foods such as whole milk and fortified cereals at the household and school level these programs ensure that children meet their daily caloric needs. However, among populations experiencing nutrition transition, and where some beneficiaries already meet the recommended daily energy allowance, universal feeding programs are likely to promote obesity.

As obesity prevention strategies are developed in developing countries, the role of supplementary nutrition programs must not be overlooked. While they are likely to continue to be necessary for segments of the population, their structure must respond to the changing nutritional reality of transitioning countries. Failing to do so will inevitably result in the execution of programs that have conflicting objectives simultaneously. Therefore, particularly in rapidly developing countries and urban areas, existing pro-poor nutrition programs should begin to identify strategies by which children continue to receive an adequate nutrition while at the same time avoiding the risk of their becoming overweight. Specifically, in geographical areas where under- and overnutrition are observed, potential strategies include the revision of the types and quality of foods offered as part of school breakfasts and lunch program menus (i.e. providing reduced fat milk and including more fruit and vegetables), a revision of national feeding practices guidelines and recommendations, and the modification of targeting mechanisms of program benefit distribution.

Conclusion

The prevalence of unhealthy weight in children is increasing in developing countries at a high rate. The potentially devastating long-term consequences of this epidemic on children's quality of life call for immediate actions and policies aimed at the prevention and control of these conditions. Although there is consensus that the caloric energy imbalance that has resulted from the simultaneous increase in consumption and decrease in levels of activity is a determining factor in the problem, the relative importance of more distal factors is still contested. Hence, the need to promote physical activity and healthy diets in a variety of different settings, particular those that children are influenced by or take part in, such as the home, school and community, is widely accepted.

At a global level, increasing children's physical activity levels and reducing energy intake will require environmental changes so that the option to make healthy choices is available. Only in environments where healthy choices are an option will communication strategies to inform and motivate reach their full potential. Producing effective interventions, particularly in developing countries, poses countless logistical challenges that require careful examination. Yet, in many cases the nature of the problem does not afford countries the luxury of conducting preliminary research. Programs and interventions need to be developed and implemented without further delay and based on the best available evidence. The key to their success lies in the implementation of thoughtful monitoring, evaluation plans and malleable structures. Only then will we be able to generate evidence-based literature to learn from—evidence that bravely documents failures, is unassuming about successes and allows all of us to draw lessons from a wide range of experiences.

References

1 Martorell R, Kettel Khan L, Hughes ML, Grummer Strawn ML: Obesity in Latin American women and children. *J Nutr* 1998; **128**(9):1464–1473.
2 Martorell R, Kettel Khan L, Hughes ML, Grummer-Strawn LM: Overweight and obesity in pre-school children from developing countries. *Int J Obes* 2000; **24**:959–967.
3 Kain J, Vio F, Albala C: Obesity trends and determinant factors in Latin America. *Cad Saúde Pública* 2003; **19** (Suppl. 1):S77–S86.
4 Amigo H: Obesity in Latin American children: situation, diagnostic criteria and challenges. *Cad Saúde Pública* 2003; **19**(Suppl. 1):S163–S170.
5 Prentice AM: The emerging epidemic of obesity in developing countries. *Int J Epidemiol* 2006; **35**:93–99.
6 Luo J, Hu FB: Time trends of childhood obesity in China from 1989 to 1997. *Int J Obes* 2002; **26**(4):553–558.

7 Jafar TH, Qadri Z, Islam M, Hatcher J, Bhutta ZA, Chaturvedi N: Rise of obesity with persistent rates of undernutrition among urban school-aged Indo-Asian children. *Arc Dis Child* 2008; **93**:373–378.

8 Kumanyika S, Jeffery RW, Morabia A, Ritenbaugh C, Atipatis VJ: Obesity prevention: the case for action. *Int J Obes* 2002; **26**:425–436.

9 Bonvecchio A, Safdie M, Monterrubio E, Gust T, Villalpando S, Rivera J: Overweight and obesity trends in Mexican children 2 to 18 years of age from 1988 to 2006: results of the National Health and Nutrition Survey. 2006.

10 Victora CG, Adair L, Fall C et al, for the Maternal and Child Undernutrition Study Group: Maternal and child undernutrition: consequences for adult health and human capital. *Lancet* 2008; **371**:340–357.

11 Long A, Reed R, Lehman G: The cost of lifestyle health risks: obesity. *J Occup Environ Med* 2006; **48**:244–251.

12 Bhutta ZA, Ahmed T, Black ER et al, for the Maternal and Child Undernutrition Study Group: Maternal and child undernutrition: what works? Interventions for maternal and child undernutrition and survival. *Lancet* 2008; **371**: 417–440.

13 Rivera JA, Sotrés-Alvarez D, Habicht JP, Shamah T, Villalpando S: Impact of the Mexican program for education, health and nutrition (Progresa) on rates of growth and anemia in infants and young children. A randomized effectiveness study. *JAMA* 2004; **291**:2563–2570.

14 Bautista-Castaño I, Doreste J, Serra-Majem L: Effectiveness of interventions in the prevention of childhood obesity. *Eur J Epidemil* 2004; **19**:617–622.

15 Summerbell CD, Waters E, Edmunds LD, Kelly S, Brown T, Campbell KJ: Interventions for preventing obesity in children. *Cochrane Database Syst Rev* 2005; (3): Art. No. CD001871. doi: 10.1002/14651858.CD001871.pub2

16 Kain J, Uauy R, Albala FV, Vio F, Cerda R, Leyton B: School-based obesity prevention in Chilean primary school children: methodology and evaluation of a controlled study. *Int J Obes* 2004; **28**:483–493.

17 Mo-suwan L, Pongprapai S, Junjana C, Puetpaiboon A: Effects of a controlled trial of a school-based exercise program on the obesity indexes of preschool children. *Am J Clin Nutr* 1998; **68**:1006–1011.

18 Safdie M, Bonvecchio A, Theodore F et al: Promoting physical activity and a healthful diet in the Mexican school system for the prevention of obesity in children. Final Report to ILSI and PAHO. 2008.

19 Jenninngs-Aburto NJ, Nava F, Bonvecchio A, Safdie M, Casanova I, Gust T, Rivera J: Physical activity during the school day in public primary schools in Mexico City. *Salud Pública Méx* 2009; **51**(2):141–147. In press.

20 Cole T, Bellizzi M: Establishing a standard definition for child overweight and obesity worldwide: international survey. *BMJ* 2000; **320**:1–6.

21 Doak C: Large-scale interventions and programmes addressing nutrition related chronic diseases and obesity: examples from 14 countries. *Public Health Nutr* 2002; **5**(1A): 275–277.

22 Zhai F, Fu D, Du S, Ge K, Chen C, Popkin BM: What is China doing in policy-making to push back the negative aspects of the nutrition transition? *Public Health Nutr* 2002; **5**:269–273.

23 Matsudo V, Matsudo S, Andrade D et al: Promotion of physical activity in a developing country: the Agita Saõ Paulo experience. *Public Health Nutr* 2002; **5**:253–261.

24 Albala C, Vio F, Kain J, Uauy R: Nutrition transition in Chile: determinants and consequences. *Public Health Nutr* 2002; **5**:123–128.

25 Rivera JA, Muñoz-Hernández O, Rosas-Peralta M, Aguilar-Salinas CA, Popkin BM, Willett WC: Consumo de bebidas para una vida saludable: recomendaciones para la población mexicana. *Salud Publica Mex* 2008; **50**:173–195.

26 Mason JB, Habicht J-P, Tabatabai H, Valverde V: Nutritional Surveillance. Geneva: WHO, 1984:1–194.

27 McGinnis JM, Harrell JA, Meyers LD: Nutrition monitoring: interface of science and policy. *J Nutr* 1990; **120**(Suppl. 11): 1437–1439.

PART 3
Evidence generation and utilization

This section covers several rapidly evolving areas in relation to obesity evidence. Laurence Moore and Lisa Gibbs review the current state of evaluating community-based obesity prevention programs. The theories and past experience of community action programs all point to the need for multi-strategy, multi-setting, community-owned interventions, but the complexity that this creates poses real challenges for program evaluators. Formative evaluation involves the development work with many stakeholders and the process evaluation has to account for many interventions applied unevenly across many settings in the true organic fashion of community development. Impact and outcome evaluations are a challenge because robust evaluation designs are usually not possible for whole-of-community programs. We need new quantitative and qualitative methods to give us confidence about the effectiveness of interventions because the risks of type 1 (false positive) and type 2 (false negative) errors are very real.

No less challenging are the economic evaluations of obesity interventions. As Marj Moodie and Rob Carter point out, the economics of obesity is moving from describing the problem in absolute dollar terms to evaluating the cost–effectiveness of interventions in terms of incremental cost–effectiveness ratios. These can be from empirical studies or modeling studies of intervention versus comparison populations. Modeling methodologies using the best available data to determine the likely cost–effectiveness (and uncertainyy intervals) of interventions are relatively new to the evidence portfolio for health researchers. However, while we await more empirical cost–effectiveness studies, we need to use these modeled results to help inform priorities for obesity prevention.

Jaap Seidell explores the importance of monitoring the childhood obesity epidemic and how these monitoring programs can help to galvanize action and evaluate impacts. In Australia, there have been only three national surveys of childhood obesity—1985, 1995 and 2007. How extraordinary it is that a wealthy country such as Australia can allow such a serious epidemic to sweep over its children without even investing in measuring it more than every 10–13 years. Imagine measuring the road toll, food poisoning, hospital admissions, or pharmaceutical bill every decade or so!

Rebecca Armstrong leads the chapter on knowledge translation and exchange, which is a rapidly emerging area, not only for obesity prevention. It took 264 years for the definitive study proving that limes prevented scurvy to be translated into British Navy policy. We are somewhat faster these days, but the lessons learned from early days of clinical guidelines are instructive—creating evidence is hard but getting it implemented is much harder. Much more effort is needed in this "back end" of the process of knowledge translation and this is particularly the case for obesity prevention because of the complexity of the many systems that need to change to reduce obesogenic environments. A major component of knowledge translation is advocacy and Jane Martin provides a clear set of guidelines about the elements of effective advocacy and the planning and implementation of successful advocacy campaigns. The obesity world has a lot to learn from successful advocacy for other issues such as tobacco, alcohol and drugs.

CHAPTER 19

Evaluation of community-based obesity interventions

Laurence Moore[1] and *Lisa Gibbs*[2]

[1] Cardiff Institute of Society and Health, School of Social Sciences, Cardiff University, Cardiff, UK
[2] Jack Brockhoff Child Health and Wellbeing Program, McCaughey Centre, Melbourne School of Population Health, University of Melbourne, Melbourne, Australia

Summary and recommendations for research

- Evaluation of complex social interventions needs to go beyond examining whether an intervention works overall in order to address the larger question, "what works, for whom, and in what circumstances?" and even better, to help us to understand "why?"

- Interventions need to have been thoroughly developed through the prior stages, which may involve theoretical development, qualitative testing, modeling, feasibility testing and an exploratory trial, prior to large-scale summative evaluation.

- Once the prototype intervention has been developed, it is important to pilot test the intervention, or at least the key components of the intervention, with a particular focus on its feasibility, acceptability and delivery, and evidence of the hypothesized causal processes being triggered as anticipated.

- It is perfectly feasible to allow variation in intervention form and composition, provided that the basic function and process of the intervention is standardized. This reproduces realistically within the trial the kind of variation that will naturally occur in real world practice.

- The RCT design ensures that systematic differences in external influences between groups do not occur and thereby ensures that an unbiased estimate of the average effect of the intervention is obtained.

- It is crucially important in an effectiveness trial of a complex community intervention to conduct a comprehensive qualitative investigation within the trial, so that variable factors can be monitored.

Introduction

This chapter attempts to provide pragmatic guidance on the key issues which need to be considered when evaluating community based action intended to prevent obesity. In seeking to provide useful guidance for evaluators, the chapter does not dwell on the many methodological and epistemological debates that have dominated the public health and health promotion literature over the vexed question of the optimal approach to evaluating complex community interventions (see Box 19.1). However, the reader is encouraged to learn from the substantial work on evaluation of complex social and public health improvement interventions that lies outside the specialized literature on obesity prevention. It is important that the developing community of multi-disciplinary obesity prevention research teams do not waste resources on repeating the mistakes and debates that have hampered progress in these other areas of significant related research and evaluation activity.

Preventing Childhood Obesity. Edited by
E. Waters, B.A. Swinburn, J.C. Seidell and R. Uauy.
© 2010 Blackwell Publishing.

Box 19.1 Methodological debate: polarization or pragmatism?

- Historically, there has been debate over the relative merits of quantitative and qualitative research methods in the evaluation of social interventions.
- The period from the late 1960s to the early 1980s was a "golden age of evaluation" with 245 "randomized field experiments" conducted in areas such as criminal justice, social welfare, education and legal policy.[5]
- Pragmatic mixed method approaches, where methods or combinations of methods are pragmatically chosen to address the specific research question,[6] has been lacking but is now developing.
- Public health is necessarily cross-disciplinary requiring the combination and integration of research methods from a diversity of contributing disciplines.[7]
- More recently, there has been a call for a transdisciplinary science approach using a shared conceptual framework to draw together the most rigorous and appropriate discipline-specific theories, models, methods and measures for the question being posed.[8]

A further lesson to be learned from experience elsewhere is that the term "evaluation" covers a wide range of activities, which vary greatly across a number of dimensions. While this chapter focuses on the evaluation of community interventions, within that focus, it is important to recognize that evaluation projects will vary according to the purpose of the evaluation, the resources available to conduct the evaluation, and the complexity of the intervention to be evaluated. We consider each of these three dimensions, with a primary focus on the evaluation of complex community interventions, and the key stages in the evaluation of such interventions.

Evaluation: purpose and resources

In planning any evaluation, it is important to consider why that evaluation is taking place. Many evaluations, particularly those carried out by practitioners rather than researchers, are undertaken primarily as an exercise in accountability, with an emphasis on documenting or measuring what happened, with possibly some attempt to identify the impact, of a particular funded activity. Such evaluations are of limited scope and are not really the concern of this chapter, as they are more appropriately conducted within a project management or performance assessment framework, rather than being considered as evaluative activities. Any true evaluation should aim to produce learning and/or improvement. A good professional ethic requires that lessons are learned regarding the process and impact of an intervention and that there is continuous ongoing assessment of whether the intervention is working as anticipated and having the desired outcomes. It is critical that the possibility that interventions can do harm is not rejected. Many well-intentioned interventions have been found to be doing more harm than good in terms of their main purpose,[1] while others have unanticipated impacts or are detrimental to subgroups of the target population. It is also important that professionals strive to improve the quality of interventions, whether by improving their reach, effectiveness, efficiency or equity.

What is evaluation?

There has been much debate as to the definition of "evaluation", and how it is distinct from "research". Shaw[2] proposes a three-level taxonomy, in which "evaluation" (which we refer to as practitioner evaluation) is characterized by a focus on practical problems with the objective of informing practice immediately and locally. It is usually undertaken by practitioners with little emphasis on scientific rigor, an enhanced form of reflexive professional practice. "Evaluation research" uses stronger methods and seeks to have an impact on practice to improve effectiveness and efficiency, with dissemination through professional and policy networks and in the grey literature. And Shaw's third level is "applied research", which is led by researchers using strong methods and is disseminated through peer-reviewed scientific papers with the aim of producing generalizable knowledge with an impact on theory and practice over a long-term period.

This chapter adopts a definition of evaluation in line with Pawson and Tilley,[3] who see the purpose of evaluation "as informing the development of policy and practice"[4] rather than focusing simply on measurement or increased understanding.

Complexity: moving beyond "what works?"

Primarily quantitative summative evaluation research methods utilize randomized controlled trials (RCT) and other experimental and quasi-experimental research designs to identify whether an intervention works better than the counterfactual, which may be no intervention, normal care or an alternative intervention. It is widely accepted that such research designs are the optimal designs to address the "what works?" question, as they eliminate or reduce potential biases in estimating intervention effects. However, in the context of complex social phenomena, the value of evaluations that focus only on "what works?" is limited,[4] since the effectiveness of interventions will vary significantly in association with variations in factors such as context, delivery and acceptability.

Whilst experimental research may show us what changes occurred following the intervention, without other forms of concurrent research activity we are left in the dark as to what the intervention actually was in its manifest form, and can only base our conclusions on the naïve assumption that the intervention was unproblematically delivered as conceived, and reproduced equally unproblematically in each context. However, it is almost certain that delivery of any complex intervention will vary. Artificial attempts at fully standardizing delivery across contexts, failing to allow any tailoring of the intervention, may not only prove unworkable in real world settings, but might also inhibit effectiveness.[9] However, acknowledgement that trials must allow an intervention to be, to some extent, "out of control"[9] brings about challenges in terms of understanding what it is about the intervention that does or does not "work".

Furthermore, social interventions do not act in an undifferentiated manner upon passive recipients. Outcomes arise through a dynamic interaction between agent and intervention, with an intervention that facilitates change for one individual or subgroup often failing for others. A key example is the tendency for health education interventions to be more effective among educated groups and, therefore, widening rather than narrowing inequalities. For these reasons, evaluation of complex social interventions needs to go beyond examining whether an intervention works at the aggregate level, in order to address the larger question, "what works, for whom, and in what circumstances?" and even better, to also help us to understand "why?"

Weiss distinguishes implementation theory and program theory.[10]

- **Implementation theory** focuses on the components of the intervention, how it was carried out and what results it produced. Implementation theory largely treats each intervention component as a black box, and does not seek to understand the mechanisms through which the intervention brings about change.
- **Program theory** additionally focuses on the causal processes and mediators[11] through which the intervention brings about its effects, and which may vary across populations, time and contexts.

Gabriel et al[12] and Pawson and Tilley[3] suggest that experimental and quasi-experimental methods can only play a limited role in addressing the "what works, for whom and in what circumstances?" question. Pawson and Tilley propose realist evaluation as an approach that can answer this question through the development of a more comprehensive program theory with particular emphasis on contexts and mechanisms. Cook[13] argues that, rather than developing alternative methods to conduct theory based evaluations, it should be possible to use theory-based methods within an experimental framework. In the main body of this chapter, we identify ways in which this may be done, as a critical part of a mixed methods approach to developing and evaluating complex community-based obesity prevention interventions.

Evaluating complex interventions—research stages and research questions

One stereotype, which is still alarmingly prevalent, is that biomedical research funders publish research calls and maintain peer-review systems that favor proposals for randomized trials of obesity prevention interventions. There is an imperative to identify effective interventions and a need to collect strong evidence of effect, so the obvious solution is to fund trials. However, Sanson-Fisher et al[14] caution that a sole focus on randomized trials as *the* method for evaluation may prevent the posing of complex questions that the method simply cannot answer, stifling innovation in intervention development. All too often, the research proposals submitted and funded are strong in terms of trial methodology, but very weak in terms of the proposed intervention, drawn up by a group of "experts" with no public involvement, and a weak and unidisciplinary theoretical and empirical basis. There is an inevitable bias towards relatively simple, individually targeted interventions rather than more complex, multi-level interventions and programs. On the other hand, complex multi-level or settings-based interventions developed in conjunction with the target audience and based on strong theory, are typically evaluated using weak research designs with either no estimate of effect due to the absence of a summative evaluation, or potentially biased effect estimates at best.

How to reorient towards helpful, rigorous evaluation designs

A helpful way to move away from this stereotype and to prevent the perpetuation of an inadequate evidence base is to recognize the different stages of research needed in the development, evaluation and implementation of complex interventions. In health promotion, there are a number of models of stages of intervention research and evaluation, including Nutbeam's six-stage development model.[15] and Green's PRECEDE/PROCEED framework,[16] which identify different research questions and the various research methods that are appropriate at each stage. The United Kingdom Medical Research Council (MRC) also published a framework for the evaluation of complex interventions[17] which identified five research stages, mirroring the stages of drug development research, of which the fourth stage was the definitive randomized controlled trial. This model has been particularly helpful in highlighting the need for interventions to have been thoroughly developed through the prior stages, which may involve theoretical development, qualitative testing, modeling, feasibility testing and an exploratory trial, prior to large-scale summative evaluation, thus limiting the reproduction of the stereotype described in the previous paragraph. Box 19.2 gives an example of an intervention that has passed through a member of research stages prior to the final trial phase.

Notwithstanding necessary simplification, we provide recommendations for selected research designs

Box 19.2 Case study: *fun 'n healthy in Moreland!*

A series of obesity prevention studies conducted in Victoria, Australia demonstrate how the different research stages can be developed. A review of the child obesity literature was conducted in 2004 and highlighted the increasing prevalence of child overweight and obesity and the complexity of environmental and socio-cultural determinants. A clear gap in the evidence base in relation to effective interventions led to the development of a pilot study conducted in three diverse primary schools—in inner urban, suburban and rural areas. This formative evaluation was conducted to test the feasibility and acceptability of a trial methodology, and a range of school, parent and child measures. As a result of this pilot study, the methodology and measures were adjusted to improve acceptability and comprehensibility and a study design was developed using a socio-environmental theoretical framework actioned by the Health Promoting in Schools Framework and culturally competent community development strategies. A five-year cluster randomized controlled trial, *fun 'n healthy in Moreland!*, was consequently implemented in 2004. This child health promotion and obesity prevention intervention and research study involves 24 primary schools in an inner-urban, culturally diverse area of Melbourne, Australia. It is being conducted in partnership with the local community health service. A comprehensive mixed method summative evaluation will allow an assessment of what worked, for whom, how, why and at what cost.[27]

for each of the two main stages of evaluation research, formative and summative. These stages can be mapped onto the three frameworks referenced above, and provide a useful classification to aid the presentation of key issues in evaluation research design. However, it is not intended to suggest that the identification of specific research questions can only be done with reference to this sequence. Indeed, as we describe below, it is likely that key questions regarding the acceptability, implementation and causal mechanisms of an intervention will need to be addressed at each of these stages.

Formative evaluation

By identifying five research stages that are comparable to the stages of drug development research, the MRC framework also helps to highlight the fact that in drug research the majority of research effort and funding goes into early stage basic science and pharmacological research, to identify disease mechanisms and potential ways to interrupt these mechanisms through the identification of active pharmacological agents. Only a small proportion of this research produces candidate therapies for drug trials.

The early research stages require a wide range of methods, which may include: epidemiological analysis of primary or secondary data to identify key modifiable correlates, including attitudes and mediating psycho-social factors; interviews and/or focus groups with key stakeholders and members of the target population to identify causal factors and potential intervention pathways; development of partnerships; discussions with key experts in the field; systematic review of the literature to identify potentially effective interventions and/or eliminate or modify candidate interventions that have previously been found unsuccessful. As a result of this early pre-intervention research and informed by theoretical perspectives ideally drawn from a range of disciplines (see Box 19.3), the composition and rationale for a prototype intervention can then be set out, identifying the key changes the intervention will directly instigate, and those that will be expected to follow as a result of the intervention. It will often be useful to map this out as a diagrammatic model, which will ideally include not only the intervention components and expected outcomes (as in an implementation model) but also a description of the mechanisms of change, key mediating factors and change mechanisms, and potential positive and negative impacts and outcomes not directly associated with the primary target variable.

Once the prototype intervention has been developed, it is important to pilot test the intervention, or at least key components of the intervention, with a particular focus on its feasibility, acceptability and delivery, and evidence of the hypothesized causal processes being triggered as anticipated. This pilot work will involve small samples and primarily qualitative research methods, but may also involve quantitative surveys among pilot study samples. An example pilot investigation was that of the Free School Breakfast Initiative in Wales,[18] where primarily qualitative case study analysis of an initial sample of schools identified important lessons for the modification of the scheme,

Box 19.3 Different forms of expertise

Comprehensive evaluations of complex community-based studies need to be conducted by a transdisciplinary team of researchers to address the complexity in both the intervention and the evaluation. For example, the *fun 'n healthy in Moreland!* study has a national team of investigators with expertise in obesity research, physical activity measures, nutrition studies, evaluation, community interventions, statistics, qualitative and mixed method approaches, body image, child and family eating habits, health economics, and cultural competency. Their depth of knowledge in their field of specialty and their interest in complex interventions makes them ideally suited to joint consideration of appropriate approaches and measures, synthesis and development of new measures and approaches, where necessary.[8] There are also strong partnerships with policy, practice and public stakeholders in various state and local government departments.

However, this does not mean that the evaluation should be "expert-driven".[12] Instead, the engagement of the community as partners and decision makers is more likely to support the development of an appropriate methodology and measures, will maximize the reach of recruitment, assist in the development of in-depth understandings of the data and meaningful findings, and assist with community dissemination and ownership of results.[29,30] In *fun 'n healthy in Moreland!*, the local community health service and the schools were partners in the intervention and research study with an active role in decision making, and cultural groups and local community organisations provided guidance and support. This approach is known as community-based participatory research in which the expertise of the community is recognized in respectful partnerships that involve mutual knowledge exchange and decisionaking at all stages of the research process.[30,31]

as well as identifying key issues to be addressed in the subsequent larger-scale evaluation. Another example was the Outreach School Garden Project implemented in two remote indigenous school communities in north-west Queensland, Australia.[19] The evaluation incorporated a descriptive qualitative approach supplemented by some quantitative data to assess feasibility, acceptability and capacity building.

The final stage of formative evaluation is to conduct an exploratory trial, in which a final draft or Beta-test version of the intervention is tested in a small-scale summative evaluation. This is not designed or powered to identify an estimate of intervention effectiveness, but is intended to further test feasibility and acceptability, identify any important remaining barriers or problems that need to be addressed, and to allow testing and estimation of key components of the summative evaluation methodology, such as outcome measurement, recruitment and retention rates. In many cases, the intervention development, pilot testing and exploratory trial phases may indicate that the intervention is not acceptable to the target population or to stakeholders in potential future implementation, or that there is no evidence that it is bringing about the anticipated changes and effects. This will lead to further modification or abandonment of the intervention. In other cases, the intervention will appear to be feasible, acceptable and potentially effective, and will thus be ready for large-scale summative evaluation.

Summative evaluation

Once a thorough process of formative evaluation has been completed, an important remaining question, which for most policy decision makers is the most important question, is whether or not the intervention works. This requires an estimate of the intervention's effect, which may then be compared to that of competing interventions, often using some form of economic analysis trading off costs and benefits of alternative programs. Pawson[20] argues that, in the case of complex social programs, it is futile to attempt an experimental evaluation, comparing a "policy on" condition with a "policy off" condition, since such programs are constantly being manipulated and renegotiated and are never stable. With such large-scale complex programs, Pawson states that "the hallowed comparison of treatment and controls is ... that between a partial and complete mystery".

It is undoubtedly the case that many large-scale interventions are not feasibly or sensibly evaluated using experimental or quasi-experimental control group designs. This will generally be the case for mass media interventions applied to whole populations, and to large-scale complex social programs that will be substantially modified during the course of their evaluation. It is also unlikely to be worth while implementing a scientifically rigorous research design of an intervention that is so politically contentious that its evaluation is "doomed to success", the political cost of a negative evaluation being too high.[21]

Efficacy and effectiveness

However, it is also very important to recognize that it is not necessary for an intervention to be highly standardized and uniformly delivered in all instances, in order for a valuable experimental summative evaluation to take place. This would be the case in an efficacy trial, which seeks to identify the impact of the intervention when delivered in ideal circumstances. However, since health promotion interventions are so dependent on context adaptation and the quality of delivery, the value of efficacy trials is limited.[22] For example, smoking education interventions have been found to work well in efficacy trials, when delivered by enthusiastic teachers with ample curriculum time, yet when implemented in the real world they have not been found to be effective.[23] In an effectiveness trial, a pragmatic approach is taken, with the intervention delivered in the trial in the same (variable) way as would realistically be achieved in the real world.

It is often argued that health promotion interventions are so dependent on the way they are implemented, and upon the context (environment, policy etc.) within which they are delivered, that context-dependent adaptation is crucial to maximize effectiveness and, therefore, randomized controlled trials are not suited to their evaluation. However, the RCT design actually has the advantage that the randomization process ensures that systematic differences in external influences between groups do not occur and thereby ensures that an unbiased estimate of the average effect of the intervention is obtained. It is, however, crucially important in an effectiveness trial of a complex community intervention to conduct a comprehensive qualitative investigation within the trial, so that these variable factors can be monitored. Thus, the qualitative research provides information on the factors that support or attenuate the effectiveness of the intervention. To undertake a trial of a complex intervention without an embedded qualitative process evaluation would be to treat the intervention as a black box, with no information on how it worked, how it could be improved, or what the crucial components of the intervention were. By including a process evaluation within the trial, data can be collected to address these questions, both to inform future development of the intervention, and also to contribute to theory and understanding of the relation between context, mechanism and outcome. Thus, it is perfectly feasible to allow variation in intervention form and composition, provided that the basic function and process of the intervention is standardized.[24] This reproduces realistically within the trial the kind of variation that will naturally occur in real world practice, and also allows assessment of key delivery and context variables that may influence intervention effectiveness and acceptability.

An example of such an effectiveness trial is a cluster randomized trial of fruit tuck shops in schools, in which intervention schools were allowed to implement the tuck shops in a variety of ways. The process evaluation assessed the alternative methods and led to the production of a booklet published by the Food Standards Agency providing guidance on alternative models.[25] The trial produced an unbiased estimate of the overall impact of fruit tuck shops on fruit consumption and norms, and also identified an important synergistic interaction between fruit tuck shops and school policy on foods that pupils were allowed to bring to schools.[26]

Control group allocation and treatment

If a summative evaluation of a community intervention is conducted without a control group, then it is impossible to attribute any measured change in outcomes to the intervention as this may in whole or in part be a change that will have occurred anyway. The measurement of outcomes in a comparison group is therefore important, although great care must be taken to minimize selection bias, whereby the two groups are different in observed or unobserved characteristics. A common source of selection bias is to implement an intervention in selected communities where key stakeholders and partnership organizations are committed to the intervention, and then to recruit randomly selected communities to act as controls. Even if these control communities are well matched in terms of socio-economic and other characteristics that may be expected to be related to obesity, it is

always very possible that greater change would have occurred in the intervention community in the absence of the intervention, owing to the commitment and interest of the key organizations and stakeholders.

Similarly, communities with high levels of obesity, compared to other comparison communities, will be more likely to experience favorable outcomes owing to regression to the mean, rather than any true intervention effect. Careful selection of intervention and control communities, and analyses that adjust for baseline differences, can mitigate the potential effects of selection bias. However, to minimize selection bias it is always preferable to allocate communities to intervention or control conditions through random allocation, in which each community has an equal chance of being allocated to the two groups. Such a design is known as a cluster randomized trial, in which randomization is undertaken at the level of the community (or other cluster such as school or workplace), rather than of individuals. Whether random or non-random allocation is used, analyses of community level interventions and sample size calculations must use appropriate statistical methods that take account of the non-independence of individuals within communities.[28]

In a controlled experimental or quasi-experimental research design, the counterfactual, or control group treatment, must be carefully determined. In an effectiveness trial of a novel community intervention, it is not necessary to require the control group to follow a highly standardized course of relative inaction. It would be ethically unacceptable to require communities to withdraw existing policies or actions. A common solution is to allow all communities within the evaluation to continue with existing policies and actions (normal care), with the intervention communities getting the extra experimental intervention or program in addition to current activities. Part of the process evaluation should be to monitor non-intervention activity in all communities, to provide data on variations in "normal care" across the two experimental groups.

Outcomes and sustainability

It would appear to be axiomatic that evaluations of obesity prevention interventions should include obesity or body mass index as a primary outcome.

However, it may be the case that the logic model underpinning the intervention does not suggest that there should be an impact on obesity within the follow-up period. Thus, effective community interventions that have substantial important impacts and outcomes should not be considered ineffective simply because there is no effect on obesity or BMI within what is usually a limited follow-up period. Equally, as was found in the context of tobacco control,[32] where there has been substantial progress in reducing smoking prevalence in many developed countries, any one intervention will be unlikely to have a statistically significant impact, given the hugely complex array of determinants of obesity. It may be possible to identify intermediate outcomes on the causal pathway, possibly including nutritional and/or physical activity outcomes, but caution should be taken regarding self-report measures where there is often substantial error and bias. Given the development of community obesity surveillance systems, such as the child measurement program in England, it may be possible to have long-term monitoring of obesity and BMI outcomes through data linkage of study participants with such datasets, although the quality of data collected in such systems remain unclear.

An important consideration in the evaluation of a community intervention is the sustainability of the intervention. Sustainability refers to the likelihood of the intervention having an ongoing impact on the community, beyond the trial follow-up period. This generally requires changes embedded in systems and structures at higher levels of the ecological framework than the individual, such as the physical environment, policies and accountability measures. There are many definitions of sustainability depending on the goals and theoretical framework of the intervention and subsequently the evaluation.[33] An intervention which targets changes in health behaviors may focus in the evaluation on sustainable health outcomes for community members, which may include anthropometry or health behaviours.[34] This is often best achieved by using repeated cross-sectional data collection within intervention and comparison communities, thus detecting sustained population effects, rather than by following up individuals over a long-term period, which will be subject to attrition, and accumulation of substantial and unmeasured exposures that will dilute and potentially bias effect estimates.

Alternatively, for an intervention conducted under a socio-ecological theoretical framework, the focus may be on the sustainability of physical and social environmental changes and/or institutionalized changes in organizational policies and programs. Measurement of environmental and organizational changes may be achieved through auditing processes, monitoring the changes objectively through photographic evidence (e.g. to show changes in the playground design to encourage active play) and organizational documents (e.g. canteen menus, organizational policy documents reflecting the introduction of drinking water policies and annual reports reflecting accountability for the changes introduced). Conversely, a community-development-based intervention may be evaluated with sustainability defined as the capacity of the community to maintain and continue to respond to the central issue on an ongoing basis. This would require an assessment of the competence and commitment of the key stakeholders.[35–37] These are all valid and important measures of sustainability and in a complex community intervention may all be required to adequately assess the sustainability of effect. If the implemented changes require ongoing additional investment of resources by the community then assessment of funding options is also critical to sustainability measures and assessment of the capacity of the community for consolidation and ongoing commitment to the changes.[38]

Evaluation funding

One of the major barriers to conducting rigorous evaluations of community interventions is the expense and scale of the interventions, a cost beyond the majority of research funders. Transdisciplinary research teams,[8] involving policy, practice and community partners are required, as exemplified in Box 19.3. There is a need to move away from the common stereotype, in which community projects funded by NGOs or state lotteries or service agencies are expected to evaluate themselves with a limited research budget, possibly 5%–15% of the program budget, and limited research expertise. Gabriel[12] cites an example in the USA of a Centre for Substance Abuse Prevention including an evaluation component in funding grants for intervention programs. Invariably, these evaluations are too ambitious in scope and, because of limitations in terms of research rigor, produce very little useful evidence to inform policy and practice change. They should either be more limited in scope, focusing on specific research questions, or there needs to be a mechanism to bring in other research funding.[34] A final option may be to redistribute these agencies' funding so that a proportion of funded projects are comprehensively evaluated, with the remainder freed from the distractions of a superficial evaluation exercise. This means that such research requires strong collaboration between academics and research funders on the one hand, and government agencies on the other.

Wales has experienced success in working with government to identify innovative policies, which have been initially implemented in an experimental fashion, allowing randomized trials to be conducted, nested within the national roll-out of both the free school breakfast initiative,[26] and the national exercise referral scheme. However, these examples remain rare, with governments generally remaining unwilling to expose novel policies to the glare of a rigorous independent controlled evaluation,[39] despite the need to take advantage of these opportunities to generate evidence of effectiveness.[40] Alternatively, policy decisions are made in parallel with the conduct of evaluations rather than being informed by the outcome of the evaluations.[39]

Conclusion

Community-based obesity prevention interventions will typically include some variability in application to accommodate different settings and populations. This presents challenges for evaluators. However, rigorous evaluation can be achieved through staged development and evaluation of the intervention program. This may progressively involve theoretical development, qualitative testing, modeling, feasibility testing and an exploratory trial. It will then be possible to conduct a large-scale intervention and summative evaluation. At this point, a randomized or cluster randomized trial is both possible and desirable to achieve an unbiased estimate of the average effect of the intervention. It is also critical to include comprehensive qualitative investigations to identify and understand the factors that influence the effectiveness of the intervention. A well developed and comprehensive approach such as this requires substantial funding as well as collaboration and commitment between researchers, funding bodies and government agencies.

Acknowledgements

Lisa Gibbs acknowledges the NHMRC Capacity Building Grant for Child and Adolescent Obesity Prevention and the Jack Brockhoff Child Health and Wellbeing Program for salary and operational funding support. The authors also acknowledge the helpful feedback provided by Andrea Sanigorski following a review of a draft of the chapter.

References

1 Macintyre S, Petticrew M: Good intentions and received wisdom are not enough. *J Epidemiol Community Health* 2000; **54**:802–803.
2 Shaw I: Qualitative Evaluation. London: Sage, 1999.
3 Pawson RD, Tilley N: Realistic Evaluation. London: Sage, 1997.
4 Tilley N. Realistic Evaluation: An Overview. 2000, from www.danskevalueringsselskab.dk/pdf/Nick%20Tilley.pdf (accessed 5 February 2007).
5 Boruch RF, McSweeney AJ, Soderstrom EJ: Randomized field experiments for program planning, development, and evaluation: an illustrative bibliography. *Eval Q* 1978; **2**: 655–695.
6 Johnson RB, Onwuegbuzie AJ: Mixed methods research: a research paradigm whose time has come. *Educ Res* 2004; **33**:14–26.
7 Baum F: Researching public health: behind the qualitative-quantitative methodological debate. *Soc Sci Med* 1995; **40**: 459–468.
8 Abrams D: Applying transdisciplinary research strategies to understanding and eliminating health disparities. *Health Educ Behav*, 2006; **33**:515–531.
9 Hawe P, Shiell A, Riley T: Complex interventions: how "out of control" can a randomised controlled trial be? *Bri Med J* 2004; **328**:1561–1563.
10 Weiss CH, ed.: Theory-based evaluation: past, present, and future. Progress and future directions in evaluation: perspectives in theory, practice and methods. In: Rog DJ, Fournier D, eds. New Directions for Evaluation. San Francisco: Jossey-Bass, 1997:41–55.
11 Baron RM, Kenny DA: The moderator-mediator variable distinction in social psychological research: conceptual, strategic and statistical considerations. *J Pers Soc Psychol* 1986; **51**:1173–1182.
12 Gabriel RM: Methodological challenges in evaluating community partnerships and coalitions: Still crazy after all these years. *J Community Psychol* 2000; **28**:339–352.

13 Cook TD: The false choice between theory-based evaluation and experimentation. *New Dir Eval* 2000; **87**:27–34.

14 Sanson-Fisher RW, Bonevski, B, Green LW, D'Este C: Limitations of the randomized controlled trial in evaluating population-based health interventions. *Am J Prev Med* 2007; **33**:155–161.

15 Nutbeam D: Evaluating health promotion—progress, problems and solutions. *Health Promot Int* 1998; **13**:27–44.

16 Green LW, Kreuter MW: Health Promotion Planning: An Educational and Ecological Approach. Mountain View, CA: Mayfield, 1999.

17 MRC: A Framework for the Development and Evaluation of RCTs for Complex Interventions to Improve Health. London: Medical Research Council, 2000.

18 Roberts J, Murphy S: A Study of the Preliminary Phase of the Welsh Assembly Government "Primary School Free Breakfast Initiative", 2005. http://wales.gov.uk/dcells/publications/info_for_learning_providers/schools/foodanddrink/freebreakfastinitiative/evaluation/firstevaluation-e.pdf?lang=en (accessed 5 October 2009).

19 Viola A: Evaluation of the outreach school garden project: building the capacity of two Indigenous remote school communities to integrate nutrition into the core school curriculum. *Health Promot J Austr* 2006; **17**:233–239.

20 Pawson R: Evidence-based Policy: A Realist Perspective. London: Sage, 2006.

21 Government Chief Social Researcher"s Office: Trying it Out: The Role of Pilots in Policy-Making. London: Cabinet Office, 2003.

22 Flay B: Efficacy and effectiveness trials (and other phases of research) in the development of health promotion programs. *Prev Med* 1986; **15**:451–474.

23 Nutbeam D, Macaskill P, Smith C et al: Evaluation of two school smoking programmes under normal classroom conditions. *Br Med J* 1993; **306**:102–107.

24 Hawe P, Shiell A, Riley T, Gold L: Methods for exploring implementation variation and local context within a cluster randomised community intervention trial. *J Epidemiol Community Health* 2004; **58**:788–793.

25 Moe J, Roberts J, Moore L: Planning and running fruit tuck shops in primary schools. *Health Educ Behav* 2001; **101**:61–68.

26 Moore L, Tapper K: The impact of school fruit tuck shops and school food policies on children's fruit consumption: a cluster randomised trial of schools in deprived areas. *J Epidemiol Community Health* 2008; **62**:926–931.

27 Waters E, Ashbolt R, Gibbs L et al: Double disadvantage: the influence of ethnicity over socioeconomic position on childhood overweight and obesity: findings from an inner urban population of primary school children. *Int J Pediatr Obes* 2008; **3**:196–204.

28 Okoumunne OC, Gulliford MC, Chinn S, Sterne JAC, Burney PGJ: Methods for evaluating area wide and organisation based interventions in health and health care: a systematic review. *Health Technol Assess* 1999; **3**:2132.

29 Israel B, Schulz A, Parker E, Becker A: Review of community-based research: assessing partnership approaches to improve public health. *Annu Rev Public Health* 1998; **19**:173–202.

30 Gibbs L, Gold L, Kulkens M, Riggs E, Van Gemert C, Waters E: Are the benefits of a community-based participatory approach to public health research worth the costs? *Just Policy* 2008; **47**:52–59.

31 RTI International—North Carolina: Community-Based Participatory Research: A Summary of the Evidence. Submitted to: Agency for Healthcare Research and Quality, Maryland, 2004.

32 Chapman S: Unravelling gossamer with boxing gloves: problems in explaining the decline in smoking. *Br Med J* 1993; **307**:429–432.

33 Gruen RL, Elliott JH, Nolan ML et al: Sustainability science: an integrated approach for health programme planning. *Lancet* 2008; **372**:1579–1589.

34 Swinburn B, King L, Bell C, Magarey A, O'Brien K, Waters E: Obesity prevention programs demand high quality evaluations. Commentary article. *Aust N Z J Public Health* 2007; **31**:305–307.

35 McLeod J: The Partnerships Analysis Tool, VicHealth. Melbourne, Australia, 2009 www.vichealth.vic.gov.au/~/media/About%20Us/Attachmentsassets/contentFiles/VHP%20part.%20tool_low%20res.pdf (accessed 5 October 2009).

36 Bush R, Dower J, Mutch A: Community Capacity Index Version 2. Centre for Primary Health Care, The University of Queensland, 2002.

37 Maclellan-Wright MF, Anderson D, Barber S et al: The development of measures of community capacity for community-based funding programs in Canada. *Health Promot Int* 2007; **4**:299–306.

38 Langberg JM, Smith BH: Developing evidence-based interventions for deployment into school settings: a case example highlighting key issues of efficacy and effectiveness. *Eval Program Plann* 2006; **29**:323–334.

39 Sowden SL, Raine R: Running along parallel lines: how political reality impedes the evaluation of public health interventions. A case study of exercise referral schemes in England. *J Epidemiol Community Health* 2008; **62**:835–841.

40 Wanless D: Securing Good Health for the Whole Population, Final Report, London: HM Treasury 2004.

CHAPTER 20

Economic evaluation of obesity interventions

Marj Moodie and *Rob Carter*
Deakin Health Economics, Deakin University, Melbourne, Victoria, Australia

Summary and recommendations for research

- To date, most health economics studies have focused on "describing" and "predicting" the magnitude of the obesity problem. This type of economic study alone does little to address the issue of obesity.
- The fight against obesity requires a "solutions-based" rather than a "problem-focused" approach. The economic evaluation of specific interventions and strategies to reduce the obesity problem offers the most valuable contribution of health economics.
- Rigorous evaluation of potential interventions is important so that policy-makers know "what works" and "what offers value for money". However, interventions with the best prospects for preventing obesity are likely to pose particular challenges for economic evaluation.
- Furthermore, economists must move beyond evaluation of single interventions to priority setting, and assist in the packaging of interventions into coordinated obesity prevention strategies.

Introduction

Why should economists work in the field of obesity prevention? What wisdom can they bring to bear on the issue that could make a difference to the prevalence and consequences of obesity? This chapter explores the role and content of economic analysis, summarizes the contribution which the discipline

Preventing Childhood Obesity. Edited by
E. Waters, B.A. Swinburn, J.C. Seidell and R. Uauy.
© 2010 Blackwell Publishing.

currently makes, and considers the contribution it could make to the fight against obesity. It draws on current research activity in the field to illustrate some of the specific methodological challenges that confront health economists working in the obesity field, and discusses the directions which economic research needs to take if the discipline is to make a positive and effective contribution to the search for solutions to the obesity crisis.

Why involve economics?

To assess the credentials of health economics to make a contribution, one must first appreciate the nature of economics and the roles which it performs. The fundamental problem addressed by economists is the allocation of scarce resources between competing demands—that is, how to maximize community welfare with available resources. In addressing resource scarcity, economists carry out four separate but interrelated tasks: "description", "prediction", "explanation" and "evaluation".[1]

Describing and projecting the cost burden of obesity

Economics enables us to "describe" current activities, health status and resource use, and to "predict" future trends in the same. To date, most of health economics' contribution to obesity prevention has centered on these two aspects. The past decade has seen a proliferation of descriptive studies which either documented the size of the disease and cost burden attributable to obesity in particular demographic groups or geographical jurisdictions, or made forecasts about the growth in the obesity problem. Whilst several writers in the 1990s[2,3] noted that such "cost of illness" (COI) studies were not particularly common in the area of obesity, more recently, authors[1,4] have referred to the growing literature documenting the economic costs of obesity. Since our earlier documentation of such COI studies of obesity,[1] there have been more studies, including for non-Western jurisdictions.[5,6]

Whilst such COI studies vary in their methodology, they generally measure costs within a prevalence-based framework.[3] The annual cost burden stemming from all cases of obesity-related disease (new or pre-existing) is measured, as the study purpose is generally to inform cost control or financial planning. This contrasts with incidence-based studies,[7] which measure the lifetime costs associated with new cases only, as a baseline against which new measures can be assessed. Most studies confine the cost burden to direct health sector costs arising from the current prevalence and treatment of obesity,[8] with few taking into consideration indirect costs arising from lost productivity[9] or diminished social functioning and quality of life.[10] The lack of consensus about obesity-related illnesses is evidenced by differences between studies in terms of the range of co-morbidities included. Studies vary in terms of the BMI cut-off points used to define obesity, as well as the perspective employed from which to measure costs. Most studies assume a national health system perspective, while some assume a narrower reference frame in terms of geographical jurisdiction[11] or target group.[12]

However, regardless of their choice of methods, these COI studies comprise essentially "descriptive" research focusing on the size of the obesity problem. They quantify the magnitude of the issue and estimate the associated disease burden in monetary terms. Such studies are premised on the basis that knowledge of the costs stemming from an illness will be important in informing decision making around resource allocation. They are considered a valuable tool when advocating for the deployment of additional resources towards obesity prevention, and have been employed by agencies such as the World Bank and the World Health Organization.

However, COI studies have also been the centre of active debate among economists.[13–15] While acknowledging that they may serve three purposes (to justify budgets, to help set funding priorities and to develop intervention programs), Rice[13] argues that the methods need to be sufficiently detailed to permit transparency and to enable the reader to assess whether the results are "fact or fiction". Byford et al[14] pose three key arguments against the conduct and use of COI studies: first, high costs do not necessarily indicate inefficiency and waste; second, the supposed "cost savings" of either fully or partially preventing a disease are likely to be overstated and partly illusory; and third, the condition may not necessarily be amenable to treatment.

More recently, there has been similar questioning about the value of such studies among economists working in the obesity field.[4,16] Roux and Donaldson[4] are highly critical of the economic credentials of such studies and conclude that they add little to the obesity debate, apart from confirming that obesity is a serious societal issue. In an earlier publication,[1] we took a more positive yet cautious approach to COI studies. While acknowledging that descriptive cost estimates can be of value to planners, we also stressed that COI estimates should not be overinterpreted. More importantly, used sensibly and carefully, COI estimates could also have a role beyond simple description and monitoring, as an input into evaluation studies and broad-based priority setting exercises.

The third task of health economics, explanation of obesity, is a relatively new and underdeveloped field. Rosin[17] recently surveyed the growing economic literature on the causes of obesity epidemic, and concluded that the key economic influences on obesity prevalence are food prices, working mothers, urbanization and technological change.

Box 20.1 Glossary of economic terms

Cost–benefit analysis: An analytical tool for estimating the net social benefit of an intervention as the incremental benefit less the incremental costs, with all benefits and costs measured in monetary terms.

Cost–effectiveness analysis: An analytic tool in which costs and benefits of a program and at least one alternative (usually current practice) are calculated and presented in a ratio of incremental cost to incremental benefit. Effects are measured as physical health outcomes (such as weight lost, BMI units saved or life years saved).

Cost-of-illness study: A type of burden of disease study that describes the relationship between current disease incidence and/or prevalence and the consequent resource implications, particularly for the structure and utilization of health services.

Direct costs: The monetary value of a resource provided to deliver medical or social services as part of the management of the disease.

Economic evaluation: A comparative analysis of the costs and outcomes of an intervention measured against a comparator.

Epidemiological modeling: Modelling is used to move from a change in behaviour (such as an increase in physical activity to a change in energy expenditure to the desired outcome (e.g. BMI) using a mix of evidence types and levels.

Incremental cost–effectiveness ratio (ICER): The ratio of the difference in net costs between two alternatives to the difference in net effectiveness between the same two alternatives.

Indirect costs: The value of a decrease in an individual's productivity as a result of the disease.

Indirect evidence: Information that strongly suggests that the evidence exists (e.g. a high and continued investment in food advertising is indirect evidence that there is positive [but propriety] evidence that food advertisement increases sales of those products).

Opportunity cost: The value of the best alternative use of a resource that is foregone as a result of its current use.

Parallel evidence: Evidence of intervention effectiveness for another public health issue using similar strategies (e.g. the role of social marketing, regulation or behavioral change initiatives in tobacco control, sun exposure, speeding, etc.).

Threshold analysis: A decision aid used to assist resource allocation decisions. A decision maker may specify an acceptable level of investment or return on an investment. This information is then used to determine which combination of parameter estimates could cause the threshold to be exceeded or achieved.

Evaluating interventions to prevent obesity

Irrespective of their views about the potential contribution of COI and causal research, most economists would agree that the fight against obesity requires a "solutions-based" rather than a "problem-focused" approach, and that it is the fourth plank of economics, "economic evaluation", which offers the potentially most valuable contribution. High quality evaluations of potential obesity interventions are required so that policy-makers know "what works" and what offers "value for money".

A full economic evaluation of a selected intervention is characterized by the incremental assessment of both its costs and benefits measured against a comparator, usually current practice.[18] This enables the analyst to answer the essential policy question of "what difference the intervention is likely to make to the disease burden and what is the net cost of doing so". The change in costs is compared with the change in outcomes and reported as an incremental cost–effectiveness ratio (ICER). Typically, with obesity interventions, the ICER will be reported as "net cost per kg of weight lost", "net cost per BMI (body mass index) unit saved", "net cost per life-year gained" or "net cost per quality-adjusted life-year saved (QALY).

To date, very few obesity interventions have been subjected to rigorous economic evaluation. It has primarily been treatment options involving either surgical or pharmacological therapies that have been economically evaluated.[1,19] These two publications between them identified only one economic evaluation of a preventive intervention[20] and seven of lifestyle treatment interventions involving diet, exercise or behaviour therapy. Furthermore, some of these were not targeted exclusively at obese persons, but at persons for whom obesity was a serious complication or subsequent disease. In a recent discussion of the literature, Cawley[21] listed four published cost–effectiveness studies of anti-obesity interventions,[20,22–24] of which only one was a preventive measure.

Our own work in assessing the cost–effectiveness of thirteen interventions targeting unhealthy weight gain in children and adolescents as part of the Assessing Cost–Effectiveness in Obesity (ACE-Obesity) project in Australia[25] is, to our knowledge, the largest body of work around the economic evaluation of obesity interventions. The interventions were evaluated using a consistent protocol to avoid methodological confounding. Some individual interventions evaluations have been published, and summarized results are available (www.health.vic.gov.au/healthpromotion/

quality/ace_obesity.htm).[26] While some interventions targeted children already overweight or obese,[27] most were of a preventive nature. They included interventions targeting either all children (reduction of TV advertising of high-fat food and high-sugar drinks to children[28]) or specific groups of children in the school (multi-faceted school-based programs), child care (Active After-school Communities program[29]) or neighborhood settings (TravelSMART Schools, Walking School Bus[30]).

The challenges in producing quality economic evaluations

The lack of economic evaluations of potential preventive interventions for obesity has been noted in the literature.[4,21] With the growing profile of obesity as a major public health issue, governments around the world are allocating funds towards obesity programs, and public health organizations, local governments and schools, and so on, are searching for solutions to the problem. However, such efforts are severely limited by the lack of information about what works, and more specifically, how to achieve the greatest "bang for the buck".[21] Cost–effectiveness analysis is a tool that can help answer this question as it facilitates intervention assessment in terms of their net costs per unit of benefit.

However, before embarking on economic evaluation, there first needs to be credible evidence that an intervention actually works (or at the very least, strong program logic built on accepted theoretical foundations that facilitate defensible assumptions about effectiveness). The evidence base around the effectiveness of programs and policies remains limited. Few obesity interventions have been rigorously evaluated, and examples of funding being directed towards measures for which there is no evidence are commonplace. The need for quality evaluations of obesity prevention initiatives has been a recent topic in the literature.[31]

Sufficiency of evidence of effectiveness was a key issue in the Australian ACE-Obesity study. Unlike previous ACE studies in other disease areas where there was sufficient evidence of effectiveness based on high quality study designs (such as randomized controlled trials, cohort studies, case-control studies), the paucity of trial-based evidence around obesity

interventions made it necessary to move from a traditional evidence classification based on epidemiologic study design to a new classification which incorporated other forms of evidence not usually captured, such as "parallel evidence", "indirect evidence" and "epidemiological modeling".

The ACE-Obesity study was criticized for its optimistic assumption about the maintenance of effect over time.[32] The study acknowledged that full maintenance of benefit was highly improbable, and aimed to be transparent in its conclusion by undertaking "threshold analysis" to determine the extent to which the 100% maintenance of benefit could be reduced before an intervention would cease to be cost-effective.[25] This assumption and the associated sensitivity analysis was a direct product of the absence of available data on which to model an alternative trajectory and the exploratory nature of the ACE-Obesity work.

But the paucity of interventions which have sufficient demonstrated evidence of effectiveness is not the only challenge to achieving quality economic evaluation. Cawley[21] raises additional issues in conducting cost–effectiveness analyses on obesity prevention interventions—flaws in using BMI to define different health states; the lack of consensus around the QALYs associated with such health states; the need for QALYs to vary by demographic variables, and for longer follow-up studies to ascertain the persistence of QALY savings over time. Cawley strongly advocates for the role of cost–effectiveness analyses in informing policy-makers and public health practitioners, and ponders the potential dangers of misallocated resources and unintended consequences which may arise from rushing ahead with interventions before establishing their effectiveness and cost–effectiveness credentials.

Another important challenge is that the type of interventions that offer the best prospects for preventing obesity are most likely to be in areas that lend themselves less readily to conventional economic evaluation methods. Effective health promotion interventions are often complex and multi-faceted, community-based rather than individual-based and inter-sectoral rather than restricted to the health sector. Further, they are likely to include policy initiatives, such as changes in taxes, subsidies or regulations, which offer their own unique difficulties for economic appraisal and establishing the evidence base. Such complex interventions not only create difficulties in outcome measurement, but also in attributing effects to different elements of the intervention and in apportioning costs, particularly where the intervention is of an organic community-based nature.

Richardson[33] addressed this issue when he proposed a four-fold classification of possible outcomes of health promotion based on a distinction between "disease cure", "individual health promotion", "community welfare" and "systemic change". While arguing that there is justification in economic theory for including all of the benefits of a health promotion program in an economic evaluation, he acknowledges that some of the current analytical tools may be of little practical use. Besides the issue of inadequate information about outcomes, the specific problem with health promotion programs is to achieve a balance between the demand for short-run accountability and the need for programs to reach sufficient maturity to achieve long-run objectives. Potentially beneficial projects may be jeopardized by premature evaluation.

Community-based interventions pose particular challenges for economic appraisal. The study design is generally of a quasi-experimental nature and interventions may not be standardized, but more of an organic nature varying and evolving according to the needs of particular communities. While challenging to evaluate, such programs are exactly the type of intervention for which research data about cost–effectiveness is currently lacking and urgently needed. Such an example is the Pacific OPIC Project (Obesity Prevention in Communities), a large multi-country project targeting adolescent obesity in Australia, New Zealand, Fiji and Tonga.[34] It involves pre and post measurement of 15,000 adolescents in intervention and control sites, and the implementation of interventions in schools, churches and villages. In such a big, complex project involving large numbers of organizational entities across four countries, it was vital that the economic evaluators were included from the initial design stage, and that the economic evaluation was adequately funded and underpinned by a clear, detailed protocol. Data collection needed to be kept manageable and tractable, given the three-year intervention timeframe, and the competing demands on the project staff and others such as teachers involved in the interventions. In large community-based interventions, the issue of measurement of "current practice" can be problematic. It is difficult to recruit schools, communities as control groups, with the expectation that they meet the same anthropometric measurement and data collection requirements, but without any investment of intervention activities.

In the ACE-Obesity project,[25] threshold analysis was used to provide additional information to policy-makers and to public health practitioners. The interventions evaluated included several existing programs, being implemented at either a national or state level, which were shown to be cost-*ineffective*. Scenario analyses were used to show how such programs could realistically be made more cost-effective through cost-cutting measures, justifiable apportionment of some costs to non-obesity objectives, or measures designed to increase recruitment and participation.[29,30]

Another contentious and problematic issue is the economist's practice of discounting future benefits and costs. For most obesity prevention programs, the discounting of the value of benefits and costs occurring in the future is likely to make the "present value" of benefits obtained after 15–20 years considerably smaller. Another issue is the potential inequity of discounting the benefits of children at the rate of time preference of adults. Richardson[33] puts forward theoretically plausible arguments for employing lower than normal discount rates for distant health benefits. It is for this reason, among others, that quality economic appraisals will report their cost–effectiveness results for a range of discount rates (e.g. 0%, 3%, 5% and 7%).

Moving beyond economic evaluation of single interventions to priority setting

Whilst the previous section discussed some of the challenges facing economists when evaluating obesity interventions, the cost–effectiveness analyses of single, stand-alone interventions are unlikely to be enough to make an effective contribution to policy decisions about strategic directions. A whole range of obesity interventions across diverse settings need to be evaluated, and given resource constraints and multiple policy objectives, decision makers need to have

Box 20.2 Key features of the assessing cost–effectiveness (ACE) approach

- Clear rationale and process for selection of interventions is to be evaluated.
- Standardized evaluation methods are used to avoid methodological confounding.
- The setting, context and comparator is common for all interventions.
- Evaluations are conducted as an integral part of the priority setting exercise.
- Country-specific data is used, wherever possible, for demography, health systems costs and disease incidence/prevalence patterns.
- Evidence-based approach is employed, with extensive use of uncertainty and sensitivity testing
- Information isvassembled by an independent research team.
- Involvement of stakeholders is required to achieve "due process".
- There is a two-stage approach to measurement of benefit.

mechanisms for combining them into effective prevention strategies for achieving healthy weight.

It is with this broader priority setting task in mind that the ACE-Obesity project set out "to assess from a societal perspective the most cost-effective options for preventing unhealthy weight gain in Australia, particularly amongst children and adolescents" in order to inform state and national policy.[25] The key features of the ACE approach to priority setting are shown in Box 2. Every effort was made to support the assumptions underpinning the economic evaluations with standardized methods and the best available evidence.[25] One distinguishing feature was the two-stage approach adopted to the measurement of benefit, to capture the broad-based nature of policy objectives. The technical cost–effectiveness results (ICERs) were placed within a broader decision-making framework, which included considerations that did not lend themselves readily to quantification. Such second stage filters, as they were termed, included "strength of evidence", "equity", "feasibility of implementation", "acceptability of stakeholders", "sustainability" and "side effects".[35] The stakeholder Working Group opted for the separate reporting of the technical results and second stage filter results, arguing that the latter infor-

mation in a qualitative format would be more transparent to policy-makers. The alternative would have been to weight the ICER results and the second filters and then combine them into a single index score.

In addition to confronting issues of how to combine the technical analyses of interventions with broader considerations of decision making, economists also need to tackle issues of how to consider, in a meaningful way, obesity outcomes with any intervention benefits of a non-health nature. For example, in the ACE-Obesity study, no attempt was made to quantify benefits of the Walking School Bus program (such as increased safety around schools, decreased traffic congestion and pollution, increased social cohesiveness, etc.) other than changes in obesity outcomes (increased walking leading to increased energy expenditure and reduced BMI). These non-obesity benefits were acknowledged and threshold analysis was undertaken to ascertain what proportion of costs would need to be attributed to them for the intervention to become cost-effective. An alternative approach would be to include a wider range of outcome measures and attempt more composite measurement approaches—such as attaching monetary values to all outcomes via a cost–benefit analysis (see Box 20.1). Such approaches are possibly more important with respect to obesity interventions than other public health areas, as many lie outside the health sector and are what Shiell[36] terms "social interventions" offering potential health and non-health benefits beyond just the reductions in BMI being measured.

Finally, to add to the complexity of the priority setting process, any budgetary constraints imposed on decision makers need also to be taken into account. Decision makers may not be able to implement the most cost-effective option(s) if the cost of implementation exceeds budgetary limits. Several approaches exist to facilitate this task of matching combinations of interventions to particular budget levels; they range from a simplistic deterministic analysis using a cost–effectiveness league table to more sophisticated methods using Generalized Cost-Effectiveness analysis,[37] stochastic league tables[38] and linear programming.[39] The more sophisticated methods are quite complex and time consuming, yet may not necessarily result in a more optimal ranking of the selected interventions than a simple deterministic cost–effectiveness league table approach. Furthermore, as discussed earlier, there are issues other than the technical cost–effectiveness results which need to be considered in the decision-making process

Conclusions

In terms of obesity prevention, health economics facilitates the performance of four separate but interrelated research tasks. Arguably, in its simplest roles, health economics enables us to "describe" current or predict future activities, health status and resource use. Most of its current contribution has centered on these two simpler aspects. However, whilst knowledge of the magnitude of the obesity problem may be of value when advocating for funds, this type of economic work alone does little to address this pressing public health issue, unless integrated with the more complex tasks of "explanation" and "evaluation".

The fight against obesity requires a "solutions-based" rather than a "problem-focused" approach. It is economic evaluation that offers the most scope for progress, but also the most challenges. Quality evaluations of potential interventions are required, so that policy-makers have reliable information about "what works" and "what offers value for money" to underpin obesity investment decisions. However, the types of interventions that offer the best prospects for preventing obesity are most likely to be in areas that lend themselves less readily to conventional evaluation methods. Furthermore, cost–effectiveness analyses of single, stand-alone interventions are not enough. Economists need to develop methodologies for combining the technical analyses of interventions with broader issues affecting decision making, and of combining, in a meaningful way, obesity outcomes with any non-health benefits. Finally, to make an effective contribution to the field, health economists must move beyond evaluation to priority setting, and assist in the packaging of interventions into coordinated obesity prevention strategies within given budget constraints.

References

1 Carter R, Moodie M: The cost–effectiveness of obesity prevention. In: Crawford D, Jeffery RW, eds. Obesity Prevention and Public Health. New York: Oxford University Press, 2005;165–204.
2 Hughes D, McGuire A: A review of the economic analysis of obesity. Br Med Bull 1997; 53(2):253–263.
3 Kortt MA, Langley PC, Cox ER: A review of cost-of-illness studies on obesity. Clin Ther 1998; 20:772–779.
4 Roux L, Donaldson C: Economics and obesity: costing the problem or evaluating solutions? Obes Res 2004; 12(2):173–179.
5 Ko GTC: The cost of obesity in Hong Kong. Obes Rev 2008; 9(Suppl. 1):74–77.
6 Zhao W, Zhai Y, Hu J et al: Economic burden of obesity-related chronic diseases in mainland China. Obes Rev 2007; 9(Suppl. 1):62–67.
7 Thompson D, Edelsberg J, Colditz GA, Bird AP, Oster G: Lifetime health and economic consequences of obesity. Arch Intern Med 1999; 159:2177–2183.
8 Allison DB, Zannolli R, Narayan KM: The direct health care costs of obesity in the United States. Am J Public Health 1999; 89:1194–1199.
9 Trogdon JG, Finkelstein EA, Hylands T, Dellea PS, Kamal-Bahl SJ: Indirect costs of obesity: a review of the current literature. Obes Rev 2008; 9(5):489–500.
10 Seidell JC: Societal and personal costs of obesity. Exp Clin Endocrinol Diabetes 1998; 106(Suppl. 2):7–9.
11 Finkelstein EA, Fiebelkorn IC, Wang G: State-level estimates of annual medical expenditures attributable to obesity. Obes Res 2004; 12:18–24.
12 Finkelstein E, Fiebelkorn C, Wang G: The costs of obesity among full-time employees. Am J Health Promot 2005; 20:45–51.
13 Rice DP: Cost-of-illness studies: fact or fiction? Lancet 1994; 344:1519–1520.
14 Byford S, Torgerson DJ, Raftery J: Cost of illness studies. Brit Med J 2000; 320:1335.
15 Akobundu E, Ju J, Blatt L, Mullins CD: Cost-of-illness studies: a review of current methods. Pharmacoeconomics 2006; 24(9):869–890.
16 Wiseman V, Mooney G: Burden of illness estimates for priority setting: a debate revisited. Health Policy 1988; 43:243–251.
17 Rosin O: The economic causes of obesity. A survey. J Econ Surv 2007; 2008:1467–6419. doi:10.1111/j00544.x
18 Drummond MF, O'Brien BJ, Stoddart GL, Torrance GW: Methods for the Economic Evaluation of Health Care Programmes, 2nd edn. New York: Oxford University Press, 1997.
19 Avenell A, Broom J, Brown TJ et al: Systematic review of the long-term effects and economic consequences of treatments for obesity and implications for health improvements. Health Technol Assess 2004; 8:1–458.
20 Wang LY, Yang Q, Lowry R, Wechsler H: Economic analysis of a school-based obesity prevention program. Obes Res 2003; 11:1313–1324.
21 Cawley J: The cost-effectiveness of programs to prevent or reduce obesity. The state of the literature and a future research agenda. Arch Pediatr Adol Med 2007; 161:611–614.
22 Maetzel A, Ruof J, Covington M, Wolf A: Economic evaluation of orlistat in overweight and obese patients with type 2 diabetes mellitus. Pharmacoeconomics 2003; 21:501–512.

23 Craig BM, Tseng D: Cost-effectiveness of gastric bypass with severe obesity. *Am J Med* 2002; **113**:491–498.

24 Roux L, Kuntz KM, Donaldson C, Goldie SJ: Economic evaluation of weight loss interventions in overweight and obese women. *Obesity* 2006; **14**:1093–1106.

25 Haby MM, Carter R, Swinburn B et al: New approaches to Assessing cost-effectiveness of obesity interventions in children and adolescents. (ACE-obesity project). *Int J Obes* 2006; **30**:1463–1475.

26 Carter R, Moodie M, Markwick A, Magnus A, Vos T, Swinburn B, Haby MM: Assessing Cost-Effectiveness in Obesity (ACE-Obesity): an overview of the ACE approach, economic methods and cost results. *BMC Public Health* 2009; **9**:419 doi:10.1186/1471-2458-9-419.

27 Moodie M, Haby M, Wake M, Gold L, Carter R. ACE: Obesity—Cost-effectiveness of a family-based GP-mediated intervention targeting overweight and moderately obese children. *Economics and Human Biology* 2008; **6**:363–376.

28 Magnus A, Haby M, Carter R, Swinburn B: The cost-effectiveness of removing television advertising of high-fat and/or high-sugar food and beverages to Australian children. *Int J Obes* 2009; **33**(10):1094–1102.

29 Moodie M, Carter R, Swinburn B, Haby M: The cost-effectiveness of Australia's Active After-School Communities Program. *Obesity* 2009. doi:10.1038/oby.2009-401.

30 Moodie M, Haby M, Galvin L, Swinburn B, Carter R: Cost-effectiveness of active transport for primary school children—Walking School Bus program. *Intl J Behavioural Nutrition and Physical Activity*, 2009; **6**:63 doi:10.1186/1479-5868-6-63.

31 Swinburn B, Bell C, King L, Magarey A, O'Brien K, Waters E: Obesity prevention programs demand high-quality evaluations. *Aust N Z J Public Health* 2007; **31**(4):305–307.

32 Segal L, Dalziel K: Economic evaluation of obesity interventions in children and adults. Letter to the Editor. *Int J Obes* 2007; **31**:1183–1184.

33 Richardson J: Economic evaluation of health promotion: friend or foe? *Aust N Z J Public Health* 1998; **22**(2): 247–253.

34 Swinburn BA, Pryor J, McCabe M, Carter R, de Courten M, Schaaf D, Scragg, R: The Pacific OPIC Project (Obesity Prevention in Communities)—objectives and design. *Health Promotion in the Pacific* 2007; **14**(2):139–146.

35 Carter R, Vos T, Moodie M, Haby M, Magnus A: Priority setting in health: Origins, description and application of the assessing cost effectiveness (ACE) initiative. *Expert Rev Pharmacoeconomics Outcomes Res* 2007; **8**(6):593–617.

36 Shiell A: In search of social value. *Int J Public Health* 2007; **52**:333–334.

37 Murray CJL, Evans DB, Acharya A, Baltussen RP: Development of WHO guidelines on generalized cost-effectiveness analysis. *Health Econ* 2000; **9**:235–251.

38 Hutubessy RCW, Baltussen RMPN, Evans DB, Barendregt JJ, Murray CJL: Stochastic league tables: communicating cost-effectiveness results to decision-makers. *Health Econ* 2001; **10**:473–477.

39 Stinnett AA, Paltiel AD: Mathematical programming for the efficient allocation of health care resources. *J Health Econ* 1996; **15**:641–653.

CHAPTER 21

Monitoring of childhood obesity

Jacob C. Seidell
EMGO Institute for Health and Care Research, Institute of Health Sciences, VU University
and VU University Medical Centre, Amsterdam, The Netherlands

Summary and recommendations for research and practice

- Definitions distinguish between monitoring and screening. Monitoring is purposive, systematic measuring to determine trends over time, variation between populations or places, and so on. Screening is purposive, systematic measurement as well but its purpose is case finding, not the determination of population trends.
- The purpose (trends, differences in populations) and value (measuring leads to action, especially if it is local data fed back to local agencies) need to be considered.
- Childhood obesity does not meet the criteria for screening (mainly because of lack of evidence of effectiveness of interventions).
- There is debate about the obligations and value of feeding (interpreted) anthropometry information back to parents (and for adolescents to them individually).
- The methodology used for monitoring is poor in most cases and, therefore, should be a priority for establishing monitoring systems.

Definitions

In this chapter I define monitoring as purposive, systematic measuring to determine trends over time, variation between populations or places, and so on. I define screening as purposive, systematic meas-

Preventing Childhood Obesity. Edited by
E. Waters, B.A. Swinburn, J.C. Seidell and R. Uauy.
© 2010 Blackwell Publishing.

urement as well, but its purpose is case finding, not the determination of population trends.

In many cases also the term surveillance is used interchangeably with monitoring. According to the Webster's dictionary, clinical surveillance refers to the monitoring of diseases or public health-related indicators by epidemiologists and public health professionals. The differences between monitoring and surveillance are often obscure, although in many instances monitoring pertains to observations and surveillance comprises observations and actions. Surveillance, for instance, includes systems to detect "events" such as infectious disease outbreaks. Frequently, however, a monitoring system is thought to be much more than just collecting and interpreting series of routinely collected data.

For instance, according to the United Nations Populations Fund a monitoring system consists of five critical elements[1]

1. definition of essential data to collect, including case definitions;
2. systematic collection of data;
3. organization and analysis of data;
4. implementation of health interventions based on the data; and
5. Re-evaluation of interventions.

According to the World Health Organization Framework Convention on Tobacco Control (WHO FCTC) surveillance is systematic ongoing collection, collation and analysis of data and the timely dissemination of information to those who need to know, so that action can be taken.[2] Tobacco control surveillance includes prevalence of tobacco use, its health and economic consequences, its socio-cultural determinants and tobacco control policy responses and tobacco industry activities.

The WHO STEPwise approach to Surveillance (STEPS) is another example of standardized international monitoring activities of risk factors for chronic diseases. It is described as a standardized method for collecting, analysing and disseminating data in WHO member countries.[3]

By using the same standardized questions and protocols, all countries can use STEPS information not only for monitoring within-country trends, but also for making comparisons across countries. The approach encourages the collection of small amounts of useful information on a regular and continuing basis.[3]

This chapter does not use the term "surveillance" but rather addresses systematic collection and analysis of data as "monitoring", and identifies individuals for interventions as "screening".

Purposes of monitoring

Monitoring of obesity trends; prediction of future prevalence and health impact

The common form of monitoring is the analyses and interpretation of routine cross-sectionally collected data on indicators of overweight and obesity. These include weight and height derived indices such as BMI or waist circumference.

The monitoring (repeated prevalence data) of BMI in children could lead to the following benefits:[4]

- describing trends in weight status over time among populations and/or subpopulations at a school, district, state or nationwide level;
- creating awareness among school and health personnel, community members, and policy makers to the extent of weight problems in specific populations;
- driving improvement in policies, practices and services to prevent and treat obesity;
- monitoring the effects of school-based physical activity and nutrition programs/policies;
- monitoring progress toward achieving national health objectives or relevant state or local health objectives related to childhood obesity.

Well-known examples of monitoring systems that have included indicators of obesity are the National Health and Nutrition Examination Surveys (NHANES) in the United States.

NHANES has been an exemplary system historically as well as currently and has some unique features so it is described in some detail. Since its inception in 1959, eight separate Health Examination Surveys have been conducted and over 130,000 people have served as survey participants.

The first three National Health Surveys—National Health Examination Survey (NHES) I, II, and III—were conducted between 1959 and 1970. In 1969 it was decided that the National Nutrition Surveillance System would be combined with the National Health Examination Survey, thereby forming the National Health and Nutrition Examination Survey, or NHANES.

Five NHANES have been conducted since 1970. NHANES I (1971–1975), NHANES II (1976–1980), the Hispanic Health and Nutrition Examination Survey (HHANES 1982–1984), NHANES III (1988–1994).

Beginning in 1999, NHANES became a continuous survey. In 1999, 64% of the US population was overweight or obese, while the prevalence of obesity among children and adolescents had more than doubled during the previous two decades. Since then, further moderate increases have been observed, but there now seems to be a gradual leveling off in the trends.

The NHANES surveys have very high response rates (94–97%) and are based on measured weights and heights rather than being self-reported. For example, the Behavioral Risk Factor Surveillance System is the basis for the maps of the USA with states changing color over time indicating an increasing prevalence of obesity. In this Survey, which is based on self-reported heights and weights in adults in a nationwide telephone survey, it was found that the prevalence of obesity in 1999 was 18.9%.[5] At the same time, the prevalence of obesity in the NHANES was 30.5%.[6] This profound difference illustrates that sampling and methodology may have important implications for assessing the problem of obesity. Misreporting of weight and heights are not only problems in surveys in adults. It has been shown that one quarter to one half of overweight adolescents would be missed if based exclusively on self-reported data.[7] Actual and

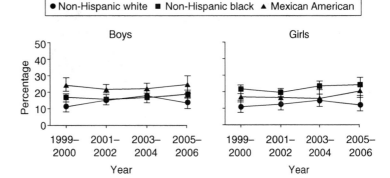

Figure 21.1 Body Mass Index for Age at or Above the 95th Percentile in the United States by Race/ Ethnicity in the period 1999–2006.[9]

perceived body size are correlated with underreporting of overweight.[8]

Figure 1 shows the time-trends of overweight and obesity in the period 1999–2006. The analyses showed no significant changes in the prevalence of obesity over the last seven years and it remained high at an overall figure of 16.3%.

Globally there are few examples of continuous monitoring systems such as NHANES. In most countries data on obesity trends are available from either a series of unrelated surveys using different sampling methods as well methodologies, or from national heath interview survey data with usually relatively low response rates and based on self-reported heights and weights. It has been shown that correction for self-reporting bias is not appropriate unless reporting bias has been assessed in the population that is being studied.[10]

Good examples of systematic surveys in Europe are the National Child Measurement Programme (NCMP).[11] The NCMP is one element of the government's work program on childhood obesity, and is operated jointly by the Department of Health (DH) and the Department for Children, Schools and Families (DCSF). The NCMP was established in 2005. Every year, as part of the NCMP, children in Reception and Year 6 are weighed and measured during the school year to inform local planning and delivery of services for children; and gather population-level surveillance data to allow analysis of trends in growth patterns and obesity. The NCMP also helps to increase public and professional understanding of weight issues in children and is a useful vehicle for engaging

with children and families about healthy lifestyles and weight issues. To encourage engagement, parents can request their child's results from their Primary Care Trusts (PCTs).

In the school year 2007/2008, 973,073 valid measurements were received for children, in England, in Reception and Year 6—about 88% of those eligible. Using sex- and age-specific percentiles to define overweight (85–95th percentile) and obesity (>95th percentile), it was observed that 14.3% and 18.3% of the children aged 10–11 (Year 6) were overweight and obese, respectively. Only 1.4% of the children could be considered underweight.

There has been a plea for an ongoing national population monitoring system covering selected ages at preschool, primary school and secondary school age in Australia.[12]

A good example of a long-standing systematic survey in Asia is the National Nutrition Survey in Japan (J-NNS),[13] an annual nationwide survey on the nutrition and diet of the Japanese people. J-NNS was started in the Tokyo Metropolitan area in 1945 following the end of the Second World War. The survey area was expanded nationwide in 1948. The current survey obtains data from more than 12,000 persons of approximately 5,000 randomly selected households. The survey consists of three parts: a physical examination, a dietary intake survey and a dietary habit questionnaire. The physical examination includes anthropometric measurements and a blood test, the dietary intake survey examines nutrient/food intake with a semi-weighed recording method, and the dietary habit questionnaire monitors nutrition/

diet-consciousness and dietary habits.[13] Recent analyses of BMI distribution curves in Japanese women over six decades of surveys showed both decreases and increases over time, depending on the different age-groups.[14]

Critical elements of appropriate monitoring

Critical elements of monitoring are:

- Representativeness of the target sample. Selected samples in towns, regions or even neighborhoods or social strata can be difficult to interpret in terms of national prevalence data.
- Size of the sample (i.e. how fine-grained the data are for analyses by subgroups of age, sex, social class, etc).
- Frequency of measurements. For some estimate of secular trends at least three measures are needed (preferably more). If a survey is done every five years this implies that 15 years will have passed before any judgement regarding time trends is possible. Continuous monitoring systems are, therefore, preferable also because the continuity of methods is more easily realized when done continuously compared to measurements with relative long time intervals.
- Participation rate and selection bias. The characteristics of non-responders are usually difficult to determine but the possibilities exist that overweight and obese children are less likely to participate in health surveys (particularly when they are also used for case finding). This may be explained by their weight status directly but also of variables related to both overweight and participation such as socio-economic status.
- Validity of measurements. The validity of self-reported heights and weights is low, thus leading to misinterpretation about body composition, fat distribution and health risks.

Monitoring of (potential) determinants and consequences of obesity

Cross-sectional analyses of associations between potential determinants or consequences of obesity may lead to interesting hypotheses but usually inferences about temporal relationships or causation should be made with caution. There are, however, examples of evaluations of interventions using monitoring systems. The interpretations become easier if, for instance, sharp changes in determinants (e.g. physical activity or diet) occur in one part of the population but not in others and are followed by changes in the health outcome (e.g. obesity prevalence) in the part of the population where the determinants changed.

Dietary habits and physical activity patterns may not only cause weight gain and obesity but obese people may also change their habits as a result of their weight status. This, for instance, can produce associations between dieting and obesity but the causal relationships are unclear. An example of this can be found in the study in adolescents in New Zealand by Utter et al.[15] Examination of the nutritional correlates of BMI in the total population found inverse relationships between BMI and consumption of high-fat/high-sugar foods and positive relationships between BMI and eating five or more fruits and vegetables a day (all significant after controlling for age, sex and ethnicity). For example, students who drank the most soft drinks or ate fruit and vegetables infrequently had the lowest mean BMI. Students' attempts to change their weight significantly moderated the relationships between most nutritional behaviors and BMI. In most cases, among students not trying to change their weight, expected relationships were observed; among students trying to lose weight, unexpected or no relationships were observed. The authors conclude that among this population of predominately overweight students, solely relying on cross-sectional findings between nutrition behaviors and BMI would misinform intervention strategies.[15]

In addition, other factors may affect associations between potential determinants and obesity. For instance, it is frequently observed that, in cross-sectionally collected survey data, increasing age is associated with higher BMI and obesity until the age of about 60–65, when it levels off, and even older ages are associated with lower BMI and obesity levels. This, as has been argued elsewhere[16] may reflect premature mortality among obese people but also true decreases in obesity in old age due to weight loss from illnesses or age-related loss of appetite. It may also reflect that older people in a survey have a different life history (i.e. they may have been born and raised in times when obesity was much less common than today). This latter explanation is called a cohort effect. In fact,

Nooyens et al recently showed that older people do have lower mean BMI compared to middle-aged people but, when followed prospectively, also, older people gain weight.[17] This example is taken from data in adults but clearly, age-period-cohort effects are also present in children and adolescents.

There are many methodological pitfalls to consider in the interpretation of secular trends in overweight and obesity, as well as risk factors and disease incidence. The associations between these trends usually depend on the strengths of the association between obesity and a particular disease, and the time lag between the onset of obesity and the incidence of disease. For instance, the rise in the prevalence of type 2 diabetes is usually related to an increase in the prevalence of obesity because of the strength of the association between the two.[18] Time trends in obesity, on the other hand, may not be related to trends in the incidence of cardiovascular disease[19,20] or cancer.[21] This is because of the relatively low risk associated with obesity, the importance of many other risk factors for these diseases that may be unrelated to changes in obesity and the long lag-time between obesity and the incidence of cardiovascular disease endpoints and different types of cancer. This means, for instance, that there is a decreasing secular trend observed in cardiovascular risk factors and the incidence of cardiovascular disease when at the same time there is an increase in the prevalence of obesity.[19,20] This is despite the fact that, on an individual basis, there is a significant association between measures of overweight such as BMI and cardiovascular risk.[19,20]

As population characteristics change over time, these changes may have an influence on relative risk estimates of obesity for diseases, such as cancer, for other exposures because of effect-measure modification. The impact of population changes on comparability between epidemiologic studies can be kept to a minimum if investigators assess obesity-disease associations within strata of other exposures, and present results in a manner that allows comparisons across studies. Effect-measure modification is an important component of data analysis that is needed to obtain a complete understanding of disease etiology.[22]

Monitoring determinants and consequences of obesity can, therefore, lead to interesting hypotheses about potential explanations of associations but are usually weak in their level of evidence for causal relationships. These methodological problems also hamper the evaluation of effectiveness of policy interventions on obesity and health.

Screening—measuring children for obesity case finding

When heights and weights are routinely monitored, there is will be individuals who meet the criteria for overweight or obesity. If the data are subsequently reported to the children and/or their parents, or are followed by referral to interventions, this would bring monitoring into the realms of screening. In essence, it would be screening for individuals who may benefit from interventions aimed at weight gain prevention or weight management, even though the primary purpose of the measurement may have been for monitoring population trends

Following the original criteria for screening by Wilson and Jungner[23] and published by WHO in 1968, there have been more extensive lists of criteria for the viability, effectiveness and appropriateness of a screening programme (see below) (Table 21.1).

Screening for obesity in different medical settings has been evaluated. Wilson and McAlpine have reviewed this for primary care.[25] Whitlock et al[26] and Westwood et al[27] have reviewed the usefulness of screening in children. In all three reviews it is argued that screening is compromised by the fact that there is little generalizable evidence for the effectiveness of primary care interventions in unselected patients.

Although there is not much scientific literature on this, there are indications that the consequences of routinely assessed weight and height in individuals in surveys may lead to differences in participation rates. If it is known in advance that routinely measured weights and heights measured at children in school are followed by a referral to an intervention requiring the participation of parents and children this may lead to a lower likelihood that parents of children who are overweight or obese and who are not interested in an intervention will give their permission for their child to be measured.

There are ethical questions surrounding the feedback of information obtained by screening. The issue is whether or not parents or (in the case of adolescents) the children themselves have a right to access the measurements taken and their interpretation. In The UK National Child Measurement Programme

Table 21.1 Criteria for appraising the viability, effectiveness and appropriateness of a screening programme 2003 by the UK National Screening Committee.[24] ($\checkmark$ condition met; p condition partially met; x condition not met (rating from reference[4]).

The condition

$\checkmark$ The condition should be an important health problem.

p   The epidemiology and natural history of the condition, including development from latent to declared disease, should be adequately understood and there should be a detectable risk factor, disease marker, latent period or early symptomatic stage.

x   All the cost-effective primary prevention interventions should have been implemented as far as practicable.

x   If the carriers of a mutation are identified as a result of screening, the natural history of people with this status should be understood, including the psychological implications.

The test

p   There should be a simple, safe, precise and validated screening test.

x   The distribution of test values in the target population should be known and a suitable cut-off level defined and agreed.

p   The test should be acceptable to the population.

x   There should be an agreed policy on the further diagnostic investigation of individuals with a positive test result and on the choices available to those individuals.

x   If the test is for mutations, the criteria used to select the subset of mutations to be covered by screening, if all possible mutations are not being tested for, should be clearly set out.

The treatment

x   There should be an effective treatment or intervention for patients identified through early detection, with evidence of early treatment leading to better outcomes than late treatment.

x   There should be agreed evidence-based policies covering which individuals should be offered treatment and the appropriate treatment to be offered.

x   Clinical management of the condition and patient outcomes should be optimized in all health care providers prior to participation in a screening program.

The screening program

x   There should be evidence from high-quality randomized controlled trials that the screening program is effective in reducing mortality or morbidity. Where screening is aimed solely at providing information to allow the person being screened to make an "informed choice" (for example, Down's syndrome and cystic fibrosis carrier screening), there must be evidence from high quality trials that the test accurately measures risk. The information that is provided about the test and its outcome must be of value and readily understood by the individual being screened.

x   There should be evidence that the complete screening program (test, diagnostic procedures, treatment/ intervention) is clinically, socially and ethically acceptable to health professionals and the public.

x   The benefit from the screening program should outweigh the physical and psychological harm (caused by the test, diagnostic procedures and treatment).

x   The opportunity cost of the screening program (including testing, diagnosis and treatment, administration, training and quality assurance) should be economically balanced in relation to expenditure on medical care as a whole (i.e. value for money).

x   There should be a plan for managing and monitoring the screening program and an agreed set of quality assurance standards.

Continued

Table 21.1 *Continued*

x	Adequate staffing and facilities for testing, diagnosis, treatment and program management should be available prior to the commencement of the screening program.
x	All other options for managing the condition should have been considered (for example, improving treatment and providing other services), to ensure that no more cost-effective intervention could be introduced or current interventions increased within the resources available.
x	Evidence-based information, explaining the consequences of testing, investigation and treatment, should be made available to potential participants to assist them in making an informed choice.
x	Public pressure for widening the eligibility criteria for reducing the screening interval, and for increasing the sensitivity of the testing process, should be anticipated. Decisions about these parameters should be scientifically justifiable to the public.
x	If screening is for a mutation, the program should be acceptable to people identified as carriers and to other family members.

(NCMP) parents of all participants in the NCMP will receive their child's results, regardless of their weight, unless they request otherwise.[11] Parents still have the opportunity to withdraw their child from the program, and children can also decide not to participate on the day. Changes were made in 2007, making it possible to access individual data, link them to names and addresses and contact the parents by mail to give them the results of the measurement. It is unclear how much of this feedback will be effective as an intervention and how parents will react to this information.

Monitoring of effects of interventions

When the effectiveness of interventions is assessed through a monitoring system, this usually means that there is no randomized controlled trial design. Usually this means that the serial assessment of outcomes (such as mean body weight, BMI or body fatness or the percentage of people with overweight or obesity) are related to the received dose of an intervention used before or during the observation period. Sometimes these can be compared to the intensity of the exposure to the intervention (intervention dose) and changes in outcome measures, such as health-related variables. For example, if one or a number of regions or states within a country implement a comprehensive obesity prevention plan including school food policies, social marketing, bans on advertising on unhealthy foods and promotion of physical activity, changes in trends of children's BMI could be compared to trends in those regions or states with no obesity prevention strategies.

Where there are no populations who can serve as controls there are limitations to such evaluations, although in many instances there are no alternatives. Randomized controlled designs may not always be a better alternative. This is partly because complex community interventions do not always lend themselves to randomization and because intense monitoring of behaviour, anthropometric measurements and health outcomes may actually serve as an effective intervention itself in the control groups. This is sometimes referred to as the Hawthorne effect.[28] It also possible that control areas or communities are contaminated though the media and adopt at least parts of the intervention. This has been documented, for instance in the Heartbeat Wales project.[29]

The evaluation of complex community interventions depends on the degree of exposure to the intervention that can be identified, and to which degree the effects of general secular trends can excluded. In the 1970s and 1980s, a series of population-based community intervention studies were carried out in high-income countries to reduce risk factors for chronic disease. These studies focused on either change in health behaviors or on risk factors such as tobacco use, bodyweight, cholesterol and blood pressure, as well as a reduction in morbidity and mortality due to cardiovascular disease. In general, they included a combination of community-wide actions as well as those focused on individuals identified as being at high risk.[30]

Gaziano et al[30] have reviewed the evidence of community interventions aimed at the prevention of chronic diseases. One of the earliest and most often cited community interventions is the North Karelia project, which began in Finland in 1972. The community-based interventions included health education, screening, a hypertension control programme and treatment. The first five years of the study saw reductions in risk factors as well as a decline in mortality owing to coronary heart disease of 2·9% per year versus a 1% per year decrease in the rest of Finland. During the next 10 years, reductions were greater in the rest of Finland. Over 25 years of follow-up, a large fall in coronary heart disease occurred in both the North Karelia region (73%) and the rest of Finland (63%). Although the overall difference in the reduction in deaths caused by coronary heart disease was not significantly greater in the study area, the reduction in tobacco-related cancers in men was significant. A similar study in the Stanford (CA, USA) area showed reductions in risk factors—for example, cholesterol (2%), blood pressure (4%), and smoking rates (13%)—when compared with sites without the intervention, but there was no effect on disease end-points. There are almost no examples of such interventions in children and adolescents.

Later, community interventions in high-income countries showed mixed results, with some showing improvements in risk factors beyond the secular decline that was occurring throughout most of the developed economies, and others showing no additional decrease. However, a meta-analysis of the randomized multiple-risk factor interventions showed net significant decreases in systolic blood pressure, smoking prevalence and cholesterol. Decreases in total mortality of 3%, and in mortality due to coronary heart disease of 4%, were not significant. The limitation with all the randomized controlled trials includes the challenge of detecting small changes that on a population level could be significant; it is possible that a 10% reduction in mortality could have been missed.[30]

Although there are comprehensive reviews on the effectiveness of obesity prevention interventions,[31] such evaluation studies on a national or regional level are as yet rare for obesity prevention. There are some examples of small local community interventions that show promising effects such as the EPODE project in France.[32] This is an expansion of the original Fleurbaix-Laventie program in two small French towns. The EPODE project is a good example of a program that needs population monitoring of trends to determine if it is effective or not because it has no comparison group. Other examples are demonstration projects in Australia, such as the one in the town of Colac.[33] The evidence base for the effectiveness of such programs using monitoring of effects needs to be expanded urgently.

Conclusions

Monitoring is an essential part in the integral approach towards evidence-based prevention of overweight and obesity in children and adolescents. In most cases, monitoring systems have severe methodological flaws and can lead to misinterpretation of prevalence and trends in obesity and its determinants. If done well it probably is the only acceptable way to evaluate the effectiveness of long-term comprehensive community approaches aimed at obesity prevention. Development of adequate monitoring systems should, therefore, be a priority for any strategic approach to health promotion interventions.

References

1 www.unfpa.org/emergencies/manual/9.htm
2 www.who.int/tobacco/surveillance/en/
3 www.who.int/chp/steps/en/
4 Wake M: Issues in obesity monitoring, screening and subsequent treatment. *Curr Opin Pediatr*. 2009 (in press).
5 Ogden CL, Carroll MD, Curtin LR, McDowell MA, Tabak CJ, Flegal KM: Prevalence of overweight and obesity in the United States, 1999–2004. *JAMA* 2006; **295**:1549–1555.
6 Mokdad AH, Ford ES, Bowman BA et al: Prevalence of obesity, diabetes, and obesity-related health risk factors, 2001. *JAMA* 2003; **289**:76–79.
7 Sherry B, Jefferds ME, Grummer-Strawn LM: Accuracy of adolescent self-report of height and weight in assessing overweight status: a literature review. *Arch Pediatr Adolesc Med* 2007; **161**:1154–1161.
8 Elgar FJ, Roberts C, Tudor-Smith C, Moore L: Validity of self-reported height and weight and predictors of bias in adolescents. *J Adolesc Health* 2005; **37**:371–375.
9 Ogden CL, Carroll MD, Flegal KM: High body mass index for age among US children and adolescents, 2003–2006. *JAMA* 2008; **299**:2401–2405.
10 Visscher TL, Viet AL, Kroesbergen IH, Seidell JC: Underreporting of BMI in adults and its effect on obesity prevalence estimations in the period 1998 to 2001. *Obesity* (Silver Spring) 2006; **14**:2054–2063.

11 www.dh.gov.uk/en/Publichealth/Healthimprovement/ Healthyliving/DH_073787

12 Swinburn B, Bell C, King L, Magarey A, O'Brien K, Waters E: Obesity prevention programs demand high-quality evaluations. *Aust NZ J Publish Health* 2007; **31**(4):305–307.

13 Katanoda K, Matsumura Y: National nutrition survey in Japan. Its methodological transition and current findings. *J Nutr Sci Vitaminol* 2002; **48**:423–432.

14 Funatogawa I, Funatogawa T, Yano E: Do overweight children necessarily make overweight adults? Repeated cross-sectional annual nationwide survey of Japanese girls and women over nearly six decades. *BMJ* 2008; **337**:a802.

15 Utter J, Scragg R, Ni Mhurchu C, Schaaf D: What effect do attempts to lose weight have on the observed relationship between nutrition behaviors and body mass index among adolescents? *Int J Behav Nutr Phys Act* 2007; **4**:40.

16 Seidell JC, Visscher TL: Body weight and weight change and their health implications for the elderly. *Eur J Clin Nutr* 2000; **54**(Suppl. 3):S33–S39.

17 Nooyens ACJ, Visscher TLS, Verschuren WMM et al: Age and cohort effects on body weight and BMI in Dutch adults: the Doetinchem cohort study. *Public Health Nutr* 2009; **12**:862–870.

18 Seidell JC: Obesity, insulin resistance and diabetes—a worldwide epidemic. *Br J Nutr* 2000; **83**(Suppl. 1):S5–S8.

19 Gidding SS, Bao W, Srinivasan SR, Berenson GS: Effects of secular trends in obesity on coronary risk factors in children: the Bogalusa Heart Study. *J Pediatr* 1995; **127**(6):868–874.

20 Chiolero A, Bovet P, Paradis G, Paccaud F: Has blood pressure increased in children in response to the obesity epidemic? *Pediatrics* 2007; **119**:544–553.

21 Vainio H, Kaaks R, Bianchini F: Weight control and physical activity in cancer prevention: international evaluation of the evidence. *Eur J Cancer Prev* 2002; **11**(Suppl. 2):S94–S100.

22 Slattery ML, Murtaugh MA, Quesenberry C, Caan BJ, Edwards S, Sweeney C: Changing population characteristics, effect-measure modification, and cancer risk factor identification. *Epidemiol Perspect Innov* 2007; **4**:10.

23 http://whqlibdoc.who.int/php/WHO_PHP_34.pdf

24 www.gp-training.net/training/tutorials/management/audit/ screen.htm)

25 Wilson AR, McAlpine DD: The effectiveness of screening for obesity in primary care: weighing the evidence. *Med Care Res Rev* 2006; **63**:570–598.

26 Whitlock EP, Williams SB, Gold R, Smith PR, Shipman SA: Screening and interventions for childhood overweight: a summary of evidence for the US preventive services task force. *Pediatrics* 2005; **116**:e125–4.

27 Westwood M, Fayter D, Hartley S et al: Childhood obesity: should primary school children be routinely screened? A systematic review and discussion of the evidence. *Arch Dis Child* 2007; **92**:416–422.

28 http://en.wikipedia.org/wiki/Hawthorne_effect

29 Nutbeam D, Smith C, Murphy S, Catford J: Maintaining evaluation designs in long term community based health promotion programmes: heartbeat Wales case study. *J Epidemiol Community Health* 1993; **47**:127–133.

30 Gaziano TA, Galea G, Reddy KS: Scaling up interventions for chronic disease prevention: the evidence. *Lancet* 2007; **370**:1939–1946.

31 Flynn MA, McNeil DA, Maloff B et al: Reducing obesity and related chronic disease risk in children and youth: a synthesis of evidence with "best practice" recommendations. *Obes Rev* 2006; **7**(Suppl. 1):7–66.

32 Romon M, Lommez A, Tafflet M, Basdevant A, Oppert JM, Bresson JL et al: Downward trends in the prevalence of childhood overweight in the setting of 12-years school- and community-based programs. *Public Health Nutr* 2009; **12**: 35–42.

33 Sanigorski AM, Bell AC, Kremer PJ, Cuttler R, Swinburn BA: Reducing unhealthy weight gain in children through community capacity-building: results of a quasi-experimental intervention program, Be Active Eat Well. *Int J Obes (Lond)* 2008; **32**(7):1060–1067. Epub 2008 Jun 10.

CHAPTER 22

Knowledge translation and exchange for obesity prevention

Rebecca Armstrong,[1] *Lauren Prosser,*[1] *Maureen Dobbins*[2] *and Elizabeth Waters*[1]

[1] Jack Brockoff Child Health and Wellbeing Program, McCaughey Centre, Melbourne School of Population Health, University of Melbourne, Melbourne, Australia

[2] School of Nursing and Department of Clinical Epidemiology and Biostatistics, McMaster University, Hamilton, Canada

Summary and recommendations for research and practice

- Knowledge translation and exchange (KTE) processes are intended to facilitate the creation and application of knowledge.
- To best support obesity prevention knowledge translation and exchange processes need to involve governments, communities (including children and their parents), practitioners and researchers who are holders of implicit and explicit knowledge.
- Tools and strategies are available to support the many purposes of KTE.
- Reflection on the application of KTE tools and strategies is necessary, in order to build the research evidence in this area and to support evidence-informed approaches to obesity prevention.

Introduction

As discussed in previous chapters, the need for an evidence-informed approach to obesity prevention is challenging but essential. Using research evidence in decision-making processes is often termed "evidence-based practice", stemming from the principles of

---

Preventing Childhood Obesity. Edited by
E. Waters, B.A. Swinburn, J.C. Seidell and R. Uauy.
© 2010 Blackwell Publishing.

evidence-based medicine (EBM). EBM typically involves the "conscientious, explicit, and judicious use of current best evidence in making decisions about the care of individual patients".[1] In more recent times, and in domains such as public health where research evidence is more complex, the term "evidence-informed" has been favoured.[2] Evidence-informed decisions should be "better matched to the context of application, more efficiently implemented, and more widely acceptable."[3] While EBM has an implied emphasis on research evidence forming the basis of decision making, "evidence-informed" decision making more clearly acknowledges that public health decisions are often informed by research evidence in combination with a range of alternative sources and influences.[4]

Obesity prevention is likely to be best supported with the use of multi-sectoral approaches across multiple disciplines. The challenge for obesity prevention is that interventions are facilitated through policies at the national, state/provincial, regional and local level. This necessarily involves the generation and synthesis of existing research evidence in combination with practitioner expertise, policy imperatives and community experiences. Given the number of key stakeholders involved in this trajectory between knowledge generation, synthesis and use, "knowledge translation and exchange" has become particularly important. The process of knowledge translation and exchange is thus, extremely complex. Initially it was believed that evidence-informed decision making could be achieved through the simple diffusion of information (e.g. development and dissemination of research reports). However, it is now acknowledged that, at a minimum, knowledge translation and exchange (KTE) must involve the building and maintenance of collaborative relationships between and among key stakeholders and researchers.[5,6]

In a more traditional sense, knowledge translation (KT) has been defined as the "exchange, synthesis and ethically sound application of research findings within a complex set of interactions among researchers and knowledge users".[7] The processes and types of knowledge used in more contemporary KTE processes refer not only to research findings or research evidence.[8] Knowledge can be viewed as either explicit or tacit. Explicit knowledge is information that can be explained in words or symbols and is often written down.[9] It can, therefore, be easily shared or copied (e.g., a program evaluation that is published in a peer-reviewed journal). Tacit knowledge is generated through experience. It is, therefore, difficult to share without some level of interpersonal contact (e.g., sharing professional expertise in identifying options for working with refugee families to promote healthy eating).[9] In obesity prevention, decision making requires the careful consideration of a number of forms of knowledge, which can be viewed as either tacit or explicit including theory, intervention research, community views, local context, policy evaluation and expert opinion. This process occurs in the "action cycle" outlined in Figure 22.1.

This chapter explores how to use research evidence within a KTE framework that considers different types of knowledge to address obesity prevention.

The characteristics of KTE needed to support obesity prevention

Interaction

It appears that an essential component of KTE is interaction between various constituents.[11,12] This may involve researchers, decision makers, policymakers, practitioners and communities. The communication of knowledge can be operationalized using a number of mechanisms, including websites, knowledge brokers, tailored or targeted messages, email, health messages, networks and formal and informal meetings.[11,13]

Multi-sectoral approach

As discussed widely in the evidence sections of this book, to be effective, action to address obesity needs to take a multi-sectoral approach. KTE processes must, therefore, acknowledge the influences (e.g. political, historical), types of knowledge and accountability requirements operating within each relevant sector. For example, some sectors may rely more heavily on types of knowledge (e.g., modeling is used within the transport sector) unfamiliar to individuals working in the health sector.[14]

The key to working across multiple sectors is communication and engagement. Part of the challenge is that those working outside the health sector may not view their work as health-related or relevant to obesity prevention. Exposure to new ideas (particular related to the determinants of health), concepts of evidence and different ways of working are essential to supporting evidence-informed decision making for obesity prevention. Those working in the health sector may begin to build these relationships by involving key partners (e.g., schools, early childhood services, transport, food supply) in health-related decision making. Other strategies may include offering to share advice in the development of policy related to the determinants of obesity prevention, sharing key publications with key contacts, summarizing research evidence likely to be of relevance or interest to these partners, and building formal networks with interested parties to support evidence synthesis and generation. It goes without saying that nurturing these relationships takes time and commitment.

Understanding context

Context refers to the "social, political and/or organizational setting in which an intervention was evaluated, or in which it is to be evaluated".[15] It must also capture the characteristics of those living and working within these settings (e.g., demographics). Understanding the context in which knowledge was originally created is as important as understanding the context where knowledge will ultimately be applied.[15,16] For example, if you were planning the implementation of a school-based intervention, it would be important to understand *why* a particular school-based intervention worked in rural New Zealand as well as considering *whether* it could be applied in metropolitan Sydney.

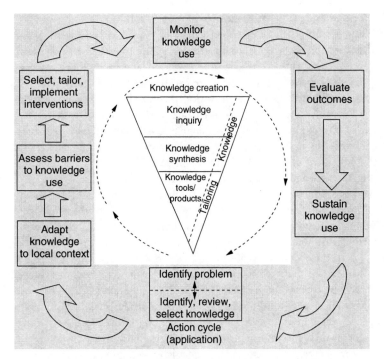

Figure 22.1 Knowledge to action process.[10]

Frameworks to support KTE

Planning for and implementing KTE strategies is complex with many barriers and challenges to be overcome. A significant issue concerns the engagement of multiple stakeholders in the KTE process, each of whom brings their unique values, perspectives and attitudes with respect to evidence-informed decision making. The challenge lies in allowing for these differences to be part of the process while promoting an environment where a common goal is sought and is achievable. Additional barriers include absence of personal contact between researchers, policy-makers and practitioners, lack of timeliness of research, mutual mistrust, power and budget struggles, poor quality of research, research that does not answer questions relevant to decision makers, political instability and debates about what constitutes evidence.[17–19] A number of models/frameworks have been developed to summarize and support these complex processes.[6,16,20]

Of particular relevance to obesity prevention is the framework developed by the Prevention Group of the International Obesity Task Force (IOTF) to support the translation of research evidence into action.[20] This

framework is practically oriented and identifies processes to be undertaken in five key stages:

1. building a case for action;
2. identifying contributory factors and points of intervention;
3. defining opportunities for action;
4. evaluating potential interventions; and
5. selecting a portfolio of specific policies, programs and actions.

Each stage is cumulative and culminates in the development of a plan to support the combination of research evidence, theoretical perspectives and contextual factors into a plan for translation into action.[20] It promotes KTE by encouraging those who use it to look not only at the research evidence but to explore the views and perspectives of decision makers and communities, to consider innovative approaches and to think outside the traditional health sector settings.

In acknowledging that there is limited research evidence to address obesity, the IOTF has suggested the development of a "promise table" as a way of helping to evaluate potential interventions.[20] It supports the consideration of interventions at varying levels of certainty of effectiveness by mapping against potential population impact (see Table 22.1). In doing so, it

Table 22.1 Mapping the research evidence: a "promise" table.[20]

Certainty of effectiveness[a]	Potential population level impact[b]		
	Low	Moderate	High
Quite high	Promising	Very promising	Most promising
Medium	Less promising	Promising	Very promising
Low	Least promising	Less promising	Promising

[a]The certainty of effectiveness is judged by the quality of the evidence, the strength of the program logic, and the sensitivity and uncertainty parameters in the modeling of the population impact.
[b]Potential population impact takes into account efficacy (impact under ideal conditions), reach and uptake, and it can be measured in a number of ways such as effectiveness, cost–effectiveness, or cost–utility.

allows decision makers to consider interventions with high levels of potential population impact where the certainty of effectiveness may be less clear.[20]

The process of integrating different types of knowledge so as to select an optimal combination of policies, programs and actions (as outlined in step 5 above) for obesity prevention is particularly challenging. Once the promise table has been completed, it is important to assess the applicability and transferability of these potential strategies to the local context. Applicability refers to whether an intervention (regardless of the outcome) could be implemented within a local setting.[21] By contrast, transferability refers to the likelihood that the intervention will be as effective within the local setting as it has been in others.[21] To support this process, Wang et al[21] have developed a series of questions that may be helpful in identifying the optimal combination of policies, programs and actions (see Table 22.2).

Options for KTE for obesity prevention

While the IOTF provides a KTE framework to support decision-making processes, KTE can operate at differing levels. For example, a researcher may be keen to build relationships with decision makers; or maybe a community member would like to become more involved in obesity prevention research and share their knowledge about local context. While there is limited research evidence to help identify the effectiveness of strategies likely to support KTE (including the IOTF example described above), a number of options have been proposed and variously tested. These include:

- face-to-face exchange (consultation, regular meetings) between decision makers and researchers;
- education sessions for decision makers;
- networks and communities of practice;
- Facilitated meetings between decision-makers and researchers
- interactive, multi-disciplinary workshops;
- capacity building within health services and health delivery organizations;
- web-based information, electronic communications;
- steering committees (to integrate views of local experts into design, conduct and interpretation of research).[13]

There has been much discussion about the use of knowledge brokers to help facilitate KTE.[22–24] Knowledge brokers work to bridge the gap between decision makers and researchers, so as to ensure that research evidence addresses the information needs of policy-makers, health care professionals, populations and patients. At the same time, they work in policy, practice and community settings to help facilitate evidence-informed decision making.

A knowledge broker may have a number of attributes, and will be:
- entrepreneurial (networking, problem solving, innovating);
- trusted and credible;
- a clear communicator;
- able to understand the cultures of both the research and decision-making environments
- able to find and assess relevant research in a variety of formats;
- facilitating, mediating and negotiating

Table 22.2 Questions to help assess the applicability and transferability of research evidence.[21]

Applicability	• Does the **political environment** of the local society allow this intervention to be implemented?
	• Is there any political barrier to implementing this intervention?
	• Would the general public and the targeted (sub)population accept this intervention? Does any aspect of the intervention go against local **social norms**? Is it ethically acceptable?
	• Can the contents of the intervention be tailored to suit the local culture?
	• Are the essential **resources** for implementing this intervention available in the local setting? (A list of essential resources may help to answer this question.)
	• Does the target population in the local setting have a sufficient **educational** level to comprehend the contents of the intervention?
	• Which organization will be responsible for the provision of this intervention in the local setting?
	• Is there any possible barrier to implementing this intervention due to the **structure of that organization**?
	• Does the provider of the intervention in the local setting have the **skill** to deliver this intervention? If not will training be available?
Transferability	• What is the **baseline prevalence** of the health problem of interest in the local setting? What is the difference in prevalence between the study setting and the local setting?
	• Are the **characteristics of the target population** comparable between the study setting and the local setting? With regards to the particular aspects that will be addressed in the intervention, is it possible that the characteristics of the target population, such as ethnicity, socio-economic status, educational level, and so on, will have an impact on the effectiveness of the intervention?
	• Is the **capacity to implement** the intervention comparable between the study setting in such matters as political environment, social acceptability, resources, organizational structure and the skills of the local providers?

• able to understand the principles of adult learning[22]

Facilitators of KTE for obesity prevention

Much of the discussion above has revolved around supporting the use of research evidence in policy or community decision-making arenas. However, it is also important to acknowledge the role or active contribution of these players in respective KTE pathways. The following examples describe how governments, researchers, practitioners and communities can all be involved in KTE.

Government

What knowledge is held: implicit and explicit
Important KTE mechanisms: driving policy-relevant research, working as a broker between researchers

and communities, using research evidence to inform decision making, undertaking natural experiments to assess policy outcomes.

Potential facilitators for KTE: existing networks and partnerships (e.g., funding bodies), skilled workforce, organizational culture conducive to research use, strong leadership, infrastructure to support KTE activities within organizations.

Potential barriers to KTE: time, resources, political agenda, limited or no leadership, no infrastructure.

Research

What knowledge is held: primarily explicit
Important KT mechanisms: generating policy-relevant research, working with communities to develop research programs to address their issues of concern, participating in decision-making processes, providing opinions to the media to inform debate.

Potential facilitators for KTE: existing relationships with decision makers, expertise in understanding and working with research evidence.

Potential barriers to KTE: may have few links with decision makers, practice and community, lack of support to participate in KTE activities beyond the scope of funded research activities, limited capacity in KTE.

Practice

What knowledge is held: implicit and explicit

Important KTE mechanisms: working as a broker between researchers and communities, using research evidence to inform decision making, working with government to help drive practice-relevant research, undertaking evaluation of programs/practice to inform the evidence base.

Potential facilitators for KTE: existing networks and partnerships (e.g., relationship with community).

Potential barriers to KTE: time, resources, workforce not skilled in KTE.

Community

What knowledge is held: primarily implicit

Important KTE mechanisms: informing research and policy that will improve health outcomes.

Potential facilitators for KTE: existing advocacy networks or identity/consumer groups.

Potential barriers to KTE: disconnected or excluded from research-policy-practice interchange.

Knowledge translation in action: translation into practice

To explain the pathways of KTE the following two case studies provide an overview of how these processes can work. The case studies provide bona fide examples for childhood obesity prevention.

Case study—obesity prevention for Pacific Island children

The Pacific Islands hold some of the highest rates of obesity in the world. In these regions, technical agencies, especially SPC (Secretariat of the Pacific Community), WHO and UNICEF work to disseminate and share information with local stakeholders to distribute the best approaches and methods based on the latest research. This process of translating knowledge is very important because most of the technical staff in-country have almost no access to scientific journals, and it is, therefore, almost impossible for them to keep up to date with current research and research findings. The technical agencies act as knowledge brokers, passing on relevant information to local stakeholders and giving them the opportunity to make more informed decisions.

The geographical location of communities in the Pacific Islands proves difficult for agencies to remain in frequent face to face contact with the local stakeholders. To ensure continual relevant and timely advice, SPC have set up an email-based information group for their multi-sectoral groups of informed stakeholders. The stakeholders receive current evidence on new and emerging projects in a brief weekly email and a quarterly newsletter containing user-friendly reviews of specific topics and training/workshops. Each of these resources contains information that is relevant to the needs of the specific regions they are working with.

In-country staff also have the opportunity to contact the agencies for advice. For example, many enquiries to a SPC nutrition adviser include requests for information about the most effective strategies to assess childhood obesity, and whether these were relevant for Pacific Island children. The SPC nutrition adviser then follows a process of giving individual advice then relaying information already stored in the email-based information and quarterly newsletters. A simple summary or factsheet of the evidence is then provided so they can work toward making a more informed decision for their community.

Case study 2—"Streets ahead" an initiative to support children to get active in their neighborhoods

Over the past two decades, there has been a decline in the number of children who walk or cycle to school. Despite most children living within 2 km of their school, a large proportion now make the journey by car. The primary reason for this trend is perceived safety issues (including road safety and neighborhood safety). In turn, this has led to increased traffic congestion and limited opportunities for children to travel around their neighborhoods independently.

The benefits lost are substantial—active transport not only increases physical activity but also provides children with knowledge of their neighborhoods, and has positive impacts on their behavioral and cognitive development, instilling significant social, physical and mental competencies.

VicHealth's "Streets Ahead" approach will enable children to become more active in their neighborhoods. The initiative aims to help communities to create supportive environments that enhance children's active transport not only to and from school but throughout other aspects of their community life (e.g., walking to the home of a friend in the neighborhood). The initiative is designed to be implemented on a place-based community level within targeted neighborhoods of a local government municipality. This initiative (implemented in July 2008) was informed by evidence from the Walking School Bus project in Victoria, Australia and other research findings, which identified the benefits of increased active transport for children becoming community led. Initially, the initiative will require the leadership of local council senior staff and a project steering group. From this, schools and local communities (children, parents, relevant groups/organizations) will be engaged to form their own groups to develop strategies that would work best within their communities to increase modes of transport. A key anticipated outcome of this project is the development of strategies that are locally driven but use knowledge translation processes to engage researchers, funding bodies, local governments and communities. The learning from these locally driven initiatives will then inform the knowledge translation and exchange process and guide further action.

Conclusion

Activities to support KTE are important in all areas of public health but are particularly pertinent in an area such as childhood obesity where solutions to problems need to be addressed through partnerships incorporating communities, decision makers, researchers and practitioners. This necessitates the use of different types of knowledge: implicit and explicit. This chapter has outlined some of the core components of KTE and outlined some tools which are intended to support KTE activities in a range of set-

tings. A number of strategies exist, which may help to facilitate the exchange of knowledge needed to address childhood obesity. As the field of KTE continues to develop, it will be important for all stakeholders to reflect on these strategies—whether they are working, how they are working, in what circumstances and what factors are needed to facilitate these processes.

References

1 Sackett DL, Rosenberg WM, Gray JA, Haynes RB, Richardson WS: Evidence based medicine: what it is and what it isn't. *BMJ* 1996; **312**(7023):71–72.

2 Davies H, Nutley S, Walter I: Why "knowledge transfer" is misconceived for applied social research. *J Health Serv Res Policy* 2008; **13**(3):188–190.

3 Canadian Health Services Research Foundation: Conceptualizing and Combining Evidence for Health System Guidance. Ottawa: Canadian Health Services Research Foundation, 2005.

4 Ciliska D, Thomas H, Buffett C: An Introduction To Evidence-Informed Public Health and a Compendium of Critical Appraisal Tools for Public Health Practice. Hamilton, ON: National Collaborating Centre for Methods and Tools, 2008.

5 Kiefer L, Frank J, Di Ruggiero E et al: Fostering evidence-based decision-making in Canada: examining the need for a Canadian population and public health evidence centre and research network. *Can J Public Health* 2005; **96**(3):Il–40 following 200.

6 Canadian Institutes of Health Research: Knowledge Translation Framework. Ottawa: Canadian Institutes of Health Research, 2003.

7 Canadian Institutes of Health Research: Knowledge Translation Strategy 2004–2009. Ottawa: Canadian Institutes of Health Research, 2004.

8 Armstrong R, Waters E, Roberts H, Oliver S, Popay J: The role and theoretical evolution of knowledge translation and exchange in public health. *J Public Health* 2006; **28**(4): 384–389.

9 The Provincial Centre of Excellence for Child and Youth Mental Health at CHEO: Knowledge Exchange: A Review of the Literature from the Perspective of Child and Youth Mental Health. Ontario, Canada: The Provincial Centre of Excellence for Child and Youth Mental Health at CHEO, 2006.

10 Graham ID, Logan J, Harrison MB et al: Lost in knowledge translation: time for a map? *J Contin Educ Health Prof* 2006; **26**(1):13–24.

11 Nutley SM, Walter I, Davies H: Using Evidence: How Research Can Inform Public Services. Bristol: The Policy Press, 2007.

12 Lavis J, Ross S, McLeod C, Gildiner A: Measuring the impact of health research. *J Health Serv Res Policy* 2003; **8**(3): 165–170.

13 Mitton C, Adair CE, McKenzie E, Patten SB, Waye Perry, B: Knowledge transfer and exchange: review and synthesis of the literature. *Milbank Q* 2007; **85**(4):729–768.

14 Armstrong R, Doyle J, Lamb C, Waters E: Multi-sectoral health promotion and public health: the role of evidence. *J Public Health (Oxford)*, 2006; **28**(2):168–172.

15 Rychetnik L, Frommer M, Hawe P, Shiell A: Criteria for evaluating evidence on public health interventions. *J Epidemiol Community Health* 2002; **56**(2):119–127.

16 Jacobson N, Butterill D, Goering P: Development of a framework for knowledge translation: understanding user context. *J Health Serv Res Policy* 2003; **8**(2):94–99.

17 Petticrew M, Whitehead M, Macintyre SJ, Graham H, Egan M: Evidence for public health policy on inequalities: 1: the reality according to policymakers. *J Epidemiol Community Health* 2004; **58**(10):811–816.

18 Innvaer S, Vist G, Trommald M, Oxman A: Health policy-makers' perceptions of their use of evidence: a systematic review. *J Serv Res Policy* 2002; **7**:239–244.

19 Elliott H, Popay J: How are policy makers using evidence? Models of research utilisation and local NHS policy making. *J Epidemiol Community Health* 2000; **54**(6):461–468.

20 Swinburn B, Gill T, Kumanyika S: Obesity prevention: a proposed framework for translating evidence into action. *Obes Rev* 2005; **6**(1):23–33.

21 Wang S, Moss JR, Hiller JE: Applicability and transferability of interventions in evidence-based public health. *Health Promot Int* 2006; **21**(1):76–83.

22 Lomas J: The in-between world of knowledge brokering. *BMJ* 2007; **334**(7585):129–132.

23 Dobbins M, DeCorby K, Twiddy T: A knowledge transfer strategy for public health decision makers. *Worldviews Evid Based Nurs* 2004; **1**(2):120–128.

24 Choi BC, Pang T, Lin V et al: Can scientists and policy makers work together? *J Epidemiol Community Health* 2005; **59**(8):632–637.

CHAPTER 23

The role of advocacy

Jane Martin
Obesity Policy Coalition, Melbourne, Australia

Summary

- Advocacy is an important component of any strategy to effect improvements in public health outcomes.
- Advocacy should challenge vested interests, promote policy solutions, engage with government and challenge community norms.
- Advocacy requires planning to identify the problems, the solutions, the policy responses, and the interested groups and individuals—including the media—that will provide access to those who make decisions or can influence decisions.
- Experts and others working in the field are well placed to act as spokespeople, disseminate research and evidence to support reforms, and to influence others to join up and support change.
- It is important to counter the arguments against obesity prevention policies from vested commercial interests and argue for the protection of the health and well-being of children to those who can effect change, as well as to the broader community.

Introduction

Advocacy is an essential element of any strategy to effect changes required to improve health outcomes brought about by poor lifestyles. The complexity of the causes of chronic disease has been a barrier to advocacy and has resulted in criticism of the public

Preventing Childhood Obesity. Edited by
E. Waters, B.A. Swinburn, J.C. Seidell and R. Uauy.
© 2010 Blackwell Publishing.

health sector as being complacent in its response to this epidemic.[1] Lang and Rayner[2] suggest that policymakers have been slow to recognize the seriousness of the issue for a number of reasons because, for example:
- the public health movement has been slow or ineffective in its advocacy work;
- the evidence is not easily transferable into policy; or
- it lacks political champions.

How can those engaged with public health be more active and challenge vested interests, promote policy solutions, engage with government and challenge community norms? This chapter outlines a strategy to develop a plan of action to advocate for prevention.

What is public health advocacy?

Public health advocacy is increasingly recognized as a key element in the promotion of public health. The World Health Organization defines advocacy as "[a] combination of individual and social actions designed to gain political commitment, policy support, social acceptance and systems support for a particular goal or program."[3]

Simon Chapman, one of public health's leading advocates, defines advocacy as a process to overcome structural (as opposed to individual or behavioral) barriers to achieving public health goals.[4] As such, it "aims to change the legislative, fiscal, physical and social environment in which individuals' knowledge and attitudes are developed and expressed, and in which behaviour changes take place."[4] This approach recognizes that improving population health requires more than just a focus on the individual and particular behaviors, but also on societal structures that work against improvements in public health.

Why do we need advocacy?

Building healthy public policy is central to the prevention of overweight and obesity. The UK Foresight report outlines the complexity of the drivers of obesity, while highlighting that most are societal issues and, therefore, require a societal response.[5] Unfortunately, action to address overweight and obesity often becomes tied up in the complexities of prevention, thereby resulting in a lack of action.

Yach[6] identified three key levers to support health policy change:

- raising the profile of the issue in the minds and on the agendas of policy-makers
- providing policy-makers with the necessary evidence to support the case for prevention
- persuading them of the need for changes in the health system away from acute care to prevention.

Advocacy is an important strategy to effect policy reform and it is important that policy-makers are provided with clear and coherent directions on which they feel that they can deliver.[2] Advocacy can be influential in setting the agenda, shaping the debate (the media is critical here), and in advancing particular policy positions.

Elements of effective advocacy

Public health advocacy requires careful planning to ensure effectiveness and often requires support from relevant organizational systems, managers and external funders—a case that, in itself, may require "advocacy".[7] It important to understand that facilitating structural change is a long-term proposition and this also needs to be considered when establishing and building capacity for advocacy.[8]

Components of an effective advocacy campaign include:[9]

- **Clear specific policy goals.** It is important to identify the problem and then propose specific policy solutions (see Box 23.1).
- **Solid research and science base for action.** Proposing evidence-based best practice helps to guide effective interventions, and adds credibility to the campaign and to the likelihood of success. Access to research, such as public opinion and local data are also important to help localize an issue and support media advocacy.

Box 23.1 Global dump soda campaign

Global Dump Soda Campaign is spearheaded by the Center for Science in the Public Interest (CSPI), and the International Association of Consumer Food Organizations (IACFO). CSPI is a leading North American non-governmental consumer advocacy organization fighting for improvements in diet and health. IACFO is a coalition of consumer organizations concerned about diet and health, food safety, and related food and agriculture policy issues. The campaign calls on governments around the world to make demands on soft drinks companies, including to: cease all marketing to children under 16; restrict products sold to children in schools; display energy content on packaging; and limit sponsorship to blind trusts. More information can be found on www.dumpsoda.org.

- **Values linked to fairness, equity and social justice.** Consideration must be given to creating rules for opportunity for engagement by others in the campaign. Equity and access issues also need to be assessed when considering policy proposals and their impact.[10]
- **Broad-based community participation.** Those affected most by the problem need to have a voice in defining solutions. However, where advocacy needs to be undertaken on behalf of children, this lends itself to be driven and supported by the public health community[11] (see Box 23.2).
- **Network and coalition building.**
[12] Building a broad but loose support base for action with groups who share the same concerns can be invaluable to advocacy. International networks of activists who focus on specific issues can provide experience and intelligence that can be translated to support an advocacy agenda. Establishing a formal coalition of agencies, respected by government, to support a particular issue can give power and credibility to its views (see Box 23.3).
- **Understanding the opposition.** Gathering strategic intelligence about the opposition is critical to countering their views and can include materials such as advertising spend, market share, advertising campaign successes and inside views from the food and advertising industry. This information can be found in advertising industry magazines, business

Box 23.2 The Parents Jury

The Parents Jury (www.parentsjury.org.au) is a national web-based network of parents who wish to improve the nutrition and physical activity environments for children in Australia. The Parents Jury began in August 2004 as an initiative of Cancer Council Victoria (CCV), Diabetes Australia (Vic) and the Australian and New Zealand Obesity Society, and membership is open to all parents, grandparents and guardians of children aged under 18. The Parents Jury seeks to improve children's health by advocating for policies that will influence the broader environment in order to support healthy eating and physical activity for children. It provides a forum for parents to voice their views on children's food and physical activity issues, and provides a channel for them to collectively advocate for the improvement of children's food and physical activity environments. This takes away the focus from that of the role of parents, to that of what others (such as the food industry or government) should be doing to support parents' efforts to raise healthy children. The Parents Jury conducts its campaigns through a number of channels, including:

- media advocacy using parents who have undertaken both media and advocacy training;
- direct delegations and submissions to key decision makers (e.g. government bureaucrats, politicians and the food industry) by the Parents Jury on behalf of its parent members;
- web-based tools and resource kits for parents to become grass-roots advocates on behalf of their children.

Box 23.3 The Obesity Policy Coalition

The Obesity Policy Coalition (OPC) was established in 2006 by four organizations with an interest in chronic disease prevention: Diabetes Australia—Victoria, Cancer Council Victoria, Victorian Health Promotion Foundation and the WHO Collaborating Centre for Obesity Prevention at Deakin University. One of the strengths of the model is that all these organizations are established, evidenced-based agencies respected by government, media and the broader community. The objectives of the OPC are to identify, analyse and advocate for evidence-based policy and regulatory initiatives to reduce overweight and obesity, particularly in children, at a local, state and national level. Staff have legal and policy expertise. Media advocacy is an important part of the work of the Coalition and support is provided through the partner organizations. Other agencies are encouraged to sign up to policy platforms and proposals, where relevant and appropriate, to broaden the support base, (www.opc.org.au).

tional trade agreements and global treaties similar to the Framework Convention on Tobacco Control.[10] At the national level, policies and regulation can support health by facilitating transport infrastructure, food subsidies and nutrition labeling, and locally by increasing the opportunity for exercise and community initiatives to promote access to healthy food.

Planning for advocacy

A framework of questions is often used to design and develop an advocacy plan for public health issues.[12–14] The main strategies of public health advocacy involve building coalitions and networks, political lobbying and media advocacy.[12] These strategic planning questions provide a process for developing effective advocacy strategies, including media advocacy.[15]

What are the goals of the advocacy effort?

Any advocacy effort must begin with a sense of its goals because government is more likely to notice clear, articulated messages. These will vary—the ulti-

and marketing sections of newspapers, food company annual reports, shareholder materials, websites, food industry newsletters, and so on.

- **Using the mass media to set the public agenda and frame issues appropriately.** This is one of the most powerful tools available to advocates and plays a dual role in informing the community about behavior changes to prevent overweight and obesity, and about what social changes are needed to support such behavioral changes. This is outlined in more detail below.
- **Using political and legislative process to create change.** The development of policies and regulations at all levels of governance can improve health. At the international level these can include interna-

mate long-term objective is to achieve comprehensive, effective, enforced obesity-prevention policies and regulation. However, because this will take some time to achieve, it is also important to set ambitious, but realistic, short-term objectives. The more specific these are, the more concrete and effective the planning will be.

Planning will also have to develop content goals (e.g. policy change) and process goals (e.g. building coalitions). These goals need to be explored and defined at the start, in a way that can launch a program, attract supporters and sustain it over time.

Who has the authority to make it happen?

It is important to identify the key decision makers because they are the people that the messages need to reach. This includes the general public, because building political will requires both government leadership and public support.[16] Government and politicians will be more likely to act if public opinion (i.e. the constituents who vote for them) is seen as supportive. Well-conducted opinion polls can provide critical evidence to persuade decision makers that proposed changes have broad community support.

The target audiences may also include individuals, such as the chairperson of a parliamentary committee examining legislative reform, or members of cabinet who are examining legislation put forward by the health minister. It is also important to consider active and influential members of the community, as these people pay attention to public affairs and can also influence key decision makers. Finally, members of the public health community are important allies. These people can be opinion leaders and, as such, can be very influential. This influence applies not just to government, but also to the broader community as many people respect the views of doctors and other health professionals over and above those of vested commercial interests.

What messages are most likely to persuade the target audience to take the recommended action?

Consideration needs to be given to the value systems and political views of the target audience when developing persuasive messages. It is easier to convince someone to act on the basis of their existing beliefs, rather than trying to convince them of something new and different.[17]

Messages should include both a core message and tailored, secondary messages to address the self-interest and concerns of the target audience. Core messages are broad, simple and direct; their aim is to tie the advocacy campaign together. Tailored messages explain how the core message can be achieved. These messages can be used to motivate political leaders, as it will be necessary to convince government that there are good reasons for them to do something, particularly if it involves taking or changing their position.

As Yussuf Saloojee, a public health advocate from South Africa said: "The clearest antidote to lack of political support is to provide politicians and society with a convincing answer to the question—what interventions work and at what social and economic cost? If clear health benefits can be realised at a reasonable cost, most politicians will support health legislation."[18] Cost needs to be framed in a way which includes the political cost (such as going against the views of the food industry). This cannot be quantified but still needs to be acknowledged as part of the equation.

How do we develop messages that speak both to the head and the heart?

It is important to ensure that messages are more than just logically persuasive and morally authoritative. Such messages will be more compelling if they are capable of evoking passion. A campaign message must speak both to the head and to the heart. Effective messages must have a simple concept, which captures the essence of a scientific idea, and must be catchy enough to capture attention. The same message can then be delivered by various messengers and diffused through the community.

Effective messages can include statistics that are both truthful and emotionally moving, that is, "creative epidemiology". How can stark, cold numbers from a study be translated into a message that evokes emotion and feeling? This is illustrated by the prevalence of Type 2 diabetes in adolescents. There are only a relatively small number of cases, but the concept that a disease stemming from unhealthy lifestyles in adults is now found in teenagers is shocking. This trend has created a much larger impact than that suggested by the data because of its emotional impact. Messages that are successful with one community may not always translate to another, owing to cultural and societal differences. To ensure success, the broader social and political cultures need to be considered when developing such messages, and it may be necessary to develop new messages that align with the values of that community.

Who can carry these messages to the target audience most effectively?

Persuading the target audience will rely as much on who delivers the message, as the message itself. Different people can have completely different credibility, power and effect. So a number of questions can be asked in order to determine the most effective messengers:

- Who is most likely to favorably influence the target audience?
- Who is the target audience politically responsive to?
- Who does that audience most want to please?
- To whom is that audience politically or financially obligated?
- Who does it respect?

For example, if the message is that "traffic light labeling on the front of packaged food will encourage healthier choices", then who could take that message to the health minister? Probably not an epidemiologist, maybe a consumer activist, but the head of the UK Food Safety Authority who has undertaken consumer research, developed a labeling system and implemented a strategy for uptake within their country, would be an ideal candidate.

It is also important to consider who the person you want to influence listens to and takes advice from, as they will also need to be reached. Often those you want to influence will be politicians so it is helpful to know how each level of government influences the policy-making process. Department staff and some ministerial advisers are extremely influential, as it is the cabinet that ultimately has to approve policy or legislative change.

Garnering support from the public health community, children's rights groups, the consumer movement and the public—particularly parents—can also provide useful voices, so it is important to identify messengers that can reach these groups and help to raise awareness and support.

What medium will be most effective in delivering the messages to the target audience?

There are two key avenues to achieve this: first, directly through lobbying legislators to do what is recommended; and second, using the media to promote the message more broadly.

Direct lobbying

Lobbying is made up of two types of approaches: inside and outside.[19] Inside lobbying is that which takes place in and around the legislature and includes a mix of strategies including:

- meeting with politicians and legislative staff; delivering information face-to-face can be very powerful. Remember to think about what is in it for them;
- providing analysis and information to committees and legislative offices;
- testifying to committees;
- negotiating with policy-makers and other lobby groups.

Outside lobbying also requires work outside, where legislation and policy is made. Some of these activities include:

- media activity including news conferences;
- building broad and diverse coalitions;
- visits to local elected representatives by their constituents;
- letter writing campaigns to legislators; and
- grass-roots activities such as rallies.

Media advocacy

Media advocacy is the "strategic use of mass media for advancing a social or public policy initiative."[20] It recognizes that publicity is not an end in itself, but asks, "How can this media initiative or opportunity best serve to advance our policy goals?"

Using the media is an extremely powerful way to advocate for change because to be successful, public health campaigns require cultural as well as political change.[21] The media provides the key channels to promote these dual aims as it reaches the general public, opinion leaders and policy-makers.

Policies to prevent obesity, like tobacco and alcohol control, often involve issues that are contested, resulting in a struggle with opposing forces. As such, the media message has to play two roles—negating the position put out by the opposition as well as advocating the particular policy position. There is also a danger in thinking that success is getting media coverage: to effect change the media interest must be harnessed to advance public policy objectives, not merely to publicize the issue.[12] A useful way to look at this is to ask three questions: What is wrong? Why does it matter? What should be done?[22]

A media advocacy campaign can be planned, but must also be flexible to enable advocates to react quickly and creatively to the changing news environment. For example, if the government releases a report on rising deaths from chronic disease, an advocacy group could put out a press release about what action government should take to address the problem.

It is important to identify the best spokesperson, which may not be the head of the organization.[23] As part of this, media training for spokespeople is a good idea; any adversaries put up by industry will be well prepared and very experienced in engaging with the media.

Media advocacy needs to be targeted to the media that is respected and used by the target audience. This is known as "narrowcasting" and is particularly useful once the campaign is advanced, such as, once you have public awareness of the problem of overweight and obesity. In order to do this it is important to know which media are most likely to influence the key decision makers and then to develop strategies to reach those media outlets. For example, politicians are more likely to read the news and editorial pages of the most widely circulated newspapers, followed by those from the region where their constituents are based. Community opinion leaders are more likely to read newspaper editorial pages, including letters to the editor and opinion editorials, than the general public.

How do we get the media to pay attention?

Stories must be newsworthy to generate media interest. Making it local and keeping it relevant are two strategies to do this. This can be done by bringing statistics from a national level down to the local level by using creative epidemiology—such as outlining the new cases of Type 2 diabetes by local government region, outlining "hot spots" and calling for action to address this problem.[24] Creating news with events is

also another strategy; this can be used to launch reports, research findings, or to publicize the visit of an international expert. This will require creative expertise to develop a "hook" to entice the media to "bite" and cover the story in the way in which you require.

How do we make sure the media tells stories that communicate the advocacy messages effectively?

How advocates and the journalists frame the issue determines how the audience decides who is responsible for the cause and solution to a problem. This is important because research around media coverage of obesity shows that the way it is reported and framed can divert attention from the structural changes required for prevention. For example, in Australia, content and framing analysis of reporting of overweight and obesity in television current affairs found that the media sees obesity as an individual problem with individual solutions.[25] The focus on the individual can give rise to a "blame the victim" approach, ignoring actions of food companies, advertisers and the effects of government policies. The emphasis on personal responsibility moves attention away from the broader environmental issues that are amenable to change.

There are several steps that advocates can take to ensure that the public health perspective resonates with the media.

- **Translate the individual problem into a social issue.** Rather than talking about behavior, talk about policies that will change the problem. The language must demonstrate that there is a wider environment in which people are trying to make healthy decisions.
- **Assign primary responsibility.** Most people assume that the individual or parents are responsible for the problem of overweight and obesity in children. However, if audiences are to understand the public health perspective, then advocates must outline the corporate, government or institutional responsibility for the problem. The body or individual responsible for taking action must be identified.
- **Present a solution.** It is not enough to speak about the problem and who is responsible. The action required also needs to be articulated in a simple and effective way.

- **Make a practical appeal.** Public health policies are usually much more effective at changing behavior than education alone. If you can demonstrate that they are also cost-effective, particularly in the short-term, that is also beneficial and worth highlighting. Outline how the policy will address the basic cause of the problem and how it will save money, enhance productivity, save lives or protect children.
- **Counter the food and advertising industry frames.** It is necessary to develop media frames to counter those of the opposition, and counter messaging is essential with an adversarial issue such as overweight and obesity. A number of common arguments are used by adversaries in the debate such as: "Parents are responsible for overseeing their children's health, particularly their diet"; "Obesity prevention is complex and there is still a lot of debate about what causes it"; "There is no evidence that food marketing is the cause of the problem or that bans on marketing are the cure"; "There are no good or bad foods, just good or bad diets"; "Individual responsibility is the key to the problem, not a heavy-handed nanny state".[26]
- **Use media bites.** These are short quotes which reporters find so appealing that they want to use them in their stories. Ideally, they provide a simplifying concept for the policy objective, they grab the attention of a journalist and gain access to a news story and they help frame the issues that points towards the policy objective. Once the media outlets have worked up the background for the story, they will look for quotes to best illustrate a particular aspect. This will often take the form of about 15 seconds in a television story, a few sentences in an article or a one-sentence grab for radio. They need to be short and sharp so that they succinctly frame the issue, for example: self-regulation of junk food marketing by the advertising and media industry is "like leaving the fox in charge of the hen house"; decisions not to regulate junk food marketing are "putting corporate wealth ahead of children's health"; high sugar breakfast cereals are "confectionery dressed up as breakfast cereal".[27]

Conclusion

Advocacy is an essential driver of meaningful change for obesity prevention. Developing a plan of action starts with a critical understanding of the problem and the solutions, identifying those who are involved with the issue, recognizing the policies related to the issue (either implemented or not), the organizations engaged with it, and the channels (including the media) that will provide access to those who make decisions, or can influence decisions.

Many countries have published expert reports, which outline the problem of overweight and obesity, along with potential solutions. These recommendations have no force unless they are implemented, which will not happen without advocacy. The public health community must acknowledge and recognize the important role that advocacy plays in the prevention of overweight and obesity. As experts, those engaged in the issue make credible spokespeople, have links to the research and evidence for obesity prevention, and are in a position to encourage others to join up and support change.

More critically, industries that may be threatened by policies and regulation to prevent obesity are, themselves, actively engaged in lobbying to ensure that their views are heard and that their economic and other contributions are recognized and supported. The alternative views on protecting the health and wellbeing of children need to be communicated and promoted to both decision makers and to the wider community. Without this action, effective policies that challenge the status quo are unlikely to be implemented and the epidemic will continue to escalate unchecked.

References

1 The Lancet. Editorial—The catastrophic failures of public health. *Lancet* 2004; **363**:745.
2 Lang T, Rayner g: Overcoming policy cacophony on obesity: an ecological public health frameworke for policymakers. *Obes Rev* 2007; **8**(Suppl. 1):165–181.
3 World Health Organization: Development Communication in Action. Report of the Inter-agency Meeting on Advocacy Strategies for Health and Development. HED/92.5. Geneva. WHO, 1995.
4 Chapman S, Lupton D: The Fight for Public Health: Principles and Practice of Media Advocacy. London: BMJ Publishing Group, 1994.
5 UK Government Office for Science: Tackling Obesities: Future Choices—Project Report, 2nd edn. London: UK Government Foresight Programme, Government Office for Science, 2007.

6 Yach D, Hawkes C, Gould CL, Hofman K: The global burden of chronic diseases—overcoming the impediments to prevention and control. *JAMA* 2004; **291**:2616–2622.

7 Public Health Alliance for the Island of Ireland (PHA): Public Health Advocacy Toolkit. Ireland: PHA Belfast, 2007.

8 Gray M: Forty years of plotting for public health. *MJA* 1997; **167**:587–589.

9 Adapted from World Health Organization: Advocacy and Public Health. Module 2, at www.euro.who.int/document/e82092_3.pdf (accessed 1 March 2008).

10 Friel S, Chopra M, Satcher D: Unequal weight: equity oriented responses to the global obesity epidemic. *BMJ* 2007; **335**:1241–1243.

11 Chapman S: Tobacco control advocacy in Australia: reflections on thirty years of progress. *Health Educ Behav* 2001; **28**(3):274–289.

12 Chapman S: Public Health Advocacy and Tobacco Control: Making Smoking History. Oxford, UK: Blackwell Publishing, 2007.

13 John Hopkins School of Public Health: A Frame for Advocacy. Baltimore USA: Population Communications Services, Centre for Communications Programs, Johns Hopkins School of Public Health, 2003; at: www.infoforhealth.org/pr/advocacy/index.shtml (accessed 3 March 2008).

14 World Health Organization: Advocacy and Public Health—Module 2, 2003; at: www.euro.who.int/document/e820892_3.pdf (accessed 24 February 2008).

15 Adapted from: American Cancer Society: Strategy Planning for Tobacco Control Advocacy. Washington, USA: American Cancer Society and International Union Against Cancer (UICC), 2003.

16 Lezine D, Reed G: Political will: a bridge between public health knowledge and action. *Am J Public Health* 2007; **97**: 2010–2013.

17 World Health Organization: Stop the Global Epidemic of Chronic Disease. A Practical Guide to Successful Advocacy. Geneva: World Health Organization, 2006.

18 American Cancer Society: Strategy Planning for Tobacco Control Advocacy. Washington, USA: American Cancer Society and International Union Against Cancer (UICC), 2003:12.

19 The Democracy Centre. Lobbying—the basics, 1997; at www.democracyctr.org/library/california/lobbying.htm (accessed 13 March 2008).

20 Pertschuk M, Wilbur P: Media Advocacy—Strategies for Reframing Public Debate. Washington, DC: Advocacy Institute, 1991.

21 Berridge V: Public health activism: lessons from history. *BMJ* 2007; **335**:1310–1312.

22 Dorfman L, Wallack L, Woodruff K: More than a message—framing public health advocacy to change corporate practices. *Health Educ Behav* 2005; **32**(3):320–336.

23 US Department of Health and Human Services: Media Strategies for Smoking Control—Guidelines. US Department of Health and Human Services, Public Health Service, National Institutes of Health, 1988.

24 Diabetes Australia—Victoria: Prevalence of Diabetes in Victoria by Local Government Area: at http://210.247.165.30/epidemic2009/index.htm (accessed 5 October, 2009).

25 Bonfiglioli C, Smith B, King L, Chapman S, Holding S: Choice and voice: obesity debates in television news. *MJA* 2007; **187**:442–445.

26 Partos L. EU food and drink industry commits to obesity challenge. 2005. at: www.foodanddrinkeurope.com/Consumer-Trends/EU-food-and-drink-industry-commits-to-obesity-challenge (accessed 6 October 2009).

27 Campaign for Commercial-Free Childhood. Frequently asked questions about the lawsuit against Viacom and Kellogg. 2005: at www.commercialexploitation.org/pressreleases/lawsuitfaq.htm (Accessed 6 October 2009).

PART 4

Policy and practice

This final section investigates the application of the existing and emerging evidence into the various settings and sectors where policy and practice can be implemented for change. Chapters 24 and 25 set the wider scene with Mark Lawrence and Boyd Swinburn defining the role of policy in obesity prevention and Phil James and Neville Rigby taking on one of the biggest challenges in obesity prevention—creating the political will for action. Policy is such an important driver for change but the role that evidence plays in the policy development process is disturbingly minor. This is a blow for health scientists who spend their lives generating the data to inform policy change only to have it swamped by other considerations—often political. No one knows this better than Phil James, President of the International Association for the Study of Obesity and former Chair of the International Obesity Taskforce. His extraordinary insights from trying to get obesity action onto government agendas around the world are laid out in Chapter 25. He also draws stark contrasts between the government responses to bovine spongiform encephalopathy with its relative apathy over obesity and chronic diseases such as coronary heart disease and diabetes.

The chapters led by Colin Bell and Annie Simmons (Chapters 26 and 27) examine some of the key approaches to whole-of-community programs—planning for sustainability and community capacity building. They draw on the experiences from the obesity projects in Victoria, Australia and the French EPODE (Ensemble Prévenons l'Obésité Des Enfants) program. A capacity building approach allows a common process to be applied with community interventions, yet gives the flexibility that is needed to incorporate the wide differences in community contexts. The EPODE program has the credentials inter-

nationally of a program which extends across many communities and several countries, and its lessons in social marketing are also used in the following chapter by Nadine Henley and Sandrine Raffin (Chapter 28). We are at the stage in social marketing for obesity prevention that we were 15 years ago for tobacco control, so we have much to learn. However, "getting the right messages" and "getting the messages right" will be a much tougher task for changing diet and physical activity patterns than changing smoking patterns.

There are several stand-out settings that must be included in any assessment of policy and practice for preventing childhood obesity. Andrea de Silva-Sanigorski leads Chapter 29 on preschool settings, which provide great opportunities for obesity prevention because the children are very environmentally dependent and the parents are relatively accessible and at a "teachable" stage of life. Schools are an obvious setting, and Goof Buijs and Sue Bowker (Chapter 30) examine the practical issues of creating health promoting schools with a focus on healthy eating and physical activity. The evidence for effectiveness is much stronger for interventions in primary schools than secondary schools and, indeed, adolescents are likely to present a challenge for prevention close to that for adults—very hard.

Interventions with minority groups in high-income countries add several more layers of complexity, including culture, migration effects, marginalization and socio-economic disadvantage. Lisa Gibbs and colleagues (Chapter 32) examine some of these issues but, in reality, we are only just scratching the surface in this vital area of research and action. Similarly, there is a rapidly rising childhood obesity epidemic in many lower-income countries, which do not have the infrastructure, funding or research capacity to manage it. As Juliana Kain and colleagues point out in Chapter 32, these countries are suffering from a double burden of undernutrition and overnutrition, which is often evident even in the same household.

Bill Dietz, who has been a pioneer in obesity research at a clinical and public health level for several decades has the final word. From this wide vantage point, he is able to draw many parallels with other epidemics about the role of grass-roots mobiliztions, the importance of policy and so on, and gazes into his crystal ball to give us his predictions for the future of obesity prevention.

CHAPTER 24

The role of policy in preventing childhood obesity

Mark Lawrence and *Boyd Swinburn*
WHO Collaborating Centre for Obesity Prevention, Deakin University, Melbourne, Australia

Summary

- Policies are statements of intent about action and they can shape the components of the food system and/or physical activity environment to help prevent obesity among children.
- The role of policy in preventing childhood obesity includes:
  - outlining a vision and "road map" for the coherent planning, implementing and evaluating of interventions;
  - communicating consistent messages about what the government values and believes throughout settings and/or organizations; and
  - institutionalizing commitments to practice and thereby ensuring sustainability of systems, processes and changes.
- The food system provides a framework for identifying opportunities and challenges for policy interventions that are systematic, coherent, comprehensive and targeted at the appropriate level and sector of government.
- Policy is political and evidence often is relegated to being just one among many inputs into the policy-making process, although there are recent moves to make policy more evidence-based.
- Policy science aims to increase our understanding of how and why policies are made to help improve policy processes and outcomes.

Preventing Childhood Obesity. Edited by
E. Waters, B.A. Swinburn, J.C. Seidell and R. Uauy.
© 2010 Blackwell Publishing.

Introduction

"Policy" is a nebulous term to describe an activity with a very practical role. Among the many definitions of policy, it is generally characterized as being a statement that captures an organization's values, beliefs and intentions towards an issue.[1] Anyone might develop a policy, though in this chapter we focus on government policy and define obesity prevention policy as:

> a statement of intent about government action to shape the components of the food system and/or physical activity environment to help prevent obesity in the population.

Policies can be broad and at a high level, such as defining national strategic directions (so-called "big P" policies), or more detailed and at a more micro level, such as school rules about accepting food company sponsorship for sporting equipment ("small p" policies). In both instances, policies are developed either in response to a problem or to proactively set out a vision. There is a rapidly evolving evidence base associated with the obesity epidemic in relation to its prevalence, its determinants, its health, social and economic implications and what interventions are most/least effective in its prevention. Against this evidence background there is an expectation for government leadership in terms of policy action to respond to the problem and to provide a vision of how obesity might be managed and reduced into the future.

In this chapter we analyse the role of policy in preventing childhood obesity. We start this analysis by examining why policy is important for obesity prevention. Our analysis covers the food system and physical activity environment but with more emphasis on the former. A brief review of policy instruments and how evidence is incorporated into policy-making is presented. Then two case studies of how evidence is, and is not, used in policy-making are outlined to provide a practical perspective on evidence-based policy development. Finally, we discuss those features that are especially important for helping to build the policy backbone for preventing childhood obesity.

Why is policy important for preventing childhood obesity?

There is a variety of competing views about the importance and role of policy for preventing childhood obesity. Certain stakeholders claim that there is little need for government policy because the food marketplace and physical activity environment is managed democratically, with people being able to demand the food and physical activity choices they want to consume or adopt, and the market then efficiently provides these for them. For instance, they point out that food manufacturers now provide abundant, safe and relatively cheap food—so what is the problem? Conversely, others (including ourselves) argue that government policy is very important because the community has an expectation that the state has a role in protecting and promoting the food system and physical activity environments as community goods. There are three particular reasons why policy is important for preventing childhood obesity.

Food system failure

Despite the impressive efficiencies of the modern food system in producing, processing and distributing food, its operation ignores the ecological fundamentals of the food and environment cyclic relationship and functions in a non-sustainable linear fashion.[2] The modern food system does not have sufficient checks and balances in place to ensure that detrimental over-consumption and environmental impacts do not happen. Indeed, the warning signs of food system failure are amply illustrated by increasing environmental damage, staple food shortages, rising food

prices and increasing obesity prevalence. This assessment is consistent with Moodie et al's observation that obesity is a sign of commercial success (increasing food sales) but a market failure because the market is failing to deliver the best outcomes for people.[3] Policy provides a statement and intentions regarding the food system structure and operation that can help avert and/or correct system failure.

People are not able to demand unencumbered what they want to consume

Generally it is an illusion that people have "free choice" and are able to demand unencumbered what food they want to consume or what physical activity they wish to participate in. In other words, all our choices are determined by individual free will. People are rarely actively involved in how the food system operates and what food products are made available or marketed to them. For instance, it is estimated that there are over 320,000 food products available in the US marketplace,[4] many of which people would not have dreamed of demanding before being persuaded by marketers. By labeling people as "consumers" we perpetuate a way of thinking about how the food system operates in terms of three "Cs"—consumption, commercialization and commodification.[5] Policy can be used to build a more engaged and informed citizenship in relation to the food system and the way it operates.

The vulnerable members of society need to be protected

Nutrition and obesity prevalence data consistently reveal that it is the most vulnerable in society and those least able to engage with the food system that are most at risk of food insecurity and obesity.[6] Engagement with the food system needs to be considered against democratic principles and rights such as participation and transparency in decision making. In this regard, Lang has also coined the term "food democracy" to refer to "the demand for greater access and collective benefit from the food system".[5] These democratic principles and attainment of food democracy can only be pursued within a food policy framework and not left to market forces and consumer demand.

The food system as a framework for analysing food policy

Food policies do not exist of their own volition. Improving policy practice and outcomes requires understanding how, why and where policy is made and implemented. The food system provides a framework to analyse the nature and scope of food issues, stakeholders, institutions, contexts and procedures associated with food policy. Typically, policy analysts describe the food system as a series of interacting subsystems extending across the production, processing, distribution, marketing, selling and consumption of food.[7-9] With a food system framework in place we are well placed to appreciate how and why food policy issues arise and who is involved, predict relationships and influences within the system, and manage the setting more effectively to influence policy processes and outcomes.

For instance, the food system can be mapped to help identify government institutional responsibilities for policies that affect the system's structure and operation. An examination of the institutional responsibilities is structured around the different levels of governance (local, national and global), or "vertical" dimension, to policy responsibilities. Within each level of governance there are various sectors (agriculture, trade, transport, education, etc.), or "horizontal" dimension, to policy responsibilities. Conceptualizing the governance influences over the food system in these two dimensions provides an approach for identifying opportunities and challenges for policy interventions that is systematic, coherent, comprehensive and targeted at the appropriate level and sector of government.[10]

The mapping of the food system in two dimensions also is important because it is frequently assumed that the health sector has primary responsibility for obesity prevention policy. Yet, a brief analysis of the food system highlights that the health sector has a limited influence on the determinants of obesity or the system's operation. Engaging non-health sectors in food policy interventions to support obesity prevention, is an illustration of "joined-up" policy or "healthy public policy",[11] and "health in all policies".[12] An example of a national joined-up approach to obesity prevention policy is *Healthy Weight, Healthy Lives: A Cross Government Strategy for England.*[13]

Irrespective of how cohesive and joined-up the policy intentions for the food system might be, the system itself does not operate in isolation. If there is to be action on the food system to create a healthier food environment for helping to make healthier food choices easier, then we need to understand the broader external circumstances and policy environment within which the food system operates, including the following.

Globalization of food trade

The term "globalization" describes how nations, businesses and people are becoming more connected and interdependent through increased economic integration and communication exchange, cultural diffusion and travel. The globalization of food trade is being linked with significant shifts in dietary patterns. For example, many developing countries are experiencing a "nutrition transition", characterized by a decline in undernutrition accompanied by a rapid increase in obesity.[14] Internationally, food trade is affected inordinately by policy developments in large trading countries, for example, the US Farm Bill, as well as by powerful sectoral interests such as the agricultural sector in the European Union. Global food trade is managed within international agreements and in particular the World Trade Organization (WTO) Agreements and other bilateral or multilateral agreements. Member countries of the WTO are obliged to abide by the rules and provisions in the WTO Agreements that set the framework for international trade liberalization and have implications for domestic food policy.

Microeconomic reform agenda of governments

The political environment within which the food system operates exerts a profound influence over the system's governance, powers and functions. Over the last few decades an explicit microeconomic reform agenda has been pursued by governments in many developed countries. The reform agenda has been characterized by reviews of the operation of components of the food system to reduce the regulatory burden on the food sector, and to examine those regulations which restrict competition, impose costs or confer benefits on business. Many public health nutritionists have argued that relaxing regulatory controls has privileged the manufacturing and marketing of highly processed food products at the expense of more basic primary foods and has not been in the interests of public health.

Environmental and social constraints on the operation of the food system

The viability and integrity of the food system is dependent on maintaining the biodiversity and carrying capacity of biological systems. Environmental and social constraints are placing "reality checks" on conventional thinking towards food policy objectives. For example, the wisdom of pursuing unfettered food production and promoting over-consumption is being increasingly questioned not just by nutritionists, but also by economists and environmentalists. Many public health nutritionists argue that rapidly increasing food prices, food security concerns and food wastage problems are symptoms of limitations with conventional thinking, that is, nature is "biting" back as environmental constraints mean that we are no longer able to sustain profligate exploitation of the food system. In the future, the environmental and social impact of food policy objectives will necessarily receive greater attention in policy planning.

The policy environment for physical activity

Physical activity levels are significantly influenced by policies. Policies on transport infrastructure, housing, urban design, neighborhood development, zoning, residential development, policing, and so on, influence the built environment, which in turn influences the amount children will walk, cycle, play outside, and take public transport.[15] Although there is some debate about the mix of individual and environmental contributions to children's physical activity levels,[16] there is an increasing consensus that environments that promote active transport and outdoor recreation are not only good for health but are also more liveable and socially connected, less polluting and more sustainable. Thus, the health advocacy for improved urban environments is in synergy with many other movements and the major barrier is the expense of retro-fitting urban environments that were built for car dependence. In comparison to the food system, the policies which influence the built environment

are more locally based and much less internationally dependent.

Policy instruments

There are a number of instruments, or tools, which governments have available for implementing policy. The primary policy instruments are: regulations and laws (rules); taxation and funding (for programs, research, monitoring and evaluation, social marketing and capacity building); services and service delivery (providing hospitals, workforce, etc.); and advocacy (to the public, private sector, and other jurisdictions). Within the contemporary political environment of many developed countries there exists a dominant ideology of neoliberalism characterized by the use of those policy instruments that place more emphasis on individual responsibility for dietary and physical activity choices and less reliance on government intervention in the environments where those choices are made.

Milio coined the terms "soft" (services, funding) and "hard" (taxation, regulations) policy instruments to distinguish among instruments in terms of their relative level of political risk.[17] Recent studies indicate that this distinction also may correlate with policy effectiveness. Brescoll et al asked nutritionists and public health policy experts to rate 51 possible child obesity prevention policies for their likely public health impact and political feasibility, respectively.[18] Results showed that strong regulatory measures such as bans on food marketing to children were regarded as being less politically feasible, but more likely to be effective in obesity prevention. Conversely, policies that focused on education and information dissemination were regarded as politically feasible, but likely to have little impact on obesity prevention.

How evidence gets incorporated into policy-making

Making policies for the prevention of childhood obesity, as with any policy, is not a linear, rational, evidence-based process. The obesity research community has been collecting large amounts of evidence, which should be informing policies for obesity prevention, but very little of it actually comes to bear on the decision-making process. Why is this? First, much of the evidence being collected is about the problem (the size, trends, determinants, mechanisms and consequences of obesity) not the solutions, and decision makers want solution-oriented evidence: what works and what does not work. Second, effective knowledge translation of evidence into policy and practice remains underwhelming, despite the fact that our knowledge of research utilization theories and practice is increasing. Researchers and policy-makers still do not have enough joint "spaces", common language and shared goals to meaningfully engage in knowledge exchange.

Although most people agree that there is a need to prevent childhood obesity, food (and, to a lesser extent, physical activity) is big business and there is a complexity implicit in gaining a commitment to develop a food-related policy, and determining what it might say and do. Food policy affects the way the food system operates and whose interests it best serves. Often there will be winners and losers emerging from policy decisions. Policy-making is highly political because it is about power relations across the food system—who can shape policy to maximize benefits and minimize risks to their interests.

The politics of power also often plays out in how evidence gets incorporated into policy-making, and this occurs in two ways.

The collection, analysis and interpretation of evidence

Human judgement is involved in setting research questions and it is not uncommon for evidence to be collected, analysed and interpreted selectively by stakeholders to privilege their particular interests. We cannot assume that all relevant evidence is made available or that the available evidence is of high quality. This applies to all sides in the debate, although there are often uneven levels of resources to obtain evidence to support and/or challenge for a particular policy position.

The translation of evidence into policies and programs

Human judgement also is involved in translating available evidence into policies and programs. Usually, experts, panels, committees and taskforces are needed to make judgements in relation to the quantity and quality of available evidence and how it might be translated into policy. For instance, one unresolved

debate is the legitimacy of evidence derived from studies using so-called less rigorous epidemiological methods such as cohort studies to inform obesity prevention policy. Whereas randomized controlled trials are widely accepted as the preferred research design for controlling potential bias (maximizing internal validity), generally, obesity prevention studies do not lend themselves to such a design or even where they do, their external validity (relevance to the real world) may be limited. This can present challenges for obtaining sufficient evidence to translate into policy. There is an evidence-based nutrition movement[19] that is striving for food policy-making to be more appropriate in assessing the evidence that is available from public health nutrition studies.

This analysis is not intended to denigrate evidence-based practice or the research being undertaken to generate evidence and improve our understanding of research utilization. Instead, it is intended to highlight that policy-making processes are political and evidence often is relegated to being just one among many inputs into the policy-making process. Evidence-based practice is an ideal we should aim for with policy-making. However, we need to move beyond focusing just on the technical details of evidence-based practice and begin analysing the political setting within which policy-making takes place if we are to improve obesity prevention policy processes and outcomes.

A future research agenda in evidence-based practice for obesity prevention policy might pursue two complementary paths. The first is the "evidence *for* policy" path that involves undertaking solution-oriented research to obtain the specific evidence needed to inform the content of obesity prevention policy. The second is the "evidence *of* policy" path that involves undertaking critical analysis (policy science) research to increase our understanding of how and why policies are made and how the evidence can be better brought to bear on those decisions: that is, improving knowledge translation processes for better policy outcomes.

Case studies of how evidence is (or is not) incorporated into policy

In this section we examine two case studies of how evidence is or is not used in policy-making. The first case study is an analysis of organizational policy, in this instance a state health department policy, to help create a healthier food environment at facilities under its jurisdiction including: canteens; kiosks; vending machines; catering at functions, meetings or special events; fundraising activities, events or prizes; and cafes or coffee shops (Box 24.1). It illustrates an orthodox evidence-based approach to policy-making. The

Box 24.1 Case study— incorporating the evidence

Queensland healthy food service policies

In 2007, Queensland Health launched "A Better Choice Healthy Food and Drink Supply Strategy for Queensland Health Facilities" (A Better Choice) with the aim of increasing the availability of healthier foods and drinks provided to staff, visitors and the general public in facilities owned and operated by Queensland Health.[20] This policy strategy, which emerged from a 2006 Queensland Obesity Summit, represents a state government department displaying leadership and setting an example for the broader community by modeling an environment that helps make healthier food choices easier food choices. The objectives of A Better Choice are to:

1. improve the availability of healthy choices (to at least 80% of foods and drinks displayed);
2. identify and promote healthy choices;
3. identify and reduce the availability of less healthy choices (to no more than 20% of foods and drinks displayed); and
4. ensure healthy choices are available at all times.

The classification of foods according to their healthiness is based on a nutrient profiling system in which foods and drinks are allocated to either green ("everyday"), amber ("choose carefully") or red ("limit") categories.[20] The authors of the policy strategy emphasize that it reflects scientific evidence drawn from 15 local, state, national and international policy documents and initiatives. They explained that the process for developing A Better Choice included:

1. a review of scientific literature;
2. an audit of food outlets across Queensland Health facilities to map foods and drinks supplied;
3. investigation into case studies of existing work within Queensland Health facilities;
4. a review of current nutrient profiling approaches;
5. the formation of a steering committee comprised of expert representatives from Queensland Health

staff, including catering and food service, nutrition, health promotion and human resources; as well as external representatives from professional associations and unions;
6. identification of scope, approach and possible implementation options;
7. the development of nutrient criteria including modeling the supply of products;
8. finalization of strategy implementation, scientific content and scope following consultation with key stakeholders.

It can be seen that the definition of "evidence" has been broad and included published literature as well as audit and program evaluation data and modeling (as recommended by the International Obesity Taskforce).[21] With that evidence and the support of a higher level policy strategy, a process was then run to bring in broad stakeholder and expert support, identify the specific policy choices and then recommend the final feasible policy plan.

second case study is national government policy towards the marketing of unhealthy food to children. It illustrates the more political nature of policy-making and, in particular, government inertia in responding to evidence and the role of lobbying and competing interests in influencing the policy process and outcome (Box 24.2).

Creating the policy backbone for obesity prevention

A strong "policy backbone" is needed to support obesity prevention efforts so that the other government and non-government actions, such as program funding and service delivery, are working to a common direction with a supportive set of "rules" to follow. What should a policy backbone include and how would the evidence be best incorporated? In weighing this question, it is important to understand the general features of the policy-making process, which are critical to its success. These are outlined in Box 24.3. First and foremost is the need for political leadership, which is only likely to materialize with concerted advocacy efforts from many quarters. Evidence of leadership can be seen in the personal role modeling of politicians, the organizational role modeling of government departments (starting with healthy food

Box 24.2 Ignoring the evidence— food marketing to children

Food marketing to children

There is strong evidence that marketing works, especially when it is specifically targeted at children and takes advantage of their credulity.[22–24] There is also strong evidence that the types of food and beverages marketed to children are overwhelmingly energy-dense and nutrient-poor. Furthermore, there is strong evidence that a high intake of energy-dense foods promotes unhealthy weight gain. Included in the evidence mix is the concept of "indirect evidence",[21] which states that there is direct evidence that marketing influences children's eating patterns but this is proprietary information not public information. However, based on their own direct evidence, food companies continue to invest billions of dollars in marketing to children so one can indirectly infer the broad findings of the proprietary studies showing the influence of marketing on children's diets.

In spite of this weight of evidence (and support from parents, professionals and the general public), policy responses are few. A few examples of policies banning food marketing to children exist but it is far less than expected, given the likely cost–effectiveness of such an intervention.[25] The reason, of course, is the vigorous pressure from the food and advertising industries on politicians not to create policies that restrict their ability to target children. Food marketing to children is a classic case of the pressure from vested interests outweighing both the evidence and public and professional calls for a tough policy response.

Box 24.3 Important features for a successful policy-making process

Political will: The level of support from senior politicians is probably the single most important determinant of successful policy-making. These may be expressed in a commitment through high-level policy strategy documents.

Policy-making structure: Is the structure cross-departmental or even cross-sectoral? Does it have high level authority to make decisions or recommendations? Does it have the responsibility (jurisdiction) to implement the policies? Does it have the capability (expertise) and capacity (resources) to create, implement and evaluate the policies?

Policy-relevant evidence: It is important that a broad definition of evidence is taken and preferably, that the modeling of the costs and benefits of the policy options have been done.

Policy development process: While there is a tendency for some government policies to be hatched in secrecy to maximize their "announceability", this process leaves little room for consultation with the key stakeholders. Ideally, for maximum buy-in and expert input, consultation needs to be an intrinsic part of the process.

services in the departments of health and hospitals), and giving the responsibility to senior ministers. Indeed, with food prices rising, potential food shortages looming, and food-related disease costs escalating, a stand-alone Ministry for Food may be warranted.

There are many possible policies that could be included in a policy backbone for obesity prevention and below we have outlined some of the key policies that could be major contributors to obesity prevention efforts.

Regulations to reduce food marketing to children: This is such a touchstone issue for obesity prevention that little progress is likely to be made at a population level while there is such an enormous marketing effort (over $10 billion/year in the USA alone)[23] undermining the health promotion efforts of the rest of society. Not only are bans on marketing obesogenic foods to children probably one of the single most effective and cost-saving strategies a government could implement,[25] but they also send a very strong message to society about what is appropriate and inappropriate food for children.

Food service policies: Government departments and government-funded organizations reach virtually everyone—they are large employers, they include many child settings, such as schools and preschools, and they feed large numbers of people in settings such as hospitals and prisons. If healthy food service policies were required of all these organizations, it would have a significant effect on actual food eaten as well as sending loud messages to a large proportion of the population about healthy food choices. Even if the food eaten in these settings is a minor proportion of the total annual food consumption, which is often the case for schools,[26] they can have a "lighthouse" effect by being highly visible and "shining their light" far and wide.

Monitoring and feedback systems: Many countries are relying on infrequent (in the case of Australia, every decade or more) surveys to monitor the changes in obesity prevalence and even then, they are usually not fine-grained enough to give meaningful data by locality, ethnicity and socio-economic disadvantage. Arkansas instituted through legislation an annual BMI check on every child in the state[27] with the information going back to parents in the form of a Health Card Report[28] and aggregate data going to each school and district. This feedback loop of regular, fine-grained monitoring to the change agents seems to have raised awareness and sparked community action throughout the state such that the rise in obesity prevalence has now flattened out.[29]

Fiscal interventions: The concept of a system of taxes and subsidies to increase the price of unhealthy foods and reduce the price of healthy choices has often been proposed.[30] This would certainly influence food purchasing behaviors if the price changes were significant, but to offset the regressive nature of such taxes, the revenue raised would be needed to support the healthy food choices. More modeling work is needed on this concept.,[31] It could not only change food choices towards the healthy options, but the extra revenue raised could be used to lift the overall funding of population prevention of chronic diseases beyond the 0.5% of the health budget, where most now languish. At the very least, the existing tax, subsidy and price control systems should be examined to see if there are perverse incentives operating, which are artificially depressing the prices of energy-dense foods (such as sugar and plant oils) and raising the prices of healthy foods (such as fruit and vegetables). Fiscal interventions, such as congestion taxes or public transport fare subsidies could have significant effects on patterns of transport, including active transport modes of walking, cycling and public transport.

Health (obesity) impact assessment: The concept of health impact assessments have been around for some years but have found footholds in only a few jurisdictions. Since many urban planning and transport infrastructure decisions have substantial impacts on the built environment and its "walkability" and "cycleability",[32] they need to take health outcomes (including obesity) into account. Other policy and funding decisions such as taxation regimes, social policies and benefits, and education policies may also have important health outcomes that need prior assessment.

Conclusion

Policy has an integral role in community-based obesity prevention. With the increasing availability and quality of evidence of the obesity epidemic and effective interventions to tackle this epidemic, there are ongoing calls for government action to translate the evidence into policy and practice. Policy demonstrates government commitment to obesity prevention and provides a road map for planning, implementing and evaluating interventions.

Despite the calls for evidence-based policy, we have shown it does not occur of its own volition or necessarily as a rational process. Policy is political. There are contested views over the evidence associated with the prevalence and distribution of the obesity epidemic, its causation and its consequences. Critically, from a policy perspective, there is heated debate over how and why the available evidence should be translated into policy activities to tackle the obesity epidemic.

Into the future, particular features of the policy-making process will be critical to support the evidence—policy relationship, namely: political will; policy-making structure; policy-relevant evidence; and policy development process. As the prevalence of obesity among children around the world increases, the need for policy will become more urgent. The five policies we have outlined represent examples of "low hanging fruit" that could be relatively easily "picked" as policy activities without further delay.

References

1 Lawrence M: Policy and politics. In: Lawrence M, Worsley A, eds. Public Health Nutrition: From Principles to Practice. Sydney: Allen & Unwin and London: Open University Press, 2007:450–476.

2 Lang T, Heasman M: Food Wars: The Global Battle for Mouths, Minds and Markets. London: Earthscan, 2004.

3 Moodie R, Swinburn B: Childhood obesity—a sign of commercial success but market failure. Int J Ped Obes 2006; 1:133–138.

4 Nestle M: Food Politics—How the Food Industry Influences Nutrition and Health. London: University California Press, 2002.

5 Lang T: Food policy for the 21st century: can it be both radical and reasonable? In: Koc M, MacRae R, Mougeot LJA, Welsh J, eds. For Hunger-Proof Cities: Sustainable Urban Food Systems. The International Development Research Centre, 1999:216–224. Available from: www.idrc.ca/en/ev-30626-201-1-DO_TOPIC.html (accessed 6 May 2008).

6 Marmot M: Social determinants of health inequalities. *Lancet* 2005; **365**:1099–1104.

7 Heywood P, Lund-Adams M: The Australian food and nutrition system: a basis for policy formulation and analysis. *Aust J Public Health* 1991; **15**:258–270.

8 Sobal J, Khan LK, Bisogni CA: Conceptual model of the food and nutrition system. *Soc Sci Med* 1998; **47**:853–863.

9 Tansey G, Worsley A: The Food System. London: Earthscan, 1995.

10 Sacks G, Swinburn B, Lawrence M: A systematic policy approach to changing the food and physical activity environments to prevent obesity. *Aust N Z J Health Policy* 2008; **5**:13–20.

11 World Health Organization: The Adelaide Recommendations on Healthy Public Policy. Geneva: World Health Organization, 1988.

12 Kickbusch I, McCann W, Sherbon T: Adelaide revisited: from healthy public policy to health in all policies. *Health Promot Int* 2008; **23**:1–4.

13 Cross-Government Obesity Unit, Department of Health and Department of Children: Schools and Families, Healthy Weight, Healthy Lives: a Cross-Government Strategy for England, 2008. Available from: www.dh.gov.uk/en/Publichealth/Healthimprovement/Obesity/DH_082383 (accessed 16 May 2008).

14 Popkin BM: Nutrition in transition: the changing global nutrition challenge. *Asia Pac J Clin Nutr* 2001; **10**:S13–S18.

15 Molnar BE, Gortmaker SL, Bull FC, Buka SL: Unsafe to play? Neighborhood disorder and lack of safety predict reduced physical activity among urban children and adolescents. *Am J Health Prom* 2004; **18**:378–386.

16 Wilkin TJ, Mallam KM, Metcalf BS, Jeffery AN, Voss LD: Variation in physical activity lies with the child, not his environment: evidence for an "activitystat" in young children. *Int J Obes* 2006; **30**:1050–1055.

17 Milio N: Nutrition Policy for Food-Rich Countries: A Strategic Analysis. Baltimore: The Johns Hopkins University Press, 1990.

18 Brescoll VL, Kersh R, Brownell KD: Assessing the feasibility and impact of federal childhood obesity policies. *Ann Am Acad Pol Soc Sci* 2008; **615**:178–194.

19 Mann J: Discrepancies in nutritional recommendations: the need for evidence based nutrition. *Asia Pac J Clin Nutr* 2002; **11**:S510–S515.

20 Queensland Health: A Better Choice Healthy Food and Drink Supply Strategy for Queensland Health Facilities. The State of Queensland, 2007. Available from: www.health.qld.gov.au/ph/Documents/hpu/32512.pdf (accessed 16 May 2008).

21 Swinburn B, Gill T, Kumanyika S: Obesity prevention: a proposed framework for translating evidence into action. *Obes Rev* 2005; **6**:23–33.

22 Dalmeny K: Food marketing: the role of advertising in child health. *Consum Policy Rev* 2003; **13**:2–7.

23 Institute of Medicine: Food Marketing to Children and Youth. Threat or Opportunity? Washington: National Academy of Sciences, 2006.

24 Hastings G, Stead M, McDermott L et al: Review of the Research on the Effects of Food Promotion to Children. Glasgow: Centre for Social Marketing, University of Strathclyde, 2003.

25 Haby MM, Vos T, Carter R et al: A new approach to assessing the health benefit from obesity interventions in children and adolescents: the assessing cost-effectiveness in obesity project. *Int J Obes* 2006; **30**:1463–1475.

26 Bell AC, Swinburn BA: What are the key food groups to target for preventing obesity and improving nutrition in schools? *Eur J Clin Nutr* 2004; **58**:258–263.

27 Ryan KW, Card-Higginson P, McCarthy SG, Justus MB, Thompson JW: Arkansas fights fat: translating research into policy to combat childhood and adolescent obesity. *Health Aff* (Project Hope) 2006; **25**:992–1004.

28 Denehy J: Health report cards: an idea whose time has come? *J Sch Nurs* 2004; **20**:125–126.

29 University of Arkansas for Medical Sciences: Year Three Evaluation: Arkansas Act 1220 of 2003 to Combat Childhood Obesity. Little Rock, Arkansas: Fay W. Boozman College of Public Health, 2005.

30 Kim D, Kawachi I: Food taxation and pricing strategies to "thin out" the obesity epidemic. *Am J Prev Med* 2006; **30**:430–437.

31 Crawford I, Leicester A, Windmeijer F: The "Fat Tax": Economic Incentives to Reduce Obesity. London: Institute for Fiscal Studies, 2003.

32 Saelens BE, Sallis JF, Black JB, Chen D: Neighborhood-based differences in physical activity: an environment scale evaluation. *Am J Public Health* 2003; **93**:1552–1558.

CHAPTER 25

Developing the political climate for action

Philip James[1,2] *and Neville Rigby*[1]
[1] International Association for the Study of Obesity, London, UK
[2] Neville Rigby & Associates, London, UK

Summary and recommendations for practice

Key elements in converting academic analyses into policy implementation

- Prepare groundwork by producing coherent evidence, reports and briefing papers, to promote public and political awareness.
- Develop a broad consensus among eminent scientific/medical leaders; anticipate poor support from many clinicians with political ambitions and little understanding of public policies.
- Engage openly with the media; focus on opinion leaders. Repeatedly explain the issues willingly and patiently.
- Be ready for confrontation from opposing viewpoints and prepare reasoned responses developing new work to answer the challenges.
- Create a movement by engaging different societal and academic groups with established political connections to agree the main consensus not the detail.
- Remember that political change takes time and depends on a crisis or incessant vocal public and expert lobbying.
- Focus on finance—health ministries are weak: other ministers or the prime minister make decisions affecting other sectors, based on economic arguments and political pressure.

Introduction

Public health initiatives require a sophisticated understanding, not only of medical concerns, but also of political issues in order to appreciate why some initiatives succeed and others do not. The national response to health needs is often delayed. Examples of this delay include the slow reaction to the HIV contamination of recombinant factor 8 plasma transfusions for hemophiliacs, and the extremely slow response to the emergence of the HIV/Aids epidemic. Similarly, the need to take action in response to the huge death and disability rates from coronary heart disease (CHD) was ignored for years by many governments, allegedly on the grounds that the scientific and medical communities could not agree that a clear link existed between CHD and high blood cholesterol levels, induced by saturated fat intakes, high blood pressure and smoking. Even if this could be proved, inaction was justified by the view that it was the individual's own responsibility to change his or her diet and lifestyle. The government's role was seen as simply providing health promotion messages to enable consumers to make "informed" food choices. The huge agricultural and food industries recognized that they had to show concern for their customers and a vague health educational message suited their interests because their profits often depended on continuing to sell high saturated fat-filled products.

Given that it has taken several decades to see major international initiatives even on tobacco, how do we create the political will for action to be taken? We conclude that the triggers owe less to a clear understanding of the science, or even evidence for the benefits of change, than to a political need to respond publicly to an issue of pressing public concern. We illustrate this from our own experience of political responses to UK and global health concerns since the mid-1970s.

Preventing Childhood Obesity. Edited by
E. Waters, B.A. Swinburn, J.C. Seidell and R. Uauy.
© 2010 Blackwell Publishing.

The contrasts in the responses to food safety and diet-related disease issues

The response to the risks of bovine spongiform encephalopathy (BSE) is instructive. Decisive action was resisted initially as there was great uncertainty about a little understood infective agent, a prion, and fairly clear evidence already that there were species barriers in the susceptibility of different species to prions. So the UK Minister of Agriculture repeatedly denied that there was any danger from eating BSE-infected meat products, for example, from some types of fast food. However, 10 years after one of the authors (WPTJ) was alerted confidentially to the development of the BSE outbreak in cattle, there was suddenly a cabinet crisis in 1996 when the head of the Expert BSE group, Professor John Pattison, insisted throughout several hours of grilling by the Prime Minister and his senior colleagues that the first 10 cases of a new strain of Creutzfeldt–Jakob disease (new variant CJD) must be assumed to arise from infected beef (personal communication). Quite dramatic moves on BSE were made by the UK Prime Minister within 24 hours because at that stage it was recognized that the agent had the potential to infect huge numbers of the population (numbered then at up to 8 million) and this would affect individuals randomly with a ghastly and inevitably fatal disease. Scientific guesswork, the presumed manipulation of evidence by ministers and the political pressure to protect the long-term interests of the farming and food sectors, magnified the alarm of the public, media, some sections of the medical profession and ministers themselves. So this was a major crisis in political, economic and social terms. The beef bans, changes in farming practice and removal of beef export licences that followed cost the UK tax payer over £6 billion and the ensuing changes in Europe cost far more.

Figure 25.1 shows the array of major factors that influence public thinking on risk in general and how these factors relate to the public's perception of the risks of BSE.

The contrast with such issues as obesity, diabetes, or coronary heart disease (CHD) is striking. Yet the draconian measures for handling BSE were taken on far less evidence than that which underlay the dietary basis for the hundreds of thousands of deaths from CHD and the contrast with the governmental effort to prevent CHD is striking. No country has spontaneously introduced major strategic changes in food policies on the basis of analyses of chronic diseases and their risk factors by government expert committees.[1] CHD is still the biggest contributor to deaths and CHD and cancers in the UK continue to account for more than two thirds of preventable UK deaths, that is, in those under 75 years. Yet the only issue which resonates in political circles is the higher death rate among the poorer classes and the failure to treat cases promptly and adequately.

The problem is that it is almost universally assumed that diet depends on an individual's choice and that while the consequences are hazardous, heart attacks and strokes occur later in life and "one has to die of something". Type 2 diabetes was seen as an unfortunate condition in the elderly and really linked to a family history of susceptibility. The dreaded risks of cancer were not linked to diet, but to pesticides and chemical carcinogens, which governments still try to understand and limit by engaging large groups of experts. Thus, the public health response to the post-war epidemic of CHD in Europe and North America has depended on groups of cardiologists initiating public debates and proposing changes. This, in turn, has stimulated the food industry to respond by producing lower-fat milks, butter and spreads, and changes in the fatty acid content of foods, thereby providing themselves with excellent marketing material! In every case where political action has been taken there has been political pressure from highly vocal individuals or groups within the academic community or civil society. Furthermore, despite the preventability of Type 2 diabetes, until very recently no effort had been made by doctors, or even by the specialist interest groups, to address its prevention. The huge charitable organizations that fund research on heart disease, stroke, diabetes and cancer, pump millions of dollars into basic research and improved treatment, but support almost nothing in prevention. Indeed, many of the heart foundations and cancer charities have either simply paid lip service to the preventive issue or even attacked preventive initiatives because they were based on crude measures or could demonstrate no "proof" of their effectiveness.

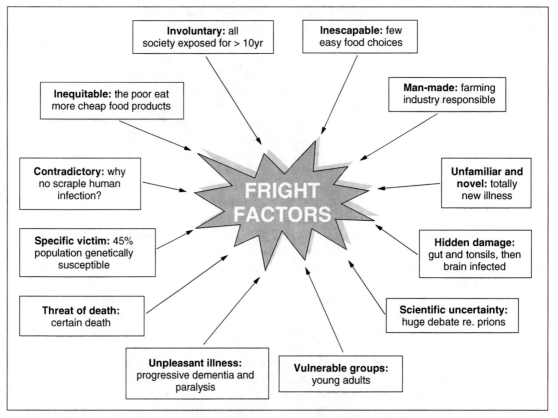

Figure 25.1 Public Perception of Risk (with examples from bovine spongiform encephalopathy risk). Key factors in the huge public response to the identification of human vCJD, acquired from Bovine Spongiform Encephalopathy in cattle, included the fear of widespread exposure through unknown sources to an indiscriminate agent which induced a terrifying and untreatable illness and certain death, particularly among the young.

Background to the obesity crisis: the reasons for its early neglect

Despite the original inclusion of obesity in the International Classification of Diseases in 1948, obesity remains a condition that even some in the medical professions fail to recognize as a disease. Yet warnings about an impending obesity epidemic came during the 1970s in the USA, with "Fogerty" conferences,[2] and in the UK with government/Medical Research Council analyses of the disease and disability likely to be induced by the growing epidemic. The UK report, with remarkable prescience, did warn in 1976: "We are unanimous in our belief that obesity is a hazard to health and a detriment to well-being. It is common enough to constitute one of the most important medical and public health problems of our time."[3]

By 1983 another UK report[4] on obesity called for public health policy changes at a time when adult obesity prevalence stood at 7%. As with the similar Royal College of Physicians reports on smoking[5] and on cardiovascular disease by Shaper,[6] these were all hailed by the College Council as being of immense political and policy importance, but had no effect because they were not locked into the political process. There was also little media coverage and lobbying by academics and civil society groups.

Putting obesity and chronic disease on WHO's agenda

The highly publicized report in the UK from the National Advisory Committee on Nutrition Education in 1983[7] led to the WHO European Regional Office asking for a major new assessment throughout Eastern, Central and Western Europe of nutritional issues, chronic diseases, (including obesity) and their prevention. This in turn led to the first global WHO/FAO report in 1990, which considered both undernutrition and chronic diseases in a coherent global context.[8] This set out far-reaching recommendations which, almost two decades later, remain the basis of widely accepted, but largely unattained, public health goals. These reports were seen by WHO as important, were referred to in major committees of ministers and were highlighted in global academic conferences. Yet despite this public recognition, public health actions were still not instigated, even though there was a clear specification of different levels of initiative required by international, national and local communities.

In fact, both WHO and FAO faced a barrage of lobbying and overt opposition from global sugar interests which dominated the US and European food industries' attitudes. The US government was persuaded by lobbyists to try to block the report's acceptance by WHO, but it failed and the scientific community endorsed the global report's new thinking at the International Congress of Nutrition in 1992.[9]

Over a period of almost 20 years, there have been numerous reports on nutritional aspects of health with, in the 1990s, specific recommendations on obesity, but again without any effect. The medical profession was then largely responsible for specifying that obesity was simply a risk factor induced by people who needed to alter their personal habits. The food industry was also totally entrenched in promoting its products and had excellent government connections, strengthened by providing financial support to political parties. As a consequence, slimming clubs flourished and tens of millions of adults have attempted repeatedly to slim, with articles on the subject guaranteeing an avid readership in women's and lifestyle magazines.

Establishing a policy focus on obesity per se

In this setting, obesity experts in 1995 asked for a public campaign to change doctors' and governments' attitudes. Given the previous experience, however, it was clearly necessary first to establish the magnitude of the problem internationally and then work out how to focus government attention to induce action. This led to the formation of the International Obesity Taskforce (IOTF). Its aim was to galvanize the scientific community to produce a comprehensive dossier of evidence to convince WHO and indeed the nutrition community, preoccupied as usual with the challenges of undernutrition, that the global scale of the obesity epidemic affected even developing countries where there was a double burden of disease. Within a year of its formation, the IOTF had presented its dossier to WHO, and helped WHO convene an expert meeting in June 1997. With unprecedented speed, an interim report was prepared and printed by May 1998.

The report would typically have languished in boxes in basement corridors, but the IOTF drew the attention of ministers to it during the World Health Assembly. One minister, the Honourable Elizabeth Thompson, then Minister of Health for Barbados and chair of the Commonwealth Health Ministers meeting, decided to make obesity one of the themes of the Commonwealth's triennial meeting over which she was to preside in Bridgetown later that year. This was significant, because the ability to address directly more than 50 health ministers should not be underestimated. Several health ministers acknowledged the problem, but they had no need to react because there was no pressure from their "constituency". There was also no ready-made toolkit for ministerial action, so IOTF had to refocus on the recommendations of the earlier controversial WHO 797 report.[8] It also had to engage the media and progressively analyse what to do in practice.

It was recognized that there were deficiencies in the original report as there was no appropriate method of assessing childhood obesity, and the economic impact of obesity was poorly assessed. The IOTF group, chaired by Bill Dietz, established the IOTF criteria for childhood obesity, and Tim Gill, Boyd Swinburn,

Shiriki Kumanyika and colleagues set out a series of approaches and proposals, which form the current framework for preventive action.

The IOTF's relocation to new headquarters in London increased its visibility and accessibility to the media, leading to the inclusion of obesity as front-cover stories in influential publications such as *Time* magazine, *Newsweek* and *Forbes*. This required thorough background briefings to journalists, who were genuinely interested in exploring in depth this new "headline" health story.

All this publicity merely accentuated the acknowledgement of the problem by politicians and, despite the systematic pressure of numerous reports—mostly based on highlighting the trends and putative problems of obesity—little was achieved. Then IOTF took part in the first WHO global analysis of the risk factors responsible for the burden of disease, which showed that excess weight gain was one of the top six risk factors for disability and premature deaths globally. This dramatic development stimulated numerous governments and health-associated groups to assess their policies, but yet again inaction prevailed. Several countries set out the principles for action, but placed the major emphasis on health educational approaches. The medical profession, without a coherent speciality for obesity comparable with, for instance, cardiology or rheumatology, remained cynical and reluctant to become too involved. The one improvement, however, was that by 2002 support among NGOs concerned with heart disease, diabetes and cancer was beginning to grow.

IOTF was then invited to take part in a WHO Western Pacific Regional meeting to discuss the prevention of chronic disease with more than 30 ministers of health. As usual, IOTF received a polite but detached hearing until the words "childhood obesity" were used as an additional issue. At that point every minister present suddenly focused and demanded to know how they should proceed to tackle this escalating problem in countries such as China, Japan and the Pacific Islands as well as Australasia. They also agreed with the "outrageous" proposition that they were actually very weak in terms of their capacity to put pressure on their government for action or special measures; health ministries constantly ask for more money to cope with their escalating medical costs but they generally lose out because the drivers of government policy are national security, economic development, foreign policy and political credibility. It became clear that ministers were anxious to focus on children because this demonstrably demanded societal action rather than invoking personal responsibility. It was also clear, however, that no minister was prepared to confront the titanic power of the agricultural/food chain industries.

WHO recognized that new initiatives were needed, and with the broad support for its development of the Framework Convention on Tobacco, WHO then decided to address the need to improve diet—a challenge that would inevitably revive conflict with the global food industry. An expert consultation was, therefore, convened to reassess the WHO 797 report. WHO adopted a public consultative process prior to the finalizing of the new expert report, which became known as the WHO "916" report.[10] This was a key part of the process of attempting to disarm an antagonistic food and beverage sector prior to the preparation of the WHO's Global Strategy on Diet, Physical Activity and Health.*

The political ramifications of these initiatives were obvious, but few academics were ready for the ferocity of the food and beverage industries' assault on WHO, led by the sugar industry. An industrial counter-offensive, which rapidly escalated from a whispering campaign to an overt denunciation of the 916 report as "bad science" made the diet strategy a major global news story. To her credit, the Director-General of WHO, Dr Gro Harlem-Brundtland, chose to launch the report in person at the FAO's headquarters in Rome, expressing her solidarity and support as she stood shoulder to shoulder with the report's vice-chair, Professor Shiriki Kumanyika.

Even within the obesity field, food lobbyists attempted to drive a wedge between researchers using those dependent on industry funding, and in the US the sugar industry embarked on *ad hominem* attacks on selected experts, while distributing sweeteners in

*Three of the editors of this book played prominent roles in the 916 group. Professor Ricardo Uauy was chair, Professor Jaap Seidell was a rapporteur, and Professor Boyd Swinburn was also a prominent member. Another IOTF working group chair, Professor Shiriki Kumanyika, was deputy chair of the expert meeting, and Professor Philip James, chair of the IOTF and chair of the original 797 report, was also a member.

Washington DC. It even managed to mobilize senators to suggest that the US government might refuse to honor its funding obligations to WHO if it did not relent over the 916 report.

Simultaneously, the sugar industry was employing scare tactics in sugar-producing developing countries, spreading rumors that their local industries would suffer if the WHO recommendation to limit added sugars to less than 10% of dietary energy was adhered to. Focusing on the agriculture ministries meant the financial "fear factor" was taken seriously, and the pressure on WHO was intensified by an elaborate and secret critique delivered to the Director-General personally by the US Department of Health and Human Services. Timely media coverage exposed the clumsy maneuvering of the DHHS Secretary, Tommy Thompson, to a barrage of protests within the USA as health professionals and NGOs recognized the unseemly response of the Bush administration to industry pressure.

The WHO's global strategy was eventually approved in Geneva in May 2004[11]—but only after an extended debate in which the USA—represented by George Bush Snr's godson, William Steiger—insisted that even a footnote referring to the WHO 916 report must be excised from the final text.

Achieving synergy among non-governmental organizations

To strengthen WHO in the implementation of its Global Strategy, the IOTF, with its own parent body, the International Association for the Study of Obesity, brought together a number of NGOs to form the Global Prevention Alliance. This consolidated the early collaboration that had developed with the International Diabetes Federation, the World Heart Federation, the International Union of Nutritional Sciences and the International Pediatric Association.

This Global Alliance paved the way for a series of initiatives to begin to galvanize national NGOs in a number of countries to engage with their governments and ministries in response to the global strategy. This catalytic action prompted groups to be formed initially in a range of countries, for example, Malaysia, Singapore, Thailand, Hong Kong and Brazil. A broader analysis also revealed that most medical leaders have little understanding of public health pol-

icy-making and often spend their time vying for preferential ministerial attention to their own speciality. Nevertheless, WHO Europe, with major NGO support, managed to convince European ministers of health to sign a charter on obesity, which included calls for many changes using legislative and regulatory measures. This is, of course, simply a charter and has no binding political significance, and similar solidly founded documents produced in countries such as the UK or Australia, which outline the dimensions and forces involved in promoting obesity, do not in themselves lead to coherent remedial action. The simple explanation is that ministers consider it unwise to take on the greatest industrial powers in the land. The "big food" corporate sector includes multinational companies that have a greater turnover than many countries.

The recent analysis of obesity, undertaken as part of the British Government's Foresight Programme,[12] has illustrated in great detail the intricate "hardwiring" of the vast array of governmental and civil society components that must be considered when attempting to deal with the multi-factorial pressures leading to obesity. This recognition of the need for an overarching "societal" approach, combined with the analysis of the projected economic burden[12] to society from obesity, was instrumental in the development of the UK Government's cross-sectoral strategy on obesity.[13] Even so, this still does not really tackle the key industrial factors which guarantee an escalating rate of obesity. The climate of opinion is beginning to move towards much higher expectations for action, and this has led initially to vague pledges by industry to improve the nutritional quality of product ranges.

They have also made limited gestures towards placing some constraints on marketing to children in an effort to evade the prospect of more stringent measures being enforced. This has been enough to draw some medical and nutritional experts into collaboration with industry, where they have the impression that they are playing an important role in the political process, so should not challenge the politicians to greater action. This requires clearly independent, media-sensitive groups to lobby for ever greater change, so that reputable advisers can legitimately press for progressive and innovative strategies to be implemented.

The next steps

Given the failure of any government to date to address the major structural changes needed to counteract obesity, one can reasonably ask: How it is possible to generate the political will to induce substantial changes in government policy? Clearly a combination of measures is needed.

First, a focus on highly visible problems with an emotional trigger is useful, such as the rise in childhood obesity, because this demands urgent government action. Second, the focus on the marketing issue is also politically valuable because it invokes major parental and public concern. Third, economic analyses are crucial, as was demonstrated in the UK response to predictions of the economic implications of obesity. The obesity community must now develop these economic analyses as effective tools for global use. Fourth, ministries of health cannot be the sole focus for influencing the agenda, as IOTF has repeatedly found.

Thus, through the Global Alliance initiative, the IOTF, using personal contacts at the highest level, has managed to help introduce obesity and the prevention of chronic diseases into the next five-year Economic and Social Development Plan for Thailand, with the strong backing of the Director General of the Economic and Social Development Board of Thailand.

Similarly IOTF was recently invited to address the 16 Caribbean presidents and prime ministers on the economic and health burden on the Caribbean populations. This was only achieved through long-standing personal contacts with a key individual, Sir George Alleyne, ex-Director of the Pan American Health Organization (PAHO), who was trusted by the leaders because they already had experience of his wisdom. Plans are now being devised locally on the basis of preliminary proposals but these, again, will need very careful monitoring if they are to be effective rather than simply politically promoting an image of action.

Conclusion

Fundamental to creating a climate for action is the need to ensure the capacity to deliver a sustained message, perhaps over many years. While many civil society groups hope for swift results, history suggests that health issues that do not convey an immediate and potentially fatal threat and which, like food quality, are seemingly under individual control, do not have staying power in terms of political priorities. As with smoking, there is a need for a medical consensus and an emotive focus combined with economic arguments, together with explicit proposals that will allow heads of government or finance ministers to change their policies on the basis of some definite political gain. Health professionals cannot afford to relax in their efforts to bring home to the public, politicians and producers the need for fundamental and long-term improvements in the nutritional quality of the whole range of products in the food supply chain if the obesity epidemic and consequent chronic diseases are to be brought under control.

References

1 James WPT, Ralph A, Bellizzi M: Nutrition policies in Western Europe: National policies in Belgium, France, Ireland, the Netherlands and the United kingdom. *Nutr Rev* 1997; **55**:S4–S20.
2 Bray GA: Fogarty Center Conference on Obesity. *American Journal of Clinical Nutrition* 1974; **27**:423–424.
3 Waterlow JC (chairman): Research on Obesity: Report of A DHSS/MRC Group. London: HMSO, 1976.
4 Royal College of Physicians. Obesity. Report by the Royal College of Physicians *J R Coll Physicians Lond* 1983; **17**(1): 1–58.
5 Smoking and Health. Summary of a Report of the Royal College of Physicians of London on Smoking in relation to Cancer of the Lung and Other Diseases. Royal College of Physicians London, 1962.
6 Prevention of coronary heart disease. Report of a joint working party of the Royal College of Physicians of London and the British Cardiac Society. *J R Coll Physicians Lond* 1976; **10**(3):213–275.
7 National Advisory Committee on Nutrition Education: A Discussion Paper on Proposals for Nutritional Guidelines for Health Education in Britain. London: Health Education Council, 1983. see: Robbins C: Implementing the NACNE report. 1. National dietary goals: a confused debate. *Lancet* 1983; **2**(8363):1351–1353. Sanderson ME, Winkler JT: Nutrition: the changing scene. Implementing the NACNE report. 2. Strategies for implementing NACNE recommendations. *Lancet* 1983; **2**:1353–1354. Walker CL: Nutrition: the changing scene. Implementing the NACNE report. 3. The new British diet. *Lancet* 1983; **2**:1354–1356. Jollans JL: Implementing the NACNE report: an agricultural viewpoint. *Lancet* 1984; **1**:382–384.
8 World Health Organization: Diet, Nutrition and the Prevention of Chronic Diseases. Report of a WHO Study Group. WHO Technical Report Series 797. Geneva: WHO, 1990.

9 FAO, WHO: Nutrition and development—a global assessment, written by FAO and WHO for the International Conference on Nutrition, 1992.

10 World Health Organization/Food and Agriculture Organization: Diet, Nutrition and the Prevention of Chronic Diseases. Report of a Joint WHO/FAO Expert Consultation. WHO Technical Report Series 916. Geneva: WHO, 2003.

11 World Health: Organization (WHO): Global Strategy on Diet, Physical Activity and Health. WHO, 2004.

12 Foresight: Tackling Obesities: Future Choices—Modelling Future Trends in Obesity & Their Impact on Health. Government Office for Science (UK), 2007.

13 Foresight: Tackling Obesities: Future Choices—Project Report, 2nd edn. Government Office for Science, 2007.

CHAPTER 26

Community interventions—planning for sustainability

Anne Simmons,[1] *Jean Michel Borys*[2] and *Boyd Swinburn*[1]
[1] WHO Collaborating Centre for Obesity Prevention, Deakin University, Geelong and Melbourne, Australia
[2] EPODE European Network, Paris, France

Summary and recommendations for research and practice

- Well-evaluated community-based obesity prevention programs are needed to provide the evidence of effectiveness of such approaches.
- Selection of priority communities for program implementation should take account of needs (e.g. level of disadvantage) as well as likelihood of success.
- A capacity building approach should underpin implementation of obesity prevention programs.
- Health promotion principles are applied to community engagement, program planning and implementation, and evaluation design, but these are inherently complex and contextual.
- Sustainability must be built in from the start, and means placing a higher priority on policies and capacity building than on events, awareness raising and education.
- Future challenges include securing sufficient investment in programs and evaluations, incorporating socio-cultural aspects, and moving from implementing individual projects to reorienting existing systems towards contributing to the obesity prevention efforts.

Introduction

Community level action to promote healthy eating and physical activity is a central component of obesity

Preventing Childhood Obesity. Edited by
E. Waters, B.A. Swinburn, J.C. Seidell and R. Uauy.
© 2010 Blackwell Publishing.

prevention efforts. Ideally, these actions should complement wider state- or national-level action, particularly policy actions needed to make environments less obesogenic.[1] In practice, programs at the community level are being established much more rapidly than policies at a state or national level. At this stage, however, the evidence base for what works and what does not work at a community level is relatively narrow,[2,3] therefore there is an imperative to properly evaluate major programs that are being implemented.[4] Establishing well evaluated demonstration projects is critical for creating the evidence about what works for whom, why, and for "what cost?"

The planning, implementation and evaluation of community intervention programs takes several years. This is especially the case if the programs are large and multi-faceted, if the structures and organizational relationships need to be built from scratch, if the stakeholder groups are numerous or require substantial relationship building, or if the resources and leadership support are low. Sustainability issues are often not high on the agenda in the early stages as people are immersed in community consultations, hiring staff, setting up governance structures, developing action plans, and so forth. However, as the evidence of long-term effectiveness of interventions emerges, the focus of choosing more sustainable action should increase.

Basic health promotion principles for the implementation of any community programs include: the need for community engagement and capacity building; program design and planning, including governance and management structures; implementation and sustainability; and evaluation. This chapter briefly expands on each of these areas, beginning with the selection of communities. Two examples of how community-wide programs are being implemented, one from France (the EPODE program) and in Australia (the Sentinel Site for Obesity Prevention), are then presented.

Selection of communities

A community's context and their existing capacity to find their own solutions to the drivers of obesity will differ enormously between communities. Building the evidence for community-based approaches to obesity prevention is in its early stages in all countries and it is, therefore, important to strike the right balance between targeting communities of highest need versus those with the highest likelihood of success. Box 26.1 highlights the characteristics of communities with a high chance of success, and these could form part of the criteria for selecting communities for community-wide obesity prevention action.

Principles of community engagement and capacity building

The principles of community engagement and capacity building are fundamental to any health promotion process. Participation is essential to sustain efforts, and community members have to be at the centre of health promotion action and the decision-making process for them to be effective.[5] To achieve sustainable outcomes, capacity building processes are required whereby the development of knowledge, skills, commitment, leadership, resources, structures and systems occur.[6–8]

Community engagement

The community engagement process for obesity prevention action in communities involves a process much like that which would occur in any health promotion process (Table 26.1). However, "obesity" is such a negative term and there is a real risk of increasing stigmatization, so obesity prevention efforts are usually framed within the community in a different manner, such as the promotion of healthy eating, physical activity and/or healthy weight.

Box 26.1 Characteristics of communities which influence the likely success of obesity prevention programs

- level of support and leadership to provide program champions and access to resources;
- amount of available resources, external and internal, within settings and organizations;
- access to target populations through sufficient settings;
- structures and partnerships of existing organizations which would provide the planning, management and implementation roles;
- ability to be evaluated (funding, access to evaluation team, meeting design criteria, sufficient numbers etc.);
- context of community interventions:
  - ownership (research-initiated, service-initiated, community-initiated)
  - stage (demonstration project, roll-out)
  - size (single/few settings to whole large community)
  - origins/aims (obesity prevention, nutrition promotion, community building, non-communicable disease prevention etc.).

The engagement process is critical for ensuring relevant organizations, settings leaders and other key stakeholders become committed to the proposed policies and programs and are able to work collaboratively around a common plan of action. Community members are usually able to provide information on

1. the needs of the community in relation to the issue;
2. the context of their community and key settings;
3. the socio-cultural dimensions; and
4. existing programs, networks and resources to support the project.

Ultimately, the stakeholders need to inform the action plan and are members of governance and management structures aligned to the implementation efforts. Establishing working coalitions and successful collaborations, with a lead agency taking the initiative and driving implementation from the grass roots, are fundamental to providing empowerment and sustainability.[8–10]

This development of partnerships and inter-sectoral collaborations need to be recognized as formal relationships between different sectors or groups in

Table 26.1 The health promotion process.

Situational analysis	Prioritization	Planning	Implementation
Technical assessment	**Elements**	**Action plan development**	**Implementation and administration of action plan monitoring and quality control**
(evidence from literature, local evidence, experience)	relating to behaviors, knowledge/skill gaps and environmental barriers to healthy eating and physical activity prioritized on importance (relevance and impact) and changeability	**Aims** (overall goal)	
and community consultation		**Objectives** (what will be achieved)	
(contextual situation, socio-cultural factors, felt needs, existing programs, resources)		**Strategies** (how the objective will be achieved)	
		Actions (what will be done by whom and when)	

Capacity building

Workforce development, leadership, partnerships/relationships, organizational development, resources

Evaluation

Formative, process, impact, outcome, dissemination

the community. They are usually more effective, efficient and sustainable in achieving intended outcomes than are organizations working alone.[7] Community ownership comes about by engaging and committing to the process and the outcomes, working collaboratively to develop a plan of action and then taking the responsibility to implement it.

Capacity building

Capacity building processes are usually required from the outset to build the knowledge, skills, commitment, leadership, resources, structures and systems to initiate and sustain implementation efforts. Figure 26.1 provides one such framework, which can be applied to obesity prevention efforts. The intent of capacity building needs to be clear from the beginning. Usually, it is best employed systematically, to build the capacity of the community to develop infrastructure, enhance program sustainability or build capabilities of community members.[11] Integrating such a framework into the action plan can assist in desired outcomes.

Principles of program design and planning

Program design

Program design begins with an assessment of contributing factors in the context of the community. Decisions can then be made about the focus and size of program, as well as about the barriers and facilitators to action.[12] The Analysis Grids of Elements Linked to Obesity(ANGELO) framework and process was specifically designed for obesity prevention, and is a useful tool for assessing a community's environment and for prioritizing information from the community to guide action.[13,14] The overall approach needs to be framed to support the community's view of the problem in order to minimize harm, stigmatization and blame.[15]

Program planning

Using a strategic plan for the program planning process can assist in attaining a balanced resource

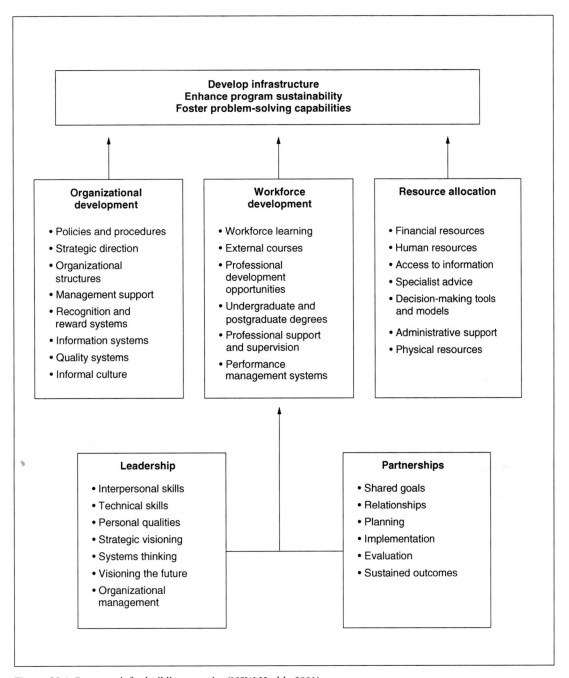

Figure 26.1 Framework for building capacity (NSW Health, 2001).

investment. The portfolio of interventions in the strategic (action) plan stems from the problem and contextual analysis of the community and should complement national, state and regional policies and plans. Essentially, the action plan guides implementation whereby objectives and strategies to achieve a stated goal are recorded, with accountability and timeframes assigned. The action plan needs to consider and build on the strengths of existing activities and partnerships in the community and use a mix of evidence-based and innovative approaches.[16] Active change processes (theories of change) need to underpin the action plan to influence environments (settings), organizations, policies and individuals.

The use of program logic models can assist all key stakeholders to understand the components and outcomes to the planned program. The path between goals, objectives and strategies are defined and the fundamentals of the program design can be checked and deemed logical.[17]

Governance and management structures

Good program management is required to implement the action plan. Governance structures and lines of accountability are essential. A structured approach to project management ensures accountability, progress and quality, and implements risk management and problem-solving strategies among project staff and key stakeholders. Partnership and organizational relationships, and lines of communication need to be specified. Progress reports/updates to funding bodies and key stakeholders are also important communication tools.

Principles of implementation and sustainability

Sustainability needs to be built into the action plan from the outset. The natural tendency for actions to be dominated by awareness-raising activities, one-off events, and educational strategies needs to be countered by a conscious effort to implement the more sustainable strategies of capacity building strategies (above), creating supportive policies, environments and social norms. Attention to the quality of implementation is also critical.

Policies and environmental change

Policies are the "set of rules" that influence the environments, which in turn influence behaviors.[1] Settings-based food service policies are a good example. School food policies that take junk food out of the school canteens, or a workplace cafeteria policy that makes low-fat milk the default choice (i.e. auto-matic option unless otherwise specified) for coffee, not only make the healthy choices easier but also signal what those healthy choices are. The policy influences the behavior indirectly by influencing obesogenic environments and sending health behavior signals. This is in contrast to seat belt or smoking policies and laws which directly mandate behaviors.

Social change

Social marketing is the application of marketing concepts, tools and techniques to any social issue.[18] Social marketing not only targets individual behavior change, but also attempts to bring about changes in the social and structural factors that impinge on an individual and their opportunities, capacities and right to a healthy and fulfilling life. The emphasis of social marketing should target community leaders who have the power and influence to make major institutional policy and legislative changes rather than focusing on voluntary health behaviors to individuals in the general population. Changing cultural norms is often difficult and controversial, but norms have powerful, sustainable effects on behaviors. Using social marketing for obesity prevention requires an integrated approach in the project's action plan and communication plan. The testing of approaches, resources, messages and images with or for the target group is imperative to ensure appropriateness, acceptability and comprehensibility.

Quality of implementation

Because little has been published on the implementation of obesity prevention efforts or the extent of effort required for change, principles for optimal implementation are still being developed. The use of process evaluation, to assess fidelity, completeness, exposure, satisfaction and reach of intervention activities, provides a good monitoring system.[19] The review and adjustment of implementation can then be achieved. Implementation efforts also need to build the capacity of all key stakeholders to ensure actions/activities are ongoing and sustained.

Responding to opportunities, often unexpected ones (e.g. emerging community requests, linking with new programs or partners) can assist with sustainability. This is especially the case where initiatives are integrated into other systems and structures and build on other areas of the community's capacity.[6]

Principles of evaluation

Evaluation is covered in Chapter 19 in detail, but some principles as they apply to the planning stages are outlined here. It is very important that the approach and framework for evaluation are developed concurrently in the program planning phase.[12] The capacity to conduct the evaluation needs to match the size and scope of the evaluation intended. The framework or evaluation plan should contain options for measuring process, impact and outcomes of the implementation. Outcome and impact evaluation correspond to changes in the program's aims and objectives. For well-evaluated demonstration projects, these would include changes in anthropometry, behaviors (skills, knowledge), environments and capacity.[4] Ideally, an economic evaluation should be conducted to contribute to the evidence of cost–effectiveness and optimal implementation. The use of standard measures and tools will enable a comparison with other programs/projects. Documenting lessons learnt is valuable in dissemination and can contribute to the evidence of what does, or does not, work. The context for evaluation needs consideration as current organizational, policy, and community contextual factors can have a major impact on the outcomes.

Evaluation findings need to be disseminated within the community in the first instance and this should occur as the findings become available so that knowledge transfer can be applied back in the community. At the next level, translation of evidence from research into policy and practice is required for a continuous response to obesity at the public health policy level.

Key challenges in establishing and sustaining community interventions

The very nature of community-based interventions creates challenges because they are inevitably complex to implement and evaluate, they are always contextual, and are usually poorly resourced. However, a few particular challenges in existing and future commu-

nity approaches to obesity prevention warrant special mention.

Sufficient investment in programs and evaluations

The time lag from the early signs of the obesity epidemic in the early 1980s to the first phase of community-based demonstration projects in a few countries in the mid-2000s was substantial and, even now, the funding investment to build the evidence base for effectiveness has remained very low. Government-funded programs traditionally provide little funding for evaluation (which may cost as much as the program itself if effectiveness and cost–effectiveness are to be measured) and research-funded programs tend to pay little attention to program sustainability and integration into existing services.

Complexity of program implementation and evaluation

There are many different approaches to program implementation but they all encounter the complexity of having to juggle multiple partners, agendas, funding constraints, and personal and organizational relationships. There is no simple formula for negotiating this complexity and the mix will be different for each context. Similarly, the evaluation of multi-sector intervention programs which are under community control are complex, especially when potential comparison populations are exposed to a variety of other local, state and national programs to promote healthy eating and physical activity. Quasi-experimental designs can be used for program evaluation but they all carry higher risks of arriving at false negative or false positive conclusions than the more rigorous controlled trials that randomize individuals or clusters (e.g. schools).

Incorporating socio-cultural components

There are significant differences in obesity prevalence rates across ethnic groups and this indicates that socio-cultural factors must be considered in any implementation program in those groups.[20,21] For example, if the over-provision and over-consumption of food is a fundamental expression of the underlying cultural values of showing care, respect and love between people, how can obesity prevention programs and messages be framed to reorient those obesogenic manifestations of positive cultural values? This is a challenge that few programs have embarked upon to date.

Moving from projects to systems

Demonstration projects have an important role to play in creating the evidence and experience about what works for whom, why, and for what cost. In the coming years, the findings, both positive and negative, will emerge from the community-based projects around the world. The next phase is not to establish more projects but to take these lessons and systematically incorporate them into the existing systems operating in schools, primary care, local government and the communities. Implementation research will be needed to work out how to ensure that existing knowledge and best practice gets converted into these systems. This knowledge exchange research and systems science are relatively new in health promotion but will need to be rapidly applied if the emerging evidence is to be converted into action.

Case study 1 the EPODE program, France

Introduction

Ensemble Prévenons l'Obésité Des Enfants (EPODE—Together, let's prevent childhood obesity) is a childhood obesity prevention community-based intervention, which was established in France in 2004. Its principles are to work with local stakeholders to influence the behavior of the whole family and to change the family's daily environments and social norms in a sustainable manner, thus contributing to the stabilization then decrease in overweight and obesity prevalence in children.

The concept was successfully piloted in the Fleurbaix Laventie Ville Santé Study (FLVS) from 1992 to 2007.[22] FLVS is now part of the EPODE program along about 200 towns across France. The program is also being adopted and implemented in Belgium, Spain, Greece, Australia and Canada.

Structure and implementation

A National Coordination team, supported by a scientific advisory board, strong political will, and public-private funding partnerships make up the four pillars

to EPODE. The FLVS non-governmental organization, which initiated the FLVS Study, is fundamental to EPODE because it receives the funding from public and private partners (about 50:50) and contracts the coordination to a professional communication company (PROTEINES®). The National Coordination/Social Marketing Team at PROTEINES® is the hub of EPODE with specialties in project management, training, social marketing, communication and public relations. It also organizes sustainable funding. Its primary role is to support the implementation of the EPODE program in local communities, towns, cities, developed to meet contextual needs (cultural, sociological, economic and political). As a resource centre, it provides all social marketing materials, tools (including a methodology book for progressive implementation), guidelines, quarterly roadmaps and a dedicated toolbox to engage key stakeholders and professional development/training to the local community. The roadmaps utilize group dynamics, decision-making processes and social policy modification to foster sustainable change in educational schemes for nutrition and physical activity. The National Coordination is advised by a scientific committee of independent experts in education, psychology, sociology, exercise and nutrition sciences.

City mayors are the point of entry into a community. In France, councils have jurisdiction over kindergartens and primary schools (core target population). The mayors are required to submit an application to be an EPODE community, to dedicate a full-time project manager and to commit at least €1 per capita for the interventions each year for five years (many commit more). The mayors act as champions for EPODE and sign a charter outlining the involvement of the city and committing to some rules.

The mayor appoints a project manager to implement EPODE using the tools provided by the National Coordination team. Their role is to establish networks, coordinate a local multi-disciplinary steering committee, and disseminate the specific tools, roadmaps and briefings to professional groups willing to be involved in the operational process.

To succeed in establishing committed local stakeholders, the project managers and their teams undertake four fundamental steps:

1. raising awareness of the obesity issue and its solutions (without stigmatization), and recruiting a

large number of stakeholders/key opinion leaders (public, private) to participate on a voluntary basis;

2. training stakeholders to convey positive messages and creative solutions guided by international recommendations, behavioral change theory, and the experience of trained local experts;

3. implementing actions in schools and towns, using the developed tools and methodologies, guided by local initiatives in keeping with EPODE's philosophy with materials being validated by the national scientific committee.

4. assessing effectiveness by measuring children's BMI, the level of stakeholders' involvement and the quality of spontaneous actions undertaken.

Financing comes from public-private partnerships, established at the national and local level. Representatives from private business (e.g. food industry, insurance sector), academia, and local and national politicians are brought together. The private support is strictly financial and they sign an ethical charter confirming their intention (supporting a public health prevention project, independent of their own agendas).

Evaluation

All EPODE communities measure and weigh children annually at school and because participation is considered the norm, the response rates are 90–95%. The data are then a virtual census and statistical tests are not required to give confidence about what is occurring in participating communities. There are no comparison populations being measured and it is, therefore, difficult to assess the impact of the program compared to having no program. The costs of obtaining comparative data and the difficulty of evaluating the influences of a multi-factorial intervention on complex behaviors are major evaluation challenges.

The monitoring of actions is an important part of evaluation. Since its launch in 2004, there have been more than 1,000 actions per year by local stakeholders in the first ten EPODE towns. A detailed monitoring chart of these actions, filled by the project managers, enables a continuous process evaluation. Economic, media and sociological aspects are also evaluated.

Sustainability

A number of factors contribute to sustainability of the project. The strong philosophy of ensuring that no stigmatization occurs ensures that perceived risks are minimized. The structure of EPODE maximizes sustainability by ensuring leadership and commitment (mayors signing on), the ongoing funding (private:public, national:local), the program quality (consistency across all towns/cities through the National Coordination team), and the local relevance and engagement (local project manager and steering committee) are built into the design and processes.

The local stakeholders develop new skills and create strong partnerships and social ties in their work. This means that they feel valued and know they are part of a large positive program for the community. Families live in an "ecological niche" (village/town, neighborhood) where events of daily life occur (education, work, shopping, medical care, leisure transport, etc.). Local stakeholders can have a strong influence in these settings, supporting families and disseminating common messages. EPODE involves the whole community creating mobilization of local resources.

Since 2000, France has had a national strategy to promote healthy lifestyles and implement supportive policies such as restricting food advertising practices. This has created a positive national context, which has facilitated the implementation of EPODE.

Transferability

The initial ten EPODE towns have created a mayors' club to promote the concept among other local authorities, explore financial, physical and human resources, extend the network to foster operational partnerships, and develop political awareness around childhood obesity. Implementation is successful from small towns (80 inhabitants) to large cities (Paris, beginning in four districts). EPODE cuts across political differences and socio-economic status. The model has also been adopted and adapted in countries outside France. Further details can be found on: www. epode.fr.

Case study 2 Sentinel site for obesity prevention, Victoria, Australia

Introduction

The Sentinel Site for Obesity Prevention established three whole-of-community demonstration projects located in the Barwon-South Western region of

Victoria, Australia. The projects were based on health promotion principles taking a community capacity building approach[23-25] and aimed to build actions, community skills and contribute to the evidence for obesity prevention.

Each project aimed to strengthen their community's capacity to promote healthy eating and physical activity, and to prevent unhealthy weight gain in children.[26] All action plans had three objectives around community capacity building, communications and evaluation, with a further 4–6 behavioral objectives and 1–2 innovative or pilot project objectives. All projects used quasi-experimental evaluation designs with parallel comparison groups and >1,000 children in each arm.[26] Funding came from multiple government and public research funding sources.

Sentinel site projects

"Romp & Chomp" targeted preschool children and their families within the City of Greater Geelong from 2005 to 2008 (~12,000 children under 5 years of age). Nineteen long day care facilities, 44 family day care centers and 38 kindergartens consented to being involved in the evaluation of the project. The project had a strong focus on developing sustainable changes in areas of policy, socio-cultural, physical and economic environments.[27]

"Be Active Eat Well" (BAEW) targeted children aged 4–12 years and their families in the rural town of Colac. Primary schools ($n = 6$) were the major setting for action but other settings such as kindergartens, neighborhoods and fast-food outlets were involved.[28] Positive anthropometric changes have been reported in this project.[29]

"It's your Move!" focused on secondary school students aged 13–17 years. All secondary schools ($n = 5$) from the East Geelong/Bellarine Peninsula area of Geelong were selected. Student ambassadors worked throughout the project as advocates and implementers. This project was part of the four-country Pacific intervention study: Obesity Prevention In Communities (OPIC).[30,31]

A research team for the Sentinel Site, based at Deakin University, supported the interventions, provided training, assisted with building capacity and, in particular, was responsible for the evaluation component of each project. The full logic model for the way the interventions were assumed to influence the

outcomes and their associated measured and modeled components is shown in Figure 26.2.

Community engagement and establishing structures and roles

The projects began by engaging key stakeholders in the target settings and relevant government and non-government agencies. Champions (people visible and influential in the community) helped cement the engagement process.

Program management, organizational structures, coordination and strategic alliances were established to support implementation. An interim steering committee with membership from stakeholders established the project and employed a project coordinator. After 6–9 months this committee was structured into a two-tiered management system (Reference Committee and Local Steering Committee) to coincide with the implementation phase. The Reference Committee's role was to provide higher-level strategic input and support and the Local Steering Committee was empowered to implement the project, including budgetary decisions. Members included project staff and those at the grass roots in the project's key settings and terms of reference were established for each committee.

Developing an action plan

The ANGELO process was used to assist each community set priorities for action, culminating in an action plan.[14] This was achieved mainly through a facilitated workshop with key stakeholders and, in the case of It's Your Move!, with members of the target group (adolescents). The "elements" in the framework refer to a list of potential target behaviors, knowledge and skill gaps, and environmental barriers developed from the literature, local evidence and experience, and specific analyses or targeted research.[32,33]

The ANGELO process had five stages as outlined in Figure 26.3, with steps 2–5 occurring within a two-day workshop.[14]

At the workshop, the situational analysis (stage 1) was presented including evidence from the literature on obesity and obesity prevention and other technical assessments, as well as information from the community engagement process (e.g. existing programs). A potential list of elements were scanned/altered by

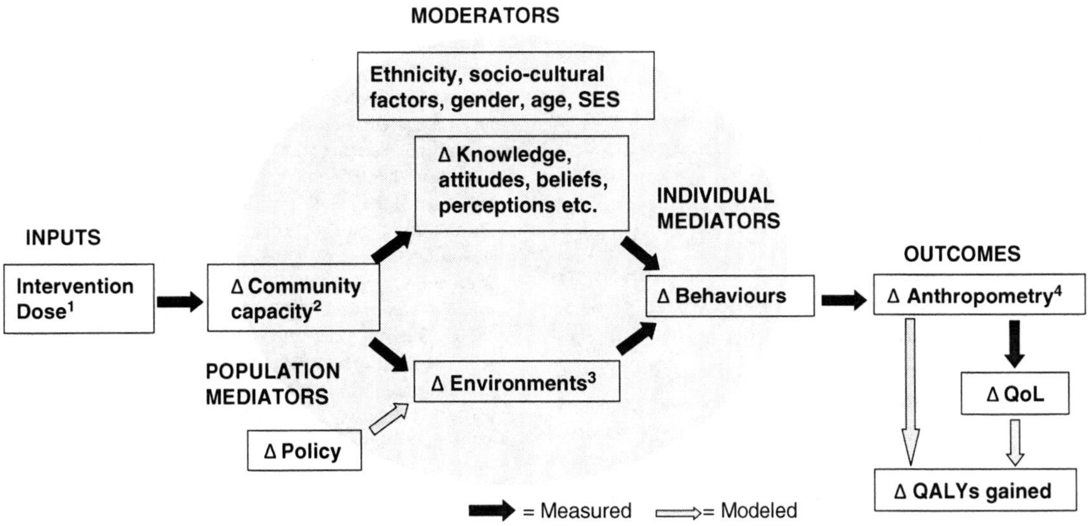

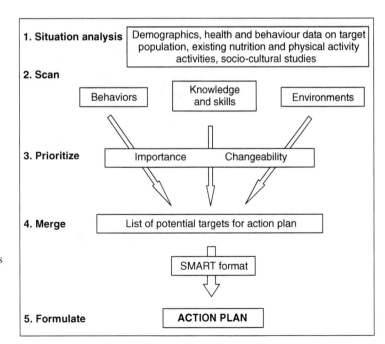

MODERATORS

Ethnicity, socio-cultural factors, gender, age, SES

Δ **Knowledge, attitudes, beliefs, perceptions etc.**

INDIVIDUAL MEDIATORS

INPUTS

Intervention Dose[1]

Δ **Community capacity[2]**

POPULATION MEDIATORS

Δ **Environments[3]**

Δ **Policy**

Δ **Behaviours**

OUTCOMES

Δ **Anthropometry[4]**

Δ **QoL**

Δ **QALYs gained**

➡ = Measured ⇨ = Modeled

Figure 26.2 General logic model for the three demonstration projects of the Sentinel Site for Obesity Prevention.
The measured components are shown in the dark arrows and modelled components in the light arrows. Δ means "change in";[1] Intervention dose is either 1 or 0 (intervention, control) or dollars (for those with economic evaluations);[2] Capacity is leadership, skills/knowledge, structures, resources;[3] Relevant environments are schools, homes, neighborhoods, churches;[4] Weight, body mass index (BMI), BMI-z score, waist, waist:height, %fat, prevalence of overweight and obesity. SES is socio-economic status. QoL is quality of life. DALYs is disability-adjusted life years saved.

1. Situation analysis | Demographics, health and behaviour data on target population, existing nutrition and physical activity activities, socio-cultural studies

2. Scan

Behaviors | Knowledge and skills | Environments

3. Prioritize | Importance | Changeability

4. Merge | List of potential targets for action plan

SMART format

5. Formulate | **ACTION PLAN**

Figure 26.3 The ANGELO (Analysis Grid for Elements Linked to Obesity) process. SMART refers to objectives which are; Specific, Measurable, Achievable, Relevant, and Time-bound.[34]

participants for appropriateness (stage 2) then prioritized according to importance and changeability (stage 3). Within settings relevant to the community (e.g. homes, early child care settings, schools, neighborhoods), environmental barriers were prioritized. A scoring and ranking process determined priorities. The merge (stage 4) integrated the highest five to seven ranked behavioral, knowledge, skill and environmental elements as targets for action. These were discussed, and in the final step, the agreed priority elements were molded into a structured action plan (stage 5). The behaviors were generally used to create the objectives with the associated knowledge gaps and environmental barriers being used to identify strategies. It was important that objectives were written in Specific, Measurable, Achievable, Relevant, Time-bound (SMART) format.[34] The action plans were further refined with the community and timelines, processes and accountability added. The action plan became a "living" document, which guided implementation and evolved through several versions during the life of the project.

Sustainability

A community capacity building approach was chosen to maximize sustainability and this was an objective on its own as well as being built into all other objectives. The extent to which this was achieved varied across the programs. Projects with champions in high places, engaged organizations with strong partnerships, experience in securing funding, and a skilled workforce were more likely to be sustainable. Where possible, integration of strategies into the organizational development domain was striven for. For example, obtaining management support from an organization to link with their strategic plan and then integrating roles and responsibilities of workers to align with the goals/objectives of the project would assist with longevity. Additionally, ensuring actions were integrated into existing policy and maximizing actions for environmental change also contributed to sustainability.

References

1 Swinburn BA: Obesity prevention: the role of policies, laws and regulations. *Aust New Zealand Health Policy* 2008; **5**:12.

2 Summerbell C, Waters E, Edmunds L, Kelly S, Brown T, Campbell K: Interventions for preventing obesity in children. *Cochrane Database Syst Rev* 2005; (3):CD001871.

3 Flynn MAT, McNeil DA, Maloff B et al: Reducing obesity and related chronic disease risk in children and youth: a synthesis of evidence with "best practice" recommendations. *Obes Rev* 2006; **7**:7–66.

4 Swinburn B, Bell C, King L, Magarey A, O'Brien K, Waters E, on behalf of the Primary Prevention Group of the Australian Childhood Obesity Research Network: Obesity prevention programs demand high quality evaluations. *Aust and NZ Public Health* 2007; **31**(4):305–307.

5 WHO: Jakarta Declaration. 1997; Available from: www.who.int/healthpromotion/conferences/previous/jakarta/declaration/en/ (accessed 4 February 2007).

6 Hawe P, Noort M, King L, Jordens C: Multiplying health gains: the critical role of capacity-building within health promotion programs. *Health Policy* 1997; **39**:29–42.

7 Smith B, Tang K, Nutbeam D: WHO health promotion glossary: new terms. *Health Promot Int* 2006; **21**(4):340–345.

8 Fleming ML, Parker E: Health Promotion: Principles and Practice in the Australian Context, 3rd edn. Sydney: Allen & Unwin, 2007.

9 Green L, Kreuter M: Health Program Planning: An Educational and Ecological Approach, 4th edn. New York: McGraw-Hill, 2005.

10 Green L: From research to "best practices" in other settings and populations. *Am J Health Behav* 2001; **25**(3):165–178.

11 NSW Health Department: A Framework for Building Capacity to Improve Health. Gladesville: Better Health Care Centre, 2001.

12 Hawe P, Degeling D, Hall J: Evaluating Health Promotion: A Health Workers Guide. Sydney: MacLennan and Petty, 1990.

13 Swinburn B, Egger G, Raza F: Dissecting obesogenic environments: the development and application of a framework for identifying and prioritizing environmental interventions for obesity. *Prev Med* 1999; **29**(6 Pt 1):563–570.

14 Simmons A, Mavoa HM, Bell AC, De Courten M, Schaaf D, Schultz J, Swinburn BA: Creating community action plans for obesity prevention using the ANGELO (Analysis Grids for Elements Linked to Obesity) Framework. *Health Promot Int* 2009; doi: 10.1093/heapro/dap029.

15 Thomas S, Hyde J, Komesaroff P: Cheapening the struggle: obese people's attitudes towards The Biggest Loser. *Obes Manag* 2007; **3**:210–215.

16 Hawe P, Shiell A: Preserving innovation under increasing accountability pressures: the health promotion investment portfolio approach. *Health Promot J Aust* 1995; **5**:4–9.

17 Pawson R, Tilley N: Realistic Evaluation. London: Sage, 1997.

18 Donovan R, Henley N: Social Marketing: Principles and Practices. Melbourne: IP Publishing, 2003.

19 Saunders RP, Evans MH, Joshi P: Developing a process-evaluation plan for assessing health promotion program implementation: a how-to guide. *Health Promot Pract* 2005; **6**(2):134–147.

20 Kumanyika S, Grier S: Targeting interventions for ethnic minority and low-income populations. *Future Child* 2006; **16**(1):187–207.

21 Waters E, Ashbolt R, Gibbs L et al: Double disadvantage: the influence of ethnicity over socioeconomic position on childhood overweight and obesity: findings from an inner urban population of primary school children. *Int J Pediatr Obes* 2008; **3**(4):196–204.

22 Romon M, Lommez A, Tafflet M et al: Downward trends in the prevalence of childhood overweight in the setting of 12-year school- and community-based programmes. *Public Health Nutr* 2008; **23**:1–8.

23 Kumanyika S, Jeffery RW, Morabia A, Ritenbaugh C, Antipatis VJ: Obesity prevention: the case for action. *Int J Obes* 2002; **26**:425–436.

24 Pate RR, Trost SG, Mullis R, Sallis JF, Wechsler H, Brown DR: Community interventions to promote proper nutrition and physical activity among youth. *Prev Med* 2000; **31**: S138–S149.

25 Swinburn B, Egger G: Preventive strategies against weight gain and obesity. *Obes Rev* 2002; **3**(4):289–301.

26 Bell AC, Simmons A, Sanigorski AM, Kremer PJ, Swinburn BA: Preventing childhood obesity: the sentinel site for obesity prevention in Victoria, Australia. *Health Promot Int* 2008; **23**(4):328–336.

27 WHO Collaborating Centre for Obesity Prevention: Romp & Chomp Obesity Prevention Project. 2009; Available from: www.deakin.edu.au/hmnbs/who-obesity/research/ssop/romp-chomp.php (accessed 15 April 2009).

28 Victorian Government Department of Human Services: Be Active Eat Well. 2009; Available from: www.goforyourlife.vic.gov.au/hav/articles.nsf/pracpages/Be_Active_Eat_Well?OpenDocument (accessed 15 April 2009).

29 Sanigorski A, Bell A, Kremer P, Cuttler R, Swinburn B: Reducing unhealthy weight gain in children through community capacity-building: results of a quasi-experimental intervention program, Be Active Eat Well. *Int J Obes* 2008; **32**(7):1060–1067.

30 Swinburn B, Pryor J, McCabe M et al: The Pacific OPIC Project (Obesity Prevention in Communities): objectives and design. *Pac Health Dialog* 2007; **14**(2):139–146.

31 WHO Collaborating Centre for Obesity Prevention: It's Your Move! Obesity Prevention Project. 2009; Available from: www.deakin.edu.au/hmnbs/who-obesity/research/ssop/its-your-move.php (accessed 15 April 2009).

32 Swinburn BA, Carter R, Haby M, Moodie M, Bell AC, Simmons A: Obesity prevention—selecting the best investments. WHO Europe—Technical Review Paper. The obesity issues in Europe: status, challenges, prospects, 2006.

33 Carter MA, Swinburn B: Measuring the: obesogenic' food environment in New Zealand primary schools. *Health Promot Int* 2004; **19**(1):15–20.

34 Round R, Marshall B, Horton K: Planning for Effective Health Promotion Evaluation. Melbourne: Victorian Department of Human Services, 2005.

CHAPTER 27

Community capacity building

Colin Bell,[1] *Eva Elliott*[2] and *Anne Simmons*[3]
[1] Department of Medicine and Public Health, University of Newcastle, Wallsend, Australia
[2] Cardiff Institute of Society and Health, School of Social Sciences, Cardiff University, Cardiff, UK
[3] Deakin University School of Population Health, Melbourne, Australia

Summary and recommendations for research and practice

- For healthy eating and physical activity to become the norm for children, the places where they live, learn and play need to foster these behaviors.
- Community capacity building for obesity prevention in children is the process of building the competencies, structures and resources in civil society required to create these environments.
- Training is an important component of community capacity building for obesity prevention, but it also involves raising community awareness of health risks, strategies to foster community cohesion, facilitating access to additional resources, developing structures to support community decision making and social and political support.
- The application of community capacity building models to obesity prevention is relatively new. However, the number of programs that incorporate its components into their designs is growing.
- At a national level, a network of creative and autonomous communities that provide local solutions to the global problem of obesity is more likely to achieve significant and sustainable behavior change than simply relying on central government.

Preventing Childhood Obesity. Edited by
E. Waters, B.A. Swinburn, J.C. Seidell and R. Uauy.
© 2010 Blackwell Publishing.

Introduction

To stem the growing epidemic of childhood obesity, what children eat and the way they physically engage with their home, school and neighborhood environments needs to change. However, for healthy eating and physical activity to become the norm, the places where children live, learn and play need to provide the cognitive, social and economic resources to foster changes in existing behavior. This will not occur if the knowledge and skills remain with the public health specialists, government officials and researchers currently driving efforts to prevent the epidemic. It will occur if the collective capacity, knowledge and resources of children, parents, residents, community sector organizations, government agencies *and* health experts are harnessed in order to understand the problem and make changes. The process of building the competencies, structures and resources in civil society, as opposed to relying on market forces or state intervention, is known as "community capacity building" and the aim of this chapter is to describe how the components of community capacity building apply to childhood obesity prevention.

What is community capacity building?

Community

Definitions and uses of the term "community" are various, and with time there has been little agreement or consistency. Over 50 years ago, the sociologist Hillery, found over 90 different meanings of the term "community" and concluded that the only commonality between the meanings was that they were about people.[1] In reference to "community capacity building" the term community has in the past been applied to a specific geographical community. However, our experience suggests, a broader definition of community is typically used and that it may or may not have a geographical boundary but may simply be a group that shares a common goal interest or identity.

Capacity building

Like community, "capacity building" also has various meanings. Hawe et al described it as one of those terms that is given to a loose or wide concept, where professionals in the field can give an impression of understanding and consensus of the concept but differ in their definition.[2] Close inspection, however, reveals similarities in the definitions. For example, NSW Health defined capacity building as "an approach to the development of sustainable skills, organizational structures, resources and commitment to health improvement in health and other sectors, to prolong and multiply health gains many times over".[3] Similarly, Bush et al defined community capacity building as "a collection of characteristics and resources which, when combined, improve the ability of a community to recognise, evaluate and address key problems … the work that is done to develop the capacity of the network of groups and organizations".[4]

Community capacity building in health promotion

Within health promotion, community capacity building has evolved from the traditions of community development. Its roots can be linked to international aid efforts and it shares its origins with the associated concepts of community organization, community action and community empowerment.[5] In essence, rather than being a mere "site" for interventions, the "community" is a resource for change. Community capacity building first became prominent in the health promotion arena in the mid-1990s, although its development can be tracked from the 1986 Ottawa Charter.[6] Elements of capacity building clearly underpin the charter's concept of empower-

Box 27.1 Capacity building definition from WHO glossary

Capacity building is "the development of knowledge, skills, commitment, structures, systems and leadership to enable effective health promotion. It involves actions to improve health at three levels: the advancement of knowledge and skills among practitioners; the expansion of support and infrastructure for health promotion in organizations, and; the development of cohesiveness and partnerships for health in communities".

ment and subsequent declarations further articulate capacity building. The Jakarta Declaration in 1997 specifically identified the need to "increase community capacity and empower the individual" and conveys both the rationale and requirements for capacity building.[7]

More recently, the Bangkok Charter called for all sectors and settings to act to "build capacity for policy development, leadership, health promotion practice, knowledge transfer and research, and health literacy" thus recognizing the need to integrate capacity building strategies into health promotion.[8] Helpfully, the term "capacity building" is now included in the World Health Organization's (WHO) Health Promotion Glossary (Box 27.1).[9] The value in such a glossary is that definitions are underpinned by a process of deliberation including a literature review and expert feedback which helps to provide at least a starting point for developing health promotion interventions.

The glossary goes on further to say that capacity building at the community level may include raising awareness about health risks, strategies to foster community identity and cohesion, education to increase health literacy, facilitating access to external resources, and developing structures for community decision making. It is noted that for action at the community level to be successful, there needs to be a social and political response to secure support for such interventions. Collectively, these components provide a means by which "stakeholders" in health promotion can consider how they may develop effective interventions that link micro-level change at the individual level, meso-level changes at the neighborhood level and macro-changes at the political and policy level.

A critic's perspective

Having arrived at a definition for community capacity building within the context of health promotion, it should be noted that the discourses have not been without their criticisms. Community capacity building has been criticised as being a smokescreen for more subtle forms of social control because proponents claim that it is an alternative to economic regeneration but does little to challenge structural forms of inequality.[10–12] For instance, concerns reflected in UK urban regeneration policy that community capacity building is about "expecting groups of people who are poorly resourced to pull themselves up by their collective bootstraps",[13] are mirrored by those who feel that similar approaches in primary health care policy in Australia depoliticize "Indigenous health, whilst legitimising and mystifying relations of white dominance".[14] Such critiques, however, give little space for collective human agency, condemning "the poor" and disenfranchised to what Bourdieu called "the weight of the world" without acknowledging that, where formal politics have failed, such approaches may provide a mechanism through which people can be authors and co-authors of transformations of their local, social, economic and cultural worlds.[15]

Why build community capacity?

The Jakarta Declaration[7] answers this question in its justification for health promotion by stating that "it improves both the ability of individuals to take action, and the capacity of groups, organisations or communities to influence the determinants of health". What can be inferred here is that health promotion principles are about increasing the ability and building the capacity to affect health determinants. Put simply, community capacity building has the power to influence individual and population health outcomes through empowering people and making changes sustainable. Although this is largely agreed upon, the rationale of empowerment and sustainability is not always made explicit.

The application of community capacity building to childhood obesity prevention

In assessing community capacity building approaches to preventing childhood obesity we find ourselves at the heart of a charged political and theoretically contested arena. Discourses on the "childhood obesity epidemic" are themselves framed, on the one hand, as problems of individual behavior and on the other, as a consequence of structural inequalities. Also, while there are a growing number of successful interventions,[16–18] we do not yet know what works to prevent overweight and obesity in children at a population level. However, we do know that multiple strategies are required in multiple settings,[19] and that this cannot be achieved in a sustainable way unless communities take on the problem themselves. Indeed, given the pervasiveness of the epidemic, it is likely that communities will not only need to take on the problem but also link with other communities and harness the support of governments so that they can overcome the sectoral (e.g. transportation) and global (e.g. fast-food franchising) contributors to the epidemic. In other words, communities need to move from the current state of disengaged awareness of childhood obesity, through recognizing and owning the problem, to accessing expertise and external resources, to intervening so that it becomes easy for children to be active and eat well. Community capacity building is the process through which this can occur.

Raising community awareness of health risks

For action to be taken on health risks, the scale of the problem needs to be meaningful for communities and they need to have an understanding of who is most at risk. In Australia, as in other Western countries, about a quarter of children are either overweight or obese and this continues to increase steadily.[20] Generally, there are minimal differences in prevalence by gender. However it is usually higher among children from lower socio-economic status backgrounds.[21] Behavioral determinants, in line with findings from other countries, include sweetened drinks, energy-dense food consumption, sedentary behavior and

environments that encourage these behaviors.[22] Owing to extensive and continued media coverage of obesity in many countries, most people are generally aware of the problem but it is difficult to demonstrate how the problem (its size, rate of increase, who it affects, determinants and consequences) applies at a community level. Unless there is a sense that the problem has relevance at this level, then it is unlikely that communities will have any interest or motivation to seek solutions, and capacity builders run the risk of "looking down" on the community.[12] This may go part way towards explaining a lack of community ownership when it comes to childhood obesity prevention, as it raises the potential for stigmatizing a community as a "problem community" and for implying blame for nurturing a generation of obese children.[23]

The problem of countering the understandable resistance of people to community capacity research initiatives was acknowledged in a Welsh government funded action research programme, the Sustainable Health Action Research Programme (SHARP), to support sustainable changes in health.[24] The problem, which cut across all seven target areas in Wales, was that local people had research and initiative fatigue.[25] People saw researchers as "parachutists" who "dropped in" from above, collected data and then disappeared without implementing any long-term change. One project site effectively overcame this fatigue and associated resistance around the chronic problem of poor diets. O'Neill et al described how a process was implemented which sought to understand how people conceptualized and experienced healthy eating and the barriers to its achievement.[26] They theorized that the meaning of food goes beyond "nutrition" and "healthier eating" but holds personal and social meanings which need to be understood in order to develop strategies for change. They then incorporated this broader meaning into both the research and intervention strategies, which were built around opportunities for engagement and mutual exchange (see Box 27.2).

The key to community engagement is a bottom-up approach involving the community in the translation of the problem[27] and in decision making regarding initial investments.[28] Communities need to be able to define the problem in their own context and contribute to how it is resolved. This approach has been

Box 27.2 The film club: a strategy designed to foster engagement and mutual exchange

One SHARP initiative was the development of a "film club" for children aged between 5 and 11 years.[26] This filled a perceived gap in social and entertainment opportunities for children on the estate and provided some respite for parents from their child care responsibilities. The club was well attended with nearly 70 children at some sessions. It also provided a platform for exchange, dialogue and education about food. The local health promotion team provided food, gradually introducing "healthy options" and gauging their response to eating fruit and vegetables that had previously been unfamiliar.

adopted in a number of community-based prevention programs in Australia where normative needs are assessed through a consultative process. This allows the community to be informed of the issues, through expert interpretation of research findings (based on local data, where possible, and expressed in terms relevant to the community) and to build a joint plan of action. (Refer to the ANGELO process in Chapter 26.) Interestingly, some communities have been happy to use the words overweight/obesity in their strategic goals while others have not because of the potential risks of stigmatization. Community input into how resources are allocated is an important part of empowerment.

Strategies to foster community identity and cohesion

In light of earlier comments, strategies to foster community identity and cohesion should clearly acknowledge the diverse definitions of community and recognize that they are influenced by self-identification, geography, politics and religion.[29] This is best achieved by allowing communities to define themselves. However, for closely evaluated demonstration projects, it does help to define a community's boundaries. This was the case for three Australian demonstration projects:[30] "Be Active Eat Well", a prevention program for primary school children in a rural town in Victoria (population ~ 11,000),[31] "Romp

& Chomp" where the community was defined as "the children attending preschool and their parents or carers" in the City of Greater Geelong, and "It's Your Move!" in five secondary schools in East Geelong. Efforts to promote healthy eating, physical activity and healthy weight were then tailored to meet the needs of that particular community. It is important to identify who can speak on behalf of the community,[32] who can provide leadership and who can become stakeholders committed to the goals of the program. There is also a need to foster program identity.[33] This brings tangibility to the program early on and fosters community ownership so that the program can become an integral part of what the community is about.

"Te Whanau Cadillac—A Waka for Change", is an example of a program that used a number of strategies to foster community identity and cohesion. This action research project from New Zealand aimed to bridge the gap between research and practice and to improve health and well-being through working with communities to increase their capacity to deal with alcohol and drug issues.[34] Central to the project, which had a strong focus on Maori youth, was an agreement that this goal could only be met through a *kaupapa* Maori (Maori worldview and philosophy) approach. This included allowing communities to operate in their own style, involving more informal meetings and having project workers who provided skills in Maori cultural practices, as well as in identifying with youth.

Education to increase health literacy

Education, or training, is fundamental to community capacity building and the aim, similar to that of a school teacher for literacy, is to give a community knowledge or competence in health. What makes it distinct from awareness-raising is the ongoing transfer of knowledge on how to do something about the problem. For example, sports coaches need to know how to ensure that every child who shows up for practice develops fundamental movement skills; while school canteen managers need to know what foods are healthy choices for children or adolescents and how best to market them. Parents need to know that watching more than two hours a day of television is

not recommended for children and what strategies can be put in place to reduce overall viewing time. "Good for Kids Good for Life" in New South Wales[35] is Australia's largest community-based program promoting healthy eating and physical activity for children up to 15 years of age.

Training on "how to" prevent obesity is central to each of the settings (preschools, schools, sports clubs, community services, health services and media) where the program is operating, and importantly, this is tailored to the specific needs of each of the settings. For example, to support the introduction of fruit and water breaks and healthier school canteen menus in primary schools, training was provided by both experts (dietitians) and education consultants for school champions (a representative from the school who would champion the program), and was designed so that it complemented and contributed to the curriculum in a range of subjects and school stages (see Box 27.3).

There is a temptation to make community capacity building synonymous with education. However, education on its own it is not enough and there is growing evidence that attention also needs to be paid to community awareness, community cohesion, facilitating access to resources, decision-making structure and social and political support aspects of capacity building.[36,37]

Box 27.3 Feedback on Good for Kids Good for Life professional development workshop for school teachers

What did you like best about the workshop?

"How to help teachers implement Nutrition lessons without "adding" to curriculum"

"[It was a] very positive approach to facilitating nutrition in schools and teaching and learning"

"How to integrate healthy eating into the curriculum"

"Curriculum resources are ready to distribute to the fellow teachers for implementing activities/lessons"

"It's made me much clearer about my role as school champion and has provided me with lots of tools to use to help devise a nutrition education policy within the school"

Facilitating access to additional resources

Additional resources are the catalyst for building the capacity of a community to create change. The resources required at the start include funding from various sources and technical expertise on obesity prevention and evaluation. Initial funding for community-based health promotion should ideally be provided by government health departments because they have the mandate to promote community health and they are the first to become aware of emerging health risks. Achieving this, however, usually requires advocacy to ensure that funding is put towards prevention rather than treatment. In addition, the funding needs to be locally rather than centrally controlled because the concepts of community empowerment and capacity building are easily lost in health department contract requirements, politics and bureaucracy. Health departments can also provide the technical expertise on obesity prevention and evaluation that communities need to take action, although universities can also fill this role, particularly where they are closely linked with the community.

The Sentinel Site for Obesity Prevention was a demonstration site in the Barwon-South West region of Victoria, Australia, that aimed to build the programs, skills and evidence necessary to attenuate and eventually reverse the obesity epidemic in children and adolescents.[30] It was based on a partnership between the region's university (Deakin University) and its health, education and local government agencies. For each of the three community-based childhood obesity prevention projects supported by the Sentinel Site, the government health department provided initial funding for the projects and the university provided technical expertise (training) and evaluated the projects.

Once the capacity building process has begun, facilitating access to additional resources becomes a process of supporting communities to reorientate existing resources towards obesity prevention. For example, in the Be Active Eat Well project which targeted children aged 4 to 12 years of age, the local government agency saw synergies between the project's goal of increasing physical activity and their own goal of supporting local sports clubs. In order to maximize these, they contributed the time and resources of their Sport and Recreation Officer to registering children's participation in an after-school activity program. It also involved supporting the community to build up core internal funding streams and to access external resources such as grants and/or sponsorship.

Most community-based programs do not seek to involve the private sector in obesity prevention, in part because of "strings" that often come with the resources they provide. However, to stay true to the idea that obesity prevention requires multiple strategies in multiple settings, and that the private sector needs to be involved, Good for Kids Good for Life has a strategy to attract sponsors to the program not only to expand the resources available but also to engage and reorientate businesses and the private sector towards creating healthier environments for children. A policy has been developed to minimize the risks associated with such commercial sponsorship (see Box 27.4).

Shape up Sommerville was a successful obesity intervention aimed at children in Massachusetts that used a community-based participatory research (CBPR) approach.[17] As part of this approach, researchers successfully helped intervention communities secure over $1.5 million from other funding sources for the interventions. In the pilot phase of a community-based obesity prevention initiative in France (Ensemble, prévenons l'obésité des enfants [EPODE] translated as "Together we can prevent obesity in children"),[38] most of their funds were received from the private sector (including the food industry) and less than a quarter from public sources such as regional councils, education, research and health departments. Currently, the mix is closer to 50:50 from the private sector (including food industry 18%, but also insurance agencies, distributors, foundations) and from public sector, mainly from the local government. The private funds are dedicated to central coordination—organizing, training, coaching, social marketing development and communications. The public funds are for the local communities to pay local project managers and for tools (personal communication, Borys JM 2008).

Developing structures for community decision making

There is a tremendous amount of creativity, innovation and know-how in communities. With adequate

Box 27.4 Excerpt from Good for Kids Good for Life sponsorship guidelines

Criteria for deciding on the appropriateness of a commercial arrangement such as sponsorship

Good for Kids Good for Life will work with other organizations in a commercial arrangement provided the following conditions are met:

1. The sponsorship or other commercial arrangement is in the name of the organization (rather than in the name of a brand or product).
2. The products or marketing practices of the organization are deemed to be appropriate by the Chief Executive or delegated officer.

Products or practices may be considered to be inappropriate in the following areas:

- products that are deemed to be contrary to public health and well-being and harmful to children (e.g. tobacco, arms, alcohol);
- a product line or marketing strategy in which the major food or beverage products are deemed to be energy-dense and micronutrient poor and thus may contribute to unhealthy weight gain;
- marketing practices which are potentially misleading or deceptive, particularly with regard to unsubstantiated claims in relation to health outcomes;
- inappropriate marketing of products to children—this could include (but is not restricted to):
  - the deliberate targeting of young children in the marketing of energy-dense, micronutrient-poor products
  - the use of inappropriate marketing techniques that take advantage of children's credulity (e.g. premiums, inducements, popular children's heroes or celebrities);
- the presentation of unbalanced or inconsistent health communications, especially where the roles of both diet and physical activity in achieving and maintaining good health are not appropriately addressed.

resources and appropriate structures this creativity can readily be applied to preventing childhood obesity. But what sorts of structures are needed to foster community decision making on childhood obesity prevention? The foundational structure may start off as a small planning committee consisting of a relatively small group of community stakeholders (for example, community health organizations and local govern-

ment) brought together by some funding opportunity. The task of the planning committee is to stimulate action in the community through a process of needs assessment, planning, implementation and evaluation. It also has the task of increasing the number of community stakeholders involved in the program and changing the way these stakeholders do business through a process of organizational change.[39] New governance structures are built around these tasks and communication structures are also required to ensure the opinions of the broader community are brought to bear on the program.

The Be Active Eat Well program in Colac, Victoria, offers an example of the kinds of structures required. In the early stages of the project, a steering committee with representatives from the funders (state health department) evaluators (university) and implementers (local health organization and local government) guided the planning and early implementation phases. As the project progressed, the governance structures also had to evolve, and the initial steering committee was replaced by a local implementation committee to guide on the ground activities, and a higher-level reference committee to provide strategic guidance, expert technical advice and broader linkages to other activities.

Moreover, as the group of stakeholders involved expanded, working parties were formed (e.g. a schools working party) that served as effector arms for the steering committee. Parents and other community members participated in some of these groups but there was also a need for communication tools or structures for broader community input. This occurred primarily through a newsletter that went home to parents from school and feedback boxes located in the schools that teachers, parents or children were encouraged to use. It also occurred through local media and, perhaps facilitated by the smallness of the township, through the presence and availability of project staff.

Examples on a larger scale are the Healthy Living Centres in the UK.[40] These were launched by the New Opportunities Fund (now know as the Big Lottery Fund or BIG) in 1998 as part of the new Labour government's strategy to improve health (in its broadest sense) and to address health inequalities. Underlying the vision for how these centres would operate was a perception that "communities" themselves would drive improvements supported by broad partnerships between health and other public, voluntary and private organizations and would themselves release resources to fund local projects and assist in sustaining them in the long term. Aimed at the most deprived areas in the UK, the healthy living centres were an excellent example of public policy that emphasized community action and partnership as mechanisms to bring about change. The process of identifying projects was competitive and, in the end, 351 projects were funded over a maximum of five years in England, Northern Ireland, Scotland and Wales. It should also be noted that by 1999 these countries had some degree of devolved decision making within their own national government assemblies since health was a policy area in which administrations could develop their own approaches. Those activities that are more likely to have survived have been ones that felt they were relevant to local concerns.[41,42]

Central to the success of EPODE has been the presence of a central coordination team to help local communities develop expertise, share best practice and develop a group dynamic between the local project managers of all the cities or communities involved and within communities.[43] Each community works with its local human and financial resources but benefits from the central framework for the training, tools, funding, political lobbying, policy-maker support and communication.

Social and political support

To maximize the impact and sustainability of a capacity building process, the systems that a community operates in also need to change and this requires social and political support. There is little value, for example, in five or six schools agreeing to implement a school canteen policy if it is not consistent with broader education department policy.

Social support refers to support given to a community for consensus building on an issue and how best to address it both within and outside the community's boundaries. One of the social support mechanisms that has been missing from efforts to prevent childhood obesity is advocacy groups. Unlike tobacco control initiatives, there have been no grass-roots lobby groups to draw attention to the problem of childhood obesity or offer advice on how to address

the problem. Recently, however, groups such as the Parents Jury[44] have emerged to give voice to parents on barriers to, and facilitators of, healthy eating and physical activity for their children.

Political support is required to ensure that existing policy provides room to accommodate the changes brought about by the program. It is also required to ensure that policy can be amended or enacted to sustain these changes, to expand their reach and to provide a benchmark against which effectiveness can be measured. Involving local Members of Parliament in the program along with relevant ministers is an obvious way of garnering political support. Having someone within or linked to the community who is familiar with relevant policies is important for getting supportive policy in place. Nu'Man et al suggest seeking commitment from top-level stakeholders, developing a national strategy, developing policies and regulations for collection of data and developing and supporting local planning groups as examples of system-level capacity building activities for HIV/Aids prevention programs that have the effect of building program sustainability, building consensus related to planning and implementation, ensuring program accountability and ensuring targeted services and programs.[39]

Incorporating the evidence

How will we know when sufficient community capacity has been built to prevent childhood obesity? The best indicator is likely to be achieving and sustaining a low overweight and obesity prevalence. A well-designed portfolio of intervention strategies in a number of settings achieves the goal and effective community capacity building sustains it. This is consistent with Hawe's suggestion that investment decisions be guided by attention to return on the investment in terms of size of health gain (e.g. reducing overweight and obesity prevalence) and by the sustainability of the outcome.[45] Unfortunately, evaluations of obesity prevention programs have largely neglected measurements of community capacity and sustainability of changes. This leaves us speculating why some programs have worked and others have not. A reason for the lack of attention to measuring community capacity building may be the long time-frames required to assess sustainability and the lack

Table 27.1 Capacity building domains from the Capacity Building Index.

Network partnerships	The relationships between groups and organizations within the project's network. This includes both the comprehensiveness and the quality of the relationships, i.e. are all of the significant groups and organizations involved and what is the nature of their involvement.
Knowledge transfer	The development, exchange and use of information within and between the groups and organizations within the project's network.
Problem solving	The ability to use well-recognized methods to identify and solve problems arising in the development and implementation of the project.
Infrastructure	The level of investment in the project by the groups and organizations that make up the project's network. Infrastructure includes both tangible and non-tangible investments such as investment in the development of protocols and policy, social capital, human capital and financial capital.

of consensus on measuring indicators of capacity building.

The Community Capacity Index (CCI),[4] however, is a useful evaluation tool and was administered for the Be Active Eat Well Project to assist in identifying baseline capacity to implement the project and increases in capacity over time. Capacity was mapped against a set of indicators within four domains (see Table 27.1).

Within the first three domains, three levels of capacity are identified, with each level measured by a set of indicators. The fourth domain, infrastructure, has four levels or sub-domains (policy, financial, human/intellectual, and social investments), also with sets of indicators. The indicators within the CCI represent the abilities, behaviors or characteristics of the project's network. At baseline, basic capacity was evident in network partnerships, knowledge transfer and problem solving. Financial infrastructure was low but social infrastructure was high. Over the three years of the project, capacity demonstrably increased in all four domains. At follow-up, similar levels of increase

in capacity were observed across the first three domains. Financial infrastructure remained relatively low while policy infrastructure made the highest gain from baseline to follow-up.

Measuring community capacity is not only important for helping us explain why an intervention did or did not work. It also reminds evaluators of the need to balance scientific evidence with community relevance,[29] to understand the value of communities being able to make use of their own data, and to contribute to the vital role of effective knowledge translation.[46]

Conclusions

Obesity in a child predicts a lifetime risk of chronic disease. Obese children have a 70–80% chance of still being obese at age 20.[47] This makes prevention paramount. The evidence suggests that the optimal approach is to have multiple strategies occurring in multiple settings to prevent childhood obesity,[19] but this cannot be achieved in a sustainable way unless communities are recognized as part of the solution. To date there are no best-practice models of community capacity building for childhood obesity prevention to help communities do this. Fortunately, however, community-based interventions are emerging that can serve as demonstration models and we have cited several examples. The next step is for these intervention programs to form networks that bring greater social and political support to community programs and foster knowledge sharing so that the obesity epidemic can be addressed more efficiently and on a progressively larger scale. In Brazil, networks of local community initiatives to promote healthy diets and active lifestyles have been described as fundamental for achieving sustainable behavior change.[48] Similar networks have been a key feature of the EPODE program which now involves almost 200 towns in France, is also running in Spain (21 communities), Belgium (18 communities) and is starting in Canada, Greece and Australia.

A community-based approach encourages creativity within communities, harnesses local passion to provide healthy environments for children, and empowers them to provide local solutions for their own contexts. For these reasons, we should be optimistic that significant and sustainable reductions in childhood obesity are possible.

References

1 Hillery GA: Definitions of community. Areas of agreement. *Rural Sociol* 1955; **20**:111–123.

2 Hawe P, King L, Noort M, Gifford S, Lloyd B: Working invisibly: health workers talk about capacity-building in health promotion. *Health Promot Int* 1998; **13**(4):285–295.

3 NSW Health Department: A Framework for Building Capacity to Improve Health. Gladesville: Better Health Care Centre, 2001.

4 Bush R, Dower J, Mutch A: Community Capacity Index Manual. Brisbane: Centre for Primary Health Care, 2002.

5 Eade D: Capacity-Building: An Approach to People-Centred Development. Oxford: Oxfam, 1997.

6 WHO: Ottawa Charter for Health Promotion. 1986; Available from: www.who.int/hpr/NPH/docs/ottawa_charter_hp.pdf (accessed 25 November 2008).

7 WHO: Jakarta Declaration. 1997; Available from: www.who.int/healthpromotion/conferences/previous/jakarta/declaration/en/ (accessed 25 November 2008).

8 WHO: The Bangkok Charter. 2005; Available from: www.who.int/healthpromotion/conferences/6gchp/bangkok_charter/en/ (accessed 26 November 2008).

9 Smith B, Tang K, Nutbeam D: WHO health promotion glossary: new terms. *Health Promot Int* 2006; **21**(4):340–345.

10 Shirlow P, Murtagh B: Capacity-building, representation and intra-community conflict. *Urban Stud* 2004; **41**(1):57–70.

11 Amin A: Local community on trial. *Econ Soc* 2005; **34**(4):612–633.

12 Craig G: Community capacity-building: something old, something new …? *Crit Soc Policy* 2007; **27**:335–359.

13 Levitas R: Community, utopia and new labour. *Local Econ* 2000; **15**(3):188–197.

14 Morrissey M: Community, social capital and indigenous health in the northern territory. *Ethn Health* 2006; **11**(3):229–246.

15 Bourdieu P: The Weight of the World: Social Suffering in Contemporary Society. Stanford University Press, 1999.

16 Taylor RW, McAuley KA, Williams SM, Barbezat W, Nielson G, Mann JI: Reducing weight gain in children through enhancing physical activity and nutrition: the APPLE project. *Int J Pediatr Obes* 2006; **1**(3):146–152.

17 Economos CD, Hyatt RR, Goldberg JP et al: A community intervention reduces BMI z-score in children: shape up Sommerville first year results. *Obesity* 2007; **15**(5):1325–1336.

18 Singh AS, Chin A, Paw MJ, Brug J, van Mechelen W: Short-term effects of school-based weight gain prevention among adolescents. *Arch Pediatr Adolesc Med* 2007; **161**(6):565–571.

19 Swinburn B, Bell AC: A comprehensive approach to obesity prevention. In: Kopelman PG, Caterson ID, Dietz WH, eds. Clinical Obesity in Adults and Children, 2nd edn. Oxford: Blackwell, 2005:456–471.

20 Sanigorski AM, Bell AC, Kremer PJ, Swinburn BA: High childhood obesity in an Australian population. *Obesity* 2007; **15**(8):1908–1912.

21 Shrewsbury V, Wardle J: Socioeconomic status and adiposity in childhood: a systematic review of cross-sectional studies 1990–2005. *Obesity* 2008; **16**(2):275–284.

22 van Zutphen M, Bell AC, Kremer PJ, Swinburn BA: Association between the family environment and television viewing in Australian children. *J Pediatr Child Health* 2007; **43**(6):458–463.

23 Puhl R, Brownell K: Bias, discrimination, and obesity. *Obes Res* 2001; **9**(12):788–805.

24 Welsh Office: Better Health Better Wales Cm 3922. Cardiff: The Stationery Office, 1998.

25 Bermingham B, Porter A: Engaging with communities. In: Cropper S, Porter A, Williams G, Carlisle S, Moore R, O'Neill R et al, eds. Community Health and Wellbeing: Action Research on Health Inequalities. Bristol: The Policy Press, 2007:105–128.

26 O'Neill M, Rebanne D, Lester C: Barriers to healthier eating in a disadvantaged community. *Health Educ J* 2004; **63**(3):220–228.

27 Coe K, Wilson C, Eisenberg M, Attakai A, Lobell M: Creating the environment for a successful community partnership. *Cancer* 2006; **107**(8 Suppl.):1980–1986.

28 Smith A, Coveney J, Carter P, Jolley G, Laris P: The Eat Well SA project: an evaluation-based case study in building capacity for promoting healthy eating. *Health Promot Int* 2004; **19**(3):327–334.

29 Judd J, Frankish J, Moulton G: Setting standards in the evaluation of community-based health promotion programmes—a unifying approach. *Health Promot Int* 2001; **16**(4):367–380.

30 Bell AC, Simmons A, Sanigorski AM, Kremer PJ, Swinburn BA: Preventing childhood obesity: the sentinel site for obesity prevention in Victoria, Australia. *Health Promot Int* 2008; **23**(4):328–336.

31 Sanigorski AM, Bell AC, Kremer PJ, Cuttler R, Swinburn BA: Reducing unhealthy weight gain in children through community capacity-building: results of a quasi-experimental intervention program, Be Active Eat Well. *Int J Obes* 2008; **32**(7):1060–1067.

32 Wiesenfeld E: The concept of "we": a community social psychology myth? *J Community Psychol* 1996; **24**(4):337–346.

33 Bell AC: Community-based approaches to prevent obesity. In: Mela D, ed. Food, Diet and Obesity. Cambridge: Woodhead, 2005:448–467.

34 Conway K, Tunks M, Henwood W, Casswell S: Te Whanau Cadillac—a waka for change. *Health Educ Behav* 2000; **27**(3):339–350.

35 NSW Health. Good for Kids Good for Life. 2008; Available from: www.goodforkids.nsw.gov.au (accessed 25 November 2008).

36 Livingstone MBE, McCaffrey TA, Rennie KL: Childhood obesity prevention studies: lessons learned and to be learned. *Pub Health Nutr* 2006; **9**(8A):1121–1129.

37 Flynn MAT, McNeill DA, Maloff B et al: Reducing obesity and related chronic disease risk in children and youth: a synthesis of evidence with "best practice" recommendations. *Obes Rev* 2006; **7**(Suppl. 1):7–66.

38 Borys Jean-Michel: Fleurbaix Laventie Ville Santé 1992–2007, 2009; Available from: www.inforelais.net/PROTEINES/200904/EPODE/page1 (accessed 7 October 2009).

39 Nu'Man J, King W, Bhalakia A, Criss S: A framework for building organizational capacity integrating planning, monitoring and evaluation. *J Public Health Manag Pract*, 2007; **13**(January Suppl.):S24–S32.

40 Great Britain Department of Health: Saving Lives: Our Healthier Nation. London: The Stationery Office, 1999.

41 Hills D, Elliott E, Kowarzik U et al: The Evaluation of the Big Lottery Fund Healthy Living Centres Programme. Final Report. London: Big Lottery Fund, 2007.

42 Elliott E, Williams G: Paper 115: Final report on the sustainability and legacy of Healthy Living Centres in Wales. Cardiff School of Social Sciences, Working Paper Series; (September) 2008, 1–84.

43 EPODE: Ensemble, Prévenons, l'obésité des enfants: 2008; Available from: www.epode.fr (accessed 24 November 2008).

44 The Parents Jury: 2008; Available from: www.parentsjury.org.au (accessed 24 November 2008).

45 Hawe P, Noort M, King L, Jordens C: Multiplying health gains: the critical role of capacity-building within health promotion programs. *Health Policy* 1997; **39**:29–42.

46 Green L, Kreuter M: Health Promotion Planning: An Educational and Ecological Approach. California: Mayfield, 1999.

47 Magarey AM, Daniels LA, Boulton TJ, Cockington RA: Predicting obesity in early adulthood from childhood and parental obesity. *Int J Obes* 2003; **27**(4):505–513.

48 Coitinho D, Monteiro CA, Popkin BM: What Brazil is doing to promote healthy diets and active lifestyles. *Public Health Nutr* 2002; **5**(1A):263–267.

Social marketing to prevent childhood obesity

Nadine Henley[1] and *Sandrine Raffin*[2]

[1] Centre for Applied Social Marketing Research, Edith Cowan University, Perth, Australia
[2] EPODE European Network, Paris, France

Summary and recommendations for research and practice

- Social marketing is one of many tools available for changing behavior; it applies commercial marketing principles to achieve socially desirable goals.
- Seven overarching communication principles should be considered before designing a social marketing campaign.
- Key marketing principles are: "getting the right message" and "getting the message right" for different target markets; the 4Ps—Product, Place, Price, Promotion, and a 5th P: Partnerships.
- The innovative French EPODE program addressing childhood obesity is used as a case study throughout this chapter to illustrate principles and process.

Introduction

This chapter first outlines the fundamental communication principles social marketers have to consider when approaching the issue of childhood obesity and then explains the marketing principles on which their decisions are based when designing a social marketing campaign to address the issue. The innovative French EPODE program is used as a case study throughout this chapter to illustrate principles and process (Box 28.1).

The term "social marketing" was first used by Kotler and Zaltman[1] to refer to the application of

Preventing Childhood Obesity. Edited by
E. Waters, B.A. Swinburn, J.C. Seidell and R. Uauy.
© 2010 Blackwell Publishing.

commercial marketing principles in the context of socially desirable goals. Andreasen[2] defined social marketing as: "the application of commercial marketing technologies to the analysis, planning, execution, and evaluation of programs designed to influence the voluntary behaviour of target audiences in order to improve their personal welfare and that of their society" (p.7). Donovan and Henley[3] modified this definition to include involuntary behaviors as there are many instances of social marketing where the individual's voluntary behavior is constrained, for example, under threat of legal sanction (drink driving) or other regulations (smoke-free venues), or where the individual's choices are restricted (e.g. government restrictions on trans-fatty acids in processed foods).

Until recently, social marketing focused primarily on persuading the individual to adopt recommended behaviors (often referred to as the "downstream" approach). However, current thinking has extended the definition of social marketing to include achieving change in the social determinants of health and safety (referred to as the "upstream" approach).[3-7] Upstream approaches attempt to bring about desired individual behavior, often without the individual's conscious cooperation.

In the present context of childhood obesity, the "upstream" advocacy role extends to working to ensure individuals have access to healthy foods (such as children's school meals) and information about nutritional value of foods (as in food labels), as well as advocacy for public facilities to encourage physical activity (such as cycle paths and parks). Other possibilities include taxes on unhealthy foods or products,

Box 28.1 The EPODE program

EPODE ('Ensemble prévenons l'obésité des enfants: Together, let's prevent childhood obesity') is an innovative program, developed in France and launched in 2004 to help prevent obesity in children. In 2010, about 200 French towns were involved in EPODE and the program is now being run out in Belgium, Spain, South Australia and Canada (Québec). The original 10 towns in the pilot program have now fulfilled their original commitment for five years and have all reaffirmed their commitment for another five years, indicating the strong sustainability of the concept.

Box 28.2 Engaging the champions

A key aspect of EPODE is its involvement of local authorities through the local mayors. In France, these local authorities have jurisdiction over kindergartens and primary schools, covering the primary target of children aged 3–12 years. Mayors are invited to submit an application to be an EPODE community; this involves signing a charter promising to employ a full-time project manager for the program, organize specific activities each month in the city, participate in national meetings of project managers and commit at least 1 euro per capita per annum for five years (although many authorities commit much more than this).

subsidies for healthy foods or products, regulating advertising to children,[8] making unhealthy foods less visible, more expensive and harder to access.[9]

It is appropriate to include advocacy elements in a social marketing strategy. Indeed, some would say that social marketers should consider environmental change first[10] and we should only attempt to persuade individuals to change their behavior when all possible environmental changes have been put in place that will make it easier for them to change. Targeting local champions is also a key social marketing strategy because they can significantly influence opinions and mobilize resources (Box 28.2).

Other chapters in this book go into more detail on strategies to change the environment so the rest of this chapter will focus on the more conventional, down-stream social marketing activities involved when trying to persuade individuals to change their behavior. Some well-accepted marketing principles are discussed later and shown how they were used in the EPODE context: "getting the right message" and "getting the message right" for different target markets; and the marketing mix. But first, we identify a number of fundamental communication principles to be considered when designing a social marketing campaign:[11]

- **The receiver is an active processor of incoming information:** A message will be received differently by different people; pre-existing beliefs, attitudes, experiences and knowledge affect the way an individual attends to, interprets and accepts a message.
- **Different target audiences may respond to different messages differently:** Target audiences must be segmented by beliefs and attitudes before the development of targeted messages.
- **Formative research, including message pre-testing is essential:** Formative research (focus groups/interviews) is conducted with the target audience to understand their different beliefs and attitudes. Messages are then pre-tested with the target audience to ensure understanding, and with secondary audiences, to ensure there are no unintended negative effects.
- **A theoretical framework increases the likelihood of success:** Campaigns guided by theoretical frameworks are more likely to be successful than those that are not. Some of the important models of attitude and behavior change include the Health Belief Model, Protection Motivation Theory, Theory of Reasoned Action and the Theory of Trying (for a summary, see Andreasen).[3]
- **Comprehensive, coordinated interventions are most successful:** Successful campaigns are comprehensive and coordinated with other environmental and on-the-ground strategies to ensure attitudinal and behavioral success.
- **Multiple delivery channels and multiple sources increase the likelihood of success:** Communication campaigns involving a number of message delivery channels and more than one source appear to be more successful than those that do not.[12]
- **Campaigns must be sustained to be effective:** Communication campaigns must be sustained over time to achieve and maintain success.

These seven overarching communication principles are fundamental to social marketing campaign decisions. The rest of this chapter discusses some of the basic social marketing principles that guide the development of successful campaigns.

Marketing principles

"Getting the right message" for different target markets

Creating effective communication messages involves a two-step process: "getting the right message" and "getting the message right".[13] The first step involves reference to three types of research:

1. Epidemiological research (using population-based statistical evidence to identify risk and protective factors in health issues), for example: What does the epidemiological evidence say about preventing obesity (e.g., 30 minutes of physical activity on most days a week has a significant effect on some indicators of adult health such as reducing cardiovascular diseases outcomes, but the evidence on the amount needed to prevent unhealthy weight gain in children is less certain and may be up to 60 minutes a day)?

2. Formative research (using qualitative methodologies such as focus groups, in-depth interviews): What do people say will motivate them to try to change behavior (e.g., to eat more fruit and vegetables) through changing attitudes and beliefs?

3. Evidence-based research (referring to available evaluations of previous strategies): What has been done before and deemed to be effective, having been rigorously evaluated against established benchmarks (e.g., which previous messages around healthy food choices resulted in measurable dietary changes)?

When trying to change behaviors relating to childhood obesity, we first have to decide what is the right message to communicate. When targeting children, we can decide on the basis of formative research with children which of the following we should be recommending: eat healthy, eat more fruit and vegetables, eat less fat, avoid soft drinks, be more physically active, be less sedentary, play outside more, sit inside watching tv/playing computer games less, watch no more than a certain number of hours on TV, and so on. Within the target market of "children", there will

be subsections. The US physical activity VERB™ campaign found that their messages around fun were more appealing to younger children and their messages around peers, competition and mastery appealed more to older children.[14]

When targeting parents, it is worth bearing in mind that parents have three roles[15] that can influence a child's nutrition and physical activity levels: they provide specific foods and physical activity options for the child; they model food consumption and activity levels; and they control (at least to some extent) the child's environment, determining the quality and diversity of experiences at mealtimes and activity times. We can decide on the basis of formative research with parents, whether it is best to recommend that mother or father or both: buy healthier food, withhold soft drinks, provide a certain number of serves of fruit and vegetables, offer smaller portions, allow fewer snacks, eat without distractions (e.g. television), persuade children to go outside to play, try different activities, accompany them on a walk to school, and so on. Within the target market of "parents", there will be subsections: different messages will be appropriate for mothers and fathers, grandparents or other carers (Box 28.3).

Box 28.3 Getting the message right

Although social marketers often think of formative research (focus groups with target audiences) as essential, it is interesting that EPODE has been developed more on evidence from the health and behavioral literature, and field experience. The primary target is families of children 0–12 years and the focus is on the adoption of healthier food choices and eating habits, and a more active lifestyle for everyone in the family. EPODE determined that children are unlikely to respond to cognitive-based strategies, for example "Eat 2 fruit a day", finding that it is better to concentrate on one simple message at a time, reinforcing it with activities, and repeating it over a long time period. For example, some of EPODE's strategies to increase fruit consumption are to suggest children try fruit compotes or fresh fruit in yoghurt, taste small pieces, participate in preparing fruit with others, and take it step by step. A key aspect is that there is never any stigma attached to a child who is reluctant to participate.

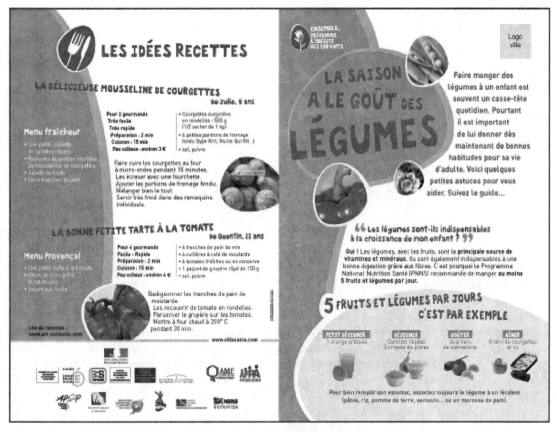

Figure 28.1 For parents: "The taste of the season" vegetables brochure.

"Getting the message right" for different target markets

The second step in creating effective communication messages, "getting the message right", involves decisions about the execution elements; how to present the message in a way that attracts attention, is believable, relevant, able to be understood, arouses appropriate emotions and does not lead to counter-argument.[16]

When targeting children, formative research is usually conducted to determine the execution elements that will appeal most to children. Generally, we would expect children to relate more to the use of stimulating execution elements, lots of colors, animation, cartoon characters, and a pictorial emphasis. It is important to use simple, easy to understand concrete (rather than abstract) concepts, suited to a child's cognitive development.[17] When targeting

parents, we would conduct formative research with parents to determine the execution elements that would be most appropriate for them. These would be likely to include more verbal communications than for children, more serious information, advice, tips, recipes, risks, etc. (Figure 28.1).

The marketing mix

The marketing mix refers to the traditional "4 Ps" of marketing: Product, Place, Price and Promotion. We have added a 5th P—Partnerships—in this chapter as the problem of childhood obesity needs to be addressed by a concerted effort of many agencies and stakeholders. Borden first used the term "marketing mix" in 1953 to compare marketing to the process of baking in which appropriate ingredients are blended in the correct proportions.[18]

Product

Product, in commercial marketing, relates to physical objects (e.g. cars, toothbrushes) and services (e.g. banking, hairdressing). In social marketing, the products are primarily ideas such as, in the context of obesity, "eat 2 fruits and 5 vegetables a day to be healthy". This product involves a tangible product component (the fruit and vegetables) but the core social product is the underlying benefit of being healthy. The recommended behavior is to eat fruits and vegetables. Performing the behavior, eating fruits and vegetables, offers the individual a way to achieve the benefit.

One of the difficulties in designing an effective social marketing strategy to prevent childhood obesity is determining what the specific core product or underlying benefit should be. What are we really "selling"? What are people most likely "to buy"? One way to decide this is to answer the following questions:

- What are the communication objectives (what do we want the target audience to know or believe)?
- What are the behavioral objectives (what do we want the target audience to do)?

On the basis of our formative research and decisions about "the right message", we may have decided that children are most likely to respond to messages about having fun or being better able to play sport or being part of a social group rather than messages relating to health. So the core product, a communication objective expressed as an underlying benefit that would appeal to children, might focus on: games at lunchtime for fun, or after school activities for staying fit and strong for sports, or walking groups for catching up with friends (Box 28.4 and Figure 28.2). The behavioral objective would be the increased physical activity involved in the lunchtime games, after-school sport skills activities or groups walking around the sports ground at lunchtime with friends.

Box 28.4 Promoting the benefits

EPODE promotes healthy behavior to children as a fun activity rather than for health benefits. For example, one theme is "Playing is already moving!" recommending fun (non-competitive) play activities. The theme is based on research that shows that playing outside with friends can significantly increase the amount of physical activity a child gets in a day.

Product considerations include concepts of branding. The American Marketing Association has defined a brand as: "a name, term, symbol, or design, or a combination of them, intended to identify the goods or services of one seller, or group of sellers and to differentiate them from those of competitors" (p. 97).[18] Key characteristics of a brand are that it should be memorable, recognizable, easy to pronounce, distinctive, and able to convey the product's benefits and appeal.[19] The US physical activity VERB™ campaign is an example of such a brand, the name chosen to connote action.[14] The brand's logo is particularly important to visually draw attention to the brand and portray an appropriate image, as exposure to the logo is often the most frequent type of contact people will have with the brand (Figure 28.3 and Box 28.5).

Place

Place (or "distribution") in marketing involves two main considerations: how to make the product conveniently available, and managing any intermediaries. Helplines and websites are used extensively in social marketing to provide a convenient "place" where the product/idea can be made more available to the consumer. Where social marketers are recommending tangible products or services, the same principles of access apply. If we want children to eat more fruit and vegetables, we need to make sure good quality, appetizing produce is available where children make food choices, such as the school cafeteria. Vending machines on school grounds, swimming pools and sports fields need to be stocked with healthy options. In social marketing, intermediaries can be health professionals, teachers, coaches, occupational health and safety officers in the workplace, and so on (Box 28.6 and Figures 28.4 and 28.5).

Price

Price is the cost of the product, both monetary and non-monetary. Price includes the concept of "exchange" where the buyer gives up something in return for the product. In commercial marketing this is primarily thought of as the monetary cost of paying for goods or services, although there may also be some non-monetary costs such as time and effort. A good place strategy can reduce time and effort costs by making the product easily accessible. In social

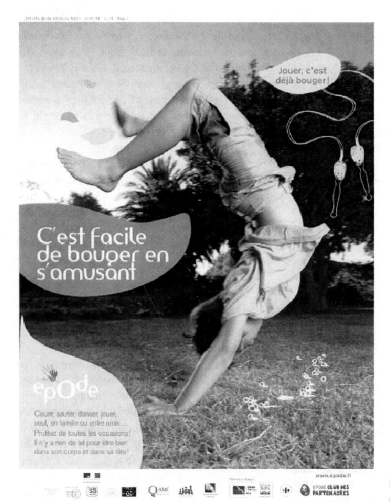

Figure 28.2 Promoting physical activity as fun.

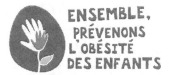

Figure 28.3 The EPODE logo.

Box 28.5 Exposing the brand

One of EPODE's branding strategies is to prominently display the city's logo in customized local materials, while minimizing the national, government and partners' logos. The EPODE name and logo are used throughout the extensive media coverage and in all local activities.

Box 28.6 Making healthy choices easy

EPODE's place strategy makes healthy choices accessible to children. They are taught the principles of nutrition and a balanced diet in school and encouraged to try healthy foods and participate in fun physical activities, including a "pedestrian school bus" to encourage walking to school. A simple strategy which illustrates the intention to make healthy decisions easy for children is that supermarkets are encouraged to present seasonal fruits, at a good price and in a place where children can pick them up themselves. EPODE builds on existing channels of distribution that already influence children's behavior, especially parents, leisure stakeholders and teachers.

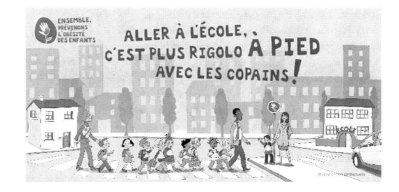

Figure 28.4 Promoting the pedestrian school bus driven by parents.

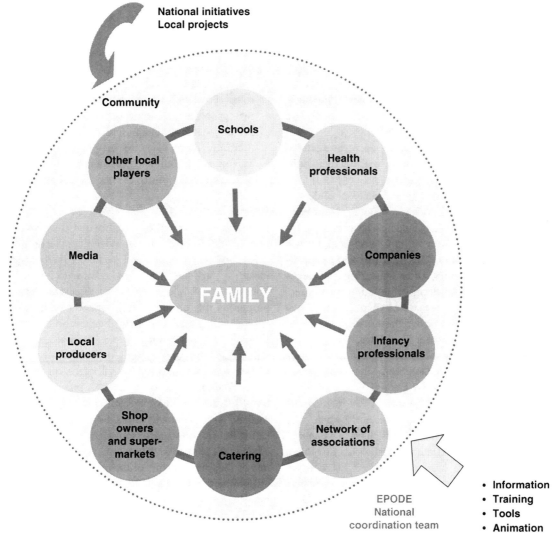

Figure 28.5 The EPODE distribution network.

marketing, there is often no monetary cost, or very little, but there is usually a substantial non-monetary cost involved in adopting a recommended behavior.

In the context of childhood obesity, we are usually asking the target audience (children) to give up the instant gratification of desired foods and soft drinks or to engage in effortful activities. We may be asking parents to deny their children desired foods and also to engage in effortful activities with their children. Persuading children and parents to adopt a physical activity routine may involve some monetary costs such as purchasing shoes, clothing or equipment. However, the major costs may relate to time, effort, physical discomfort and possibly guilt.

The key consideration when designing a pricing strategy is the concept of exchange: the target audience will weigh up the costs and benefits based on what we present to them and their previous experience. When they do this cost–benefit analysis, we need them to clearly see: "What's in it for me?" (known in marketing as "the WIIFM"). There are three ways to help people identify the WIIFM:

1. **Minimize the costs of taking up recommended behaviors.** For example, in a physical activity campaign this could mean showing how easy it is to fit 30 minutes of activity into your daily schedule; this has been the main pricing strategy in recent years of Western Australia's "Find Thirty" campaign.

2. **Maximize the costs of not taking up recommended behaviors.** This is the threat appeal strategy used in many social marketing campaigns where the consequences of not adopting the recommended behavior may be shown. This approach has not been used much in the nutrition and physical activity arena, to our knowledge, despite strong evidence in the research that fear does motivate people to avoid problems and can be used effectively when efficacy levels are high, that is, when people believe they are capable of performing the behavior ("self efficacy"); and when they believe that the behavior will have a beneficial effect ("response efficacy").[20] However, this threat appeal strategy has perhaps been overused in health promotion[6,21] and is not recommended here as an appropriate strategy to address childhood obesity.

3. **Maximize the benefits of taking up recommended behaviors.** In a physical activity campaign, this

Box 28.7 Reducing the "cost" and maximizing the benefits

EPODE's pricing strategy has been to stress the benefits of a healthier lifestyle, including the family value of preparing and eating healthy food together and doing physical activities together; at the same time, the program finds ways to make healthy products less expensive by working with supermarkets, school canteens, and so on. EPODE has rejected the strategy of maximizing the consequences of not following the recommended behaviors, believing that people are much more likely to respond to positive messages highlighting pleasurable taste sensations and enjoyable family life experiences rather than negative messages producing feelings of guilt and shame.

could involve focusing on the fun, fitness and social benefits as well specific health benefits, including mental health, concentration, sleep patterns, and so on (Box 28.7). A Western Australia study found that people were unable to name many specific health benefits although those who could were significantly more likely to be physically active.[22] Maximizing health benefits could enhance uptake of recommendations in the obesity context.

Promotion

Promotion is the range of activities that create awareness of the product (or reminder that the product exists) and its attributes, and persuades the buyer to make the purchase.[23] Decisions relating to a promotion strategy should be based on three criteria: the purpose of the communication; what the target audience would prefer; and how much it will "cost".[23] Promotional tools include advertising, personal selling, sales promotion and publicity. Advertising (for example, via mass media, billboards, direct mail, telemarketing, point of purchase, internet, blogs, SMS)[23] is the most visible element of the marketing mix and is often thought of as synonymous with marketing but it is only one of four elements in the range of activities relating to Promotion, which itself is only one of the four elements of the marketing mix.

Commercial marketers usually have much larger budgets to spend on advertising their product than social marketers, but social marketing products often attract publicity more easily than commercial products; for example, new campaign strategies are often

Box 28.8 Multiple promotion approaches

Many of EPODE's promotion activities are focused at the local level, advertising local initiatives and events, using personal selling through, for example, doctors and teachers to promote the message. However, the extensive publicity the program has received is seen as encouraging more towns to enter the program. It could also have the effect of reinforcing a social norm around the program's activities which would encourage families to be involved.

Box 28.9 Public–private partnerships

A key element of EPODE is the public–private partnership. Funding for the program comes from a mix of public and private partnerships at the national and local levels. National private sponsors have, to date, come primarily from the food industry, insurance and distribution sectors. These partners sign a charter to confirm their intention to support this public health project focusing on preventing childhood obesity, promising that the program will not be referred to in any product promotion, and that they will not intervene in any way in the program content and will refer to their involvement only in corporate communications.

aired on prime-time news broadcasts. Personal selling is important in commercial sales of items like computers and cars but can be equally effective when one-on-one selling is included in the social marketing strategy to sell the idea of a health behavior, for example, using teachers, coaches and doctors. Perhaps one area that social marketers could consider more is that of sales promotions. In commercial marketing this refers to free samples, discounts or gift. Sales promotions in social marketing are "incentives" or "facilitators". Offers for a week's free trial at a gym or prizes available for those entering a competition would fall into the category of "sales promotions". The EPODE program uses many of these approaches to promotion (Box 28.8).

Partnerships

In the context of obesity, "Partnerships" is a fifth essential marketing mix element as the problem can only be solved by an integrated effort involving numerous agencies and stakeholders[24] including education departments, schools, teachers, parents, health departments and health professionals, regulatory bodies, the food industry, commercial marketing industry, and so on. Combining public and private partners in a common endeavor is a powerful strategy for engagement, particularly if there is joint funding. However, there are important considerations in defining those relationships to ensure that the content and delivery of public health programs or messages are not influenced commercial factors (Box 28.9).

Incorporating the evidence

The many decisions made in the development of any social marketing campaign need to be supported by

evidence, whether formative research with the primary and secondary target audiences, or, as in the case of EPODE, evidence from scientific literature and field experience. In addition, there is (and should be) an element of the marketers' judgement about what will work: "We must allow hunch and common sense and—above all, vision" (p. 7).[6]

Conclusion

Effective social marketing requires coordinated approaches both upstream (environmental, policy changes) and downstream (individual behavior changes). In practice, social marketing campaigns need to be sustained over time to create change at a cultural or societal level. We have been successful in recent years in changing normative attitudes, for example, towards drinking and driving, and making smoking less cool. We have also had successes in the challenging public health fields of HIV/Aids, cot deaths and some cancers.[25] We are now trying to create social norms that physical activity and healthy eating are desirable. This will require commitments from governments for strategic, long-term funding, "measured in decades not years" (p. 192)[26] for comprehensive, innovative and properly evaluated interventions.[25]

Knowledge alone is not enough to change people's behavior. The principles of social marketing are not intellectually difficult or necessarily expensive but they do provide "intelligent solutions"[5] to important social problems. The art of social marketing is to apply these principles in a coordinated, sustained and innovative effort, such as is seen in the EPODE case study. The target audience comes to recognize the recommended behavior as a worthwhile product, with more benefits than costs, that is easily obtainable and satisfies an internal need or desire.

References

1 Kotler P, Zaltman G: Social marketing: an approach to planned social change. *J Mark* 1971; **35**:3–12.

2 Andreasen AR: Marketing Social Change: Changing Behavior to Promote Health, Social Development, and the Environment. San Francisco: Jossey-Bass Publishers, 1995.

3 Donovan RJ, Henley N: Social Marketing: Principles and Practice. Melbourne: IP Communications, 2003.

4 Andreasen AR: Social Marketing in the 21st Century. Thousand Oaks, London and New Delhi: Sage, 2006.

5 Hastings G, Saren M: The critical contribution of social marketing. *Mark Theory* 2003; **3**(3):305–322.

6 Hastings G: Ten promises to Terry: towards a social marketing manifesto. *Soc Mark Qual* 2006; **12**(2):59–62.

7 Wilkinson R, Marmot M: Social Determinants of Health. The Solid Facts, 2nd edn. Copenhagen: World Health Organization Europe, 2003; Available from: www.euro.who.int/document/e81384.pdf (accessed 13 June 2008).

8 Moodie R, Swinburn B, Richardson J, Somaini B: Childhood obesity—a sign of commercial success, but a market failure. *Int J Pediatr Obes* 2006; **1**(3):133–138.

9 Hoek J: Marketing communications and obesity: a view from the dark side. *NZ Med J* 2005; **118**:1220. Available from 28. /www.nzma.org.nz/journal/118-1220/1608/ (accessed 1 February 2008).

10 Smith B: Forget messages … Think about structural change first. *Soc Mark Qual* 1998; **4**(3):13–19.

11 Henley N, Donovan R, Francas M: Developing and implementing communication messages. In: Doll L, Bonzo S, Mercy J, Sleet D, eds. Handbook of Injury and Violence Prevention. New York: Springer, 2007:433–447.

12 Lefebvre C, Olander C, Levine E: The impact of multiple channel delivery of nutrition messages on student knowledge, motivation and behavior: results from the Team Nutrition pilot study. *Soc Mark Qual* 2000; **5**(3):90–98.

13 Egger G, Donovan R, Spark R: Health and the Media. Principles and Practices for Health Promotion. Sydney: McGraw-Hill Book Company, 1993.

14 Huhman M, Potter LD, Wong FL, Banspach SW, Duke JC, Heitzler CD: Effects of a mass media campaign to increase physical activity among children: year-1 results of the VERB campaign. *Pediatrics* 2005; **116**:e277–e284.

15 Pettigrew S: To whom should messages be tailored? Facilitating change in children's nutritional behaviors. Proceedings of Tailoring Health Messages Conference, 2005 July 6–10; Locarno Switzerland, 2005.

16 Donovan R: Public health advertising: execution guidelines for health promotion professionals. *Health Promot J Aust* 1991; **1**:40–45.

17 Wang C, Henley N: Why do children change their minds about smoking? Child development theory applied to social marketing practice. Proceedings of the Australia and New Zealand Marketing Academy Conference, Massey, NZ, 2001.

18 Sargeant A: Marketing Management for Nonprofit Organizations. Oxford: Oxford University Press, 1999.

19 Kotler P, Roberto N, Lee N: Social Marketing: Improving the Quality of Life. Thousand Oaks, CA: Sage, 2002.

20 Witte K, Allen M: A meta-analysis of fear appeals: Implications for effective public health campaigns. *Health Educ Behav* 2000; **27**(5):591–615.

21 Henley N, Donovan R: Unintended consequences of arousing fear in social marketing. Proceedings of the Australia & New Zealand Marketing Academy Conference, Sydney, 1999.

22 Henley N, Ganeshasundaram R, Nosaka K: Promoting physical activity with "response efficacy" strategies: Convincing people that being physically active will have specific, beneficial effects on their health. Report to Faculty of Business & Law, Centre for Applied Social Marketing Research, Edith Cowan University, Perth, Western Australia; 2007.

23 Thackeray R, Neiger BL, Hanson CL: Developing a promotional strategy: important questions for social marketing. *Health Promot Pract* 2007; **8**:332–336.

24 Ayadi K, Young B: Community partnerships: Preventing childhood obesity. *Young Consumers: insights and ideas for responsible marketers* 2006; **7**(4):35–40.

25 Swinburn BA: The obesity epidemic in Australia: can public health interventions work? *Asia Pac J Clin Nutr* 2003; **12**(Suppl. S7).

26 Stead M, Hastings G, McDermott L: The meaning, effectiveness and future of social marketing. *Obes Rev* 2006; **8** (Suppl. 1):189–193.

CHAPTER 29

Obesity in early childhood and working in pre-school settings

Andrea M. de Silva-Sanigorski,[1,2] *Camila Corvalán*[3] and *Ricardo Uauy*[4,5]

[1] WHO Collaborating Centre for Obesity Prevention, Deakin University Geelong, Australia
[2] Jack Brockoff Child Health and Wellbeing Program, The McCaughey Centre, Melbourne School of Population Health, The University of Melbourne, Melbourne, Australia
[3] School of Public Health, University of Chile, Santiago, Chile
[4] Institute of Nutrition and Food Technology, University of Chile, Santiago, Chile
[5] Nutrition and Public Health Intervention Research Unit, London School of Hygiene and Tropical Medicine, London, UK

Summary and recommendations for research and practice

- The new WHO growth standards for children aged 0–5 years are a major improvement on previous reference standards.
- The risk of obesity is related to children's growth, development, behaviors and environments in the early years of their lives.
- Appropriate nutrition requirements should be used to guide education directed at parents of infants, and policy-based requirements are needed in care settings.
- With more young children going into child care earlier, it is important that there should be regulation regarding the nutritional quality of the foods and drinks provided, and the opportunities for physical activity in these settings.
- Adequate structured and unstructured active play is needed for children to maintain a healthy weight and also to develop the skills needed for lifelong participation in physical activity.
- Physical inactivity is also an issue in young children and strategies to limit or reduce screen-based activities in the home and child care settings are needed.

Preventing Childhood Obesity. Edited by
E. Waters, B.A. Swinburn, J.C. Seidell and R. Uauy.
© 2010 Blackwell Publishing.

Introduction

This chapter examines several issues on obesity in early childhood that have direct practical relevance to supporting healthy weight gain in this critical period of life. The first fundamental issue for child health nursing practice is the definition of normal growth in early childhood, which leads directly into an examination of the assessment of at-risk growth patterns and other risk factors for later childhood (and adult) obesity. Appropriate feeding practices are fundamental to healthy weight gain in early childhood and these recommendations are reviewed as well as the importance of active play, motor skill development and reduced television viewing time. Patterns for all human behaviors are highly influenced by environments, and this is most true in the early childhood years. Thus, the many preschool settings outside the home environment are also examined as opportunities for implementing the policies and practices needed to promote healthy eating and active play.

Growth and excess weight assessment in early childhood

Historically, good health and nutrition in childhood have been defined by the capacity to support normal growth. Existing national and international standards have defined normal growth based on the weight and length gain observed in apparently "healthy" children. This has led in practice to support the notion that "bigger is better". This is a reasonable approach if the objective is to enhance survival in infancy and early childhood in areas where malnutrition and infection in synergy claim the lives of infants and young children. However, it is certainly not the case in countries where deaths of young children are rare and the concern has shifted to the prevention of obesity and related burden of chronic disease.[1] Moreover, there is also mounting evidence that exposure to undernutrition during early life (i.e. in utero and the first two years of life) may have long-term consequences for adult body composition and health if there is a mismatch between early nutritional deprivation and later nutritional conditions that may support rapid weight gain in childhood.[2-4] Thus, the definition of "normal" growth is of paramount importance to secure normal health and nutrition of both individuals and populations in developed and developing countries.

Growth references and standards to define growth in early childhood

The reference/standards used to assess growth are fundamental for both clinical practice and to establish public health recommendations. Normative gender and age specific data of weight, height, weight/height, and BMI have been used as indicators of nutritional adequacy in infancy, childhood and adolescence.

Most of the available growth charts are based on the observed growth for a normal reference population rather than recommended growth based on health outcomes throughout the life course. Until 2006, the growth charts most commonly used were based on the USA National Center for Health Statistics (NCHS) The NCHS growth reference, which originally served as the basis for the WHO international growth standards for infants aged 0–36 months, was derived from children growing in an affluent rural society in the town of Yellow Springs, Ohio.[2] However, these references had major flaws because they were derived from a non-representative sample of the population and the infants included were predominantly formula fed and received energy-dense complementary foods. Thus, the NCHS distributions of normal weight-for-age and weight-for-length are skewed towards higher values, relative to those observed in predominantly breastfed infants and this may have been a contributory factor

to the increase in childhood obesity, since normal-sized children may have been considered underweight and prescribed additional energy.

Aware of these limitations, in 2006 the WHO launched the Multi-country (Brazil, Norway, India, Ghana, USA and Oman) Growth Reference Standard (MGRS). The MGRS was developed based on the growth of infants and children from diverse geographical regions, whose mothers were non-smokers of middle to high income so that environmental conditions were not restrictive for growth, and care givers followed the established WHO feeding recommendations (i.e. infants were predominantly breastfed for 4–6 months and fed appropriate complementary foods after weaning).[3] The new international growth reference provides a scientifically reliable descriptor of physiologic growth and a powerful tool for advocacy in support of good health and nutrition. Most importantly, this reference is based on the growth of the breastfed infant as the normative standard.

Definitions of overweight and obesity in children

In children, there is a lack of consistency in the use of the terms "overweight" and "obesity". All recommendations take into account two levels of excess weight, but use of different definitions and terminology may lead to confusion in interpreting results and comparing prevalence across populations. This is further complicated by the lack of evidence on the most appropriate anthropometric indices and cut-off points that best predict long-term adverse health outcomes. BMI has been used to define categories of excess weight so that there is concordance with adult assessment, although for children the definitions are age and sex specific. The 2000 CDC growth charts provide BMI-for-age curves for the US population over 2 years of age[4] and define children with a BMI ≥ 95th percentile as "overweight" and children with BMI between the 85th and the 95th percentile as "at risk of overweight".[5] The WHO growth standards for 0–5-year-olds in combination with the new WHO reference for 5–18-year-olds provide an international reference from birth to 18 years.[6] The terminology for body size categories (thinness, normal weight, overweight, obesity) using the WHO and International Obesity Task Force charts ensures concordance between adults and children because the childhood BMI curves were anchored at age 18 years to the agreed adult cut-off points (18.5, 25, 30 kg/m² for thinness, overweight and obesity respectively).[7,8]

Developmental origins of obesity

The relationship between low birth weight and the later occurrence of obesity and central obesity has been documented in a number of epidemiological studies conducted mostly in industrialized countries,[9,10] and in follow-up studies of historic cohorts from transitional countries.[11] In most developing regions low birth weight, and underweight and stunting in young children, coexists with overweight and obesity in older children, adolescents and the adult population;[12] thus, it is likely that the effect of low birth weight in these countries will be higher than that of developed countries. Analyses of the five existing cohort studies from developing countries (India, Guatemala, South Africa, Brazil and the Philippines) have reported that in India, Guatemala and Brazil, birth weight was positively associated with BMI at age 25–30, yet the associations were stronger for lean mass than for fat mass.[11]

Macrosomia or high birth weight (greater than 4,000 g) is also a potential problem with long-term consequences. Excessive intrauterine growth in this case is driven by elevated maternal glucose and insulin levels due to gestational diabetes and/or maternal overweight.[13] Several studies of macrosomic children have shown that high birth weight is a risk factor for later development of obesity and diabetes.[14–17]

The importance of the existence and timing of a period of rapid childhood growth in potentiating the relationship between fetal undernutrition and later obesity is a matter of current debate,[18,19] partly because of the rapid changes in the environment associated with progressive increase in the prevalence of obesity. Older cohorts have subtle changes. The systematic review by Monteiro and Victora[20] identified 16 studies that presented data on the role of rapid childhood growth as a possible determinant of obesity in adulthood, 13 of which reported significant associations, although they also noted the significant lack of standardization between studies making interpretation difficult. The degree to which rapid infant growth represents a risk may depend on whether it occurs in the context of recovery from fetal growth restriction and

results in normalization of body weight and length, or whether excess growth is predominantly ponderal with constrained linear gain, thus leading to excess weight for length.[11,21]

The effect of rapid weight gain in early life may also depend on prenatal and postnatal characteristics such as exposure to tobacco *in utero*, maternal overweight or obesity, the type of early feeding, or the amount of fat in the diet.[22,23] Overall, the effect of rapid infant weight gain on later development of overweight seems to be relevant. In relatively contemporary cohorts of children from USA it has been reported that the population risk for overweight at 4 or 7 years attributable to infant weight gain (0 to 4–6 months) in the highest quintile is around 20%.[24,25] Another study in a non-contemporary cohort of African-Americans reported that almost 30% of the risk of overweight at 20 years was due to a rapid weight gain (over one standard deviation above the mean value) from 0 to 4 months of age.[26] Given the actual increase in obesity among children and adults, is likely that the attributable risk might even be higher.

The age at adiposity rebound (age at which the BMI increases after its nadir in early childhood) is another period in which childhood growth seems to be critical for later obesity.[27] On average, this normally happens between the ages of 5 and 7 but it has been shown that an earlier adiposity rebound is associated with increased fatness later in life.[28] For example, one study reported that adults who had their adiposity rebound by 4.8 years had a 6 times higher risk of having a BMI > 27 kg/m² than adults who had their adiposity rebound after 6.2 years.[29] There remains some uncertainty, however, over whether the apparent negative effect of an early adiposity rebound is independent of early life BMI or BMI percentile crossing.[30,31]

Energy intakes and feeding patterns in young children

Recommended energy intakes

Energy recommendations for infants and children published by FAO/WHO/UNU in 2004 are based on actual measurements and estimates of total daily energy expenditure, either by the doubly labeled water method or estimates based on heart rate monitoring during active periods coupled to individual calibrations of oxygen consumption[32] The energy needs for tissue deposition related to growth in case of infants, children and adolescents were added to the estimate of daily energy expenditure. The recommendations also include a need for physical activity to maintain fitness and health, and to reduce the risk of developing obesity and diseases associated with sedentary lifestyles. Moreover, different requirements are given for populations with lifestyles that involve different levels of habitual physical activity, starting at 6 years of age.

In the case of infants, the new recommendations are based on breastfed infants rather than those who are formula fed; for the first year of life the mean values for the former are 5–10% lower than figures for formula-fed babies. The present recommendations based on expenditure are also substantially lower for children up to age 10 years in comparison to those derived on observed food intake as used in 1985 by FAO/WHO/UNU.

Breastfeeding

The new recommendations will serve to strongly support exclusive breastfeeding since, as energy needs drop, the sufficiency of breast milk energy supply is prolonged. Recent meta-analyses of published observational studies have suggested that breastfeeding is associated with a lower prevalence of obesity[33] and BMI later in life[34] in a dose-dependent way (i.e. longer duration of breastfeeding is associated with lower risk of overweight).[35] The mechanisms by which breastfeeding would decrease the risk of obesity could be broadly summarized in three categories: nutritional components of milk; growth pattern of breastfed babies; and behavioral. There is some concern that the association between breastfeeding and obesity may not be causal but confounded by unmeasured factors,[36,37] and the only available randomized controlled trial based on an intervention to promote exclusive and prolonged breastfeeding showed that the intervention increased duration and exclusivity of breastfeeding but did not reduce adiposity at age 6.5 years.[38]

Other early life-risk factors for obesity

A number of other potential early life predictors of obesity have been identified in studies conducted mainly in developed countries. The most consistent associations point to a role of maternal overweight, maternal feeding behaviors, low physical activity levels, low socio-economic status, and obesogenic environments.[39]

Physical activity and inactivity in young children

Physical activity

Physical activity in childhood years has been identified as a key factor in the prevention and control of overweight and obesity.[40–48] Benefits include improvement in children's general health status, their ability to maintain normal growth and development, and delay prevent the onset of obesity.[49,50] Evidence shows that patterns of physical activity established early can carry over into adulthood[49,51] and a positive relationship has been shown between being physically active during preschool years and lower weight gain by early adolescence,[41] confirming the importance of the early years. Additional benefits of physical activity during childhood are enhanced psychological well-being, self-esteem, moral and social development, developing an active lifestyle and decreasing the prevalence of chronic disease factors.[52]

Physical activity for children may be planned (structured) or incidental (unstructured). The activity of day-to-day living can be described as unstructured, whereas structured activities include more formal sporting games and activities.[49,50,53] Although young children have a natural tendency to be somewhat physically active, there is evidence to show that over recent decades, children have become less so.[50–52]

Physical activity is important for maintaining normal growth and development during childhood and adolescence[50] and the 2005 US national physical activity guidelines for preschool-aged children recommended at least two hours of physical activity a day, half in structured physical activity and half in unstructured, free play settings.[54]

Play is the "spontaneous activity in which children engage to amuse and occupy themselves" and is critically important for preschool children.[55] Movement and activity can satisfy a child's curiosity, promote good feelings and happiness, enhance problem-solving skills and assist in developing lifelong attitudes towards physical activity.[56] Children are also able to gain success through activity challenges and enhance social interaction through games and activities. Learning and mastering the fundamental motor skills

(FMS) in early childhood, has a positive effect on involvement in physical activity such as organized sports later in life.[57] And a positive reinforcer for increasing participation in physical activity has been shown to be successful motor performance.[58]

To ensure that young children participate sufficiently, physical activities need to be well integrated into children's daily routines.[59] The activities should promote the necessary skills to facilitate enjoyment and enable children to develop an appreciation of physical movement, which will most likely track through adolescence and into adulthood. One way to ensure that children in day care settings engage in adequate physical activity is to add structured play to their daily program as well as providing more time for free play in environments which facilitate physical activity.[60]

Physical inactivity

The development of childhood obesity is complicated and multi-factorial, however, screen time has been identified as an independent modifiable risk factor for the development of childhood obesity,[61–65] with high amounts of screen time associated with less physical activity and higher child BMI.[61,63–65]

The American Academy of Pediatrics recommends no television viewing for children under the age of 2 years, and that children older than 2 years watch no more than 1–2 hours of TV and video per day.[66,67] It has been shown that preschoolers who watch more than 3 hours of TV/day are 50% more likely to become obese than children who watch <2 hours/day[68] and 3 main mechanisms by which TV impacts weight gain have been proposed:[69]

1. TV displaces time spent doing physical activity.
2. TV promotes in-between meal snacking, thus increasing daily caloric intake.
3. TV food advertising influences children's food choice, attitudes and beliefs.

A recent study of children in the USA has shown that two thirds of the children aged under 2 years, and over 80% of 3–4-year-olds watched television on a typical day. On that typical day, the average time spent watching television by children of all ages was 1 hour and 19 minutes. In addition, approximately one third of the children watched videos or DVDs on a typical day, for an average of 1 hour and 18 minutes.[70] About one fifth of 0–2-year-olds and more than one third of the 3–4-year-olds and the 5–6-year-olds also had a television in their bedroom, which was related to higher levels of viewing, most notably for the youngest age group.[70]

Environments and early childhood settings

Child care settings

The ecological model has been utilized to examine the range of influences that alter the ability of children to maintain a healthy weight.[71] In addition to the home, child care settings are recognized as important environments that can have an impact on children's weight through the nutritional quality of the foods provided and children's access to opportunities for physical activity while in day care.

The proportion of mothers returning to the workforce before their children reach school age is increasing and children are going into child care at younger ages. Therefore, child care arrangements (either outside their own homes or by others within their homes) are becoming increasingly important settings for child development.

Early childhood settings and services vary widely around the world as shown in a comprehensive review of child care services across 29 countries in 1993.[72] Although the terminology varies, common types of formal care can be summarized. Day care centers (also sometimes known as crèche or nursery) provide up to a full day of care for groups of children in a non-residential setting such as a business, church or school. Family day care (also known as family- or home-based care) provides a full day of care for small groups of children (usually up to six) in the care provider's home, or a large family of group child care homes usually have two care providers caring for seven to twelve children in a provider's home. Home care is typically provided by a non-relative such as a nanny or au pair in the family home and informal (or "kith and kin") care is provided by a relative, neighbor, friend or babysitter.[72,73]

Parents, therefore, choose from a range of child care options and some countries have day care systems dominated by family day care, whereas other countries emphasize center-based care. Children can enter day care from six weeks of age and can be in care for up to 40 hours per week until they reach school age.

A study in the USA found that 18% of preschool children were not in child care, 16% were in care for 1 to 14 hours per week, 25% for 15 to 34 hours per week and 41% for 35 hours or more per week.[74] Across the USA, approximately 80% of children aged under 5 years who had working mothers were found to be in a child care arrangement (both formal and informal) for about 40 hours per week.[73]

Similarly, in Australia, the predominant types of formal care are center-based long day care and family day care. A recent study has shown that the use of formal child care has increased from about 15% in 1966 to about 23% in 2005. In 2005 the usage of formal care increased from 7% for children up to 12 months, to 31% at the age of 1 year, and 53% for children aged up to 3 years.[75] Of all children aged 0–12 in the survey who used formal care, about half were in care for 10 hours or less and about 30% were in care for 10 to 20 hours.

The increased participation of women in the labor force and the increased number of children with both parents working is viewed as a major change in family life over the last thirty years.[76] In recent years there has been a paradigm shift from a view that child care is an exclusively family responsibility to acceptance of a shared responsibility and recognition that a significant proportion of the child raising process is now a public concern. This paradigm shift is seen as the legitimization of out-of-home child socialization. It necessitates an effectively integrated early childhood education and care system and the concept of extra-familial care and education as shared family and state responsibility.[72]

Child care and obesity risk

A study on the effect of maternal employment on childhood obesity demonstrated that a 10-hour increase in average hours worked per week over a child's lifetime increased the probability of childhood obesity by 1 percentage point[77] Although the mechanisms are unclear, it appears that the relationship is dependent more on the intensity of work rather than working per se. Women who work less intensive hours may also have time to participate in active play with their child, prepare nutritious meals, walk to/from school with their child and even have higher breastfeeding rates and duration—all factors thought to be related to a child's risk of being overweight or obese.[76]

Despite the increasing usage of formal care for young children, insufficient attention has been paid to the relationship between child care and childhood obesity.[71,73] The nutrition and physical activity environments in child care settings have not been extensively studied, and the little evidence that does exist indicates that the meals provided are often nutritionally inadequate and the level of physical activity by children in day care may also be insufficient.

The food environments in early childhood settings

It has been suggested that young children attending day care may have less adult modeling and encouragement for eating healthier foods, as well as less control on portion sizes, than children receiving individual attention.[78] It is also known that as children spend more time in child care, maternal influence on children's diet diminishes and other care givers play a more critical role in children's nutrition.[79] This represents a missed opportunity to promote healthy weight in young children.

In the USA, between 1977 and 1998 the diet of preschool children (3–5 years) increased in the consumption of added sugars, juices and total energy.[80] In the case of infants and toddlers (4–24 months) energy intakes were higher than recommended, up to a third of children ate no vegetables or fruit on the day of the dietary recall, and, for children 15 to 18 months, the vegetable most commonly eaten was French fries.[81]

Energy, macronutrient and micronutrient contents of the diets provided at day cares should be based on daily recommendations for each age and the FAO 2004 energy recommendations,[32] depending on the amount of waking hours that children expend in the day care. However, the acceptability of the food offered at the day cares should be considered when trying to achieve these dietary recommendations. Also, attention should be paid to feeding practices of child care providers because they have a direct impact on the development of eating behaviors of preschool children[82] which, in turn, may be related to later obesity.[83]

For children below 6 months, exclusive breastfeeding should be recommended followed by mixed breastfeeding until at least 12 months.[84] Day care centers should ensure that working mothers have a supportive breastfeeding environment (e.g. availability of breast pumps at the centers, a place for mothers to breastfeed, adequate breast milk storage). Appropriate content of vitamins and minerals of weaning foods provided at the day care should be ensured without exceeding energy, protein and fat recommendations. Examples of interventions conducted in early childhood settings are provided in Chapter 8.

The physical activity environments in early childhood settings

Environments are a major contributing factor to children's physical activity participation and facilities, equipment and the amount and type of physical space all have the potential to influence a child's engagement in physical activity.[53,59] In early childhood settings it is important that children have access to sufficient indoor and outdoor space to move about freely, enabling them to use their bodies actively. Children's physical activity participation has been shown to increase with participation in outdoor activities.[85]

Children who spend significant time in day care and kindergarten settings may have their participation in physical activity limited or enhanced largely by the setting's inclusion of physical activity in the program. A reduction in children's free playtime between 1981 and 1997 has been associated with an increase in the amount of time children spend in structured settings such as school and day care.[86] Brown et al conducted a study on the amount of physical activity that American children participated in during preschool attendance. This study found that 80% of the children's time was spent on sedentary activities (e.g. transition, snack and nap time) and only 5% in moderate to vigorous physical activity.[87] This indicates a need to enhance opportunities for children to be active, which includes evaluating the amount of time allocated to free and structured physical activity/play in care settings. A recent study found that children in child care centers with supportive physical environments achieved higher participation in moderate to vigorous physical activity, spent less time in sedentary activities and had higher average physical activity levels when compared to less supportive centers.[88]

As so many young children attend child care, these settings can be a major influence in shaping children's physical activity participation and, therefore, contrib-

ute to combating the childhood obesity epidemic.[73,89] Early childhood staff who work in long day care settings have a unique opportunity to encourage and facilitate an active lifestyle among children. Engaging with these workers to develop solutions to overcoming barriers in care settings will be important before sustainable changes can be implemented.

Conclusions

The new WHO standards for growth have been a major step forward in creating credible reference standards for normal growth and definitions of obesity, overweight and thinness. This will strengthen the emerging evidence on the growth-related risk factors for future obesity. There are also continuing improvements in the standards and recommendations for energy intake, physical activity and sedentary behaviors for early childhood. The existing patterns of breastfeeding, dietary intake, active play and television viewing in preschool children suggest that there are major opportunities for shifting towards healthier and less obesogenic patterns of these behaviors. While the home environment is paramount for promoting these healthy behaviors, the increasing use of child care provides an excellent opportunity for those settings to take a leading role to model healthy eating and active play in this critically important age group.

References

1 Popkin BM, Gordon-Larsen P: The nutrition transition: worldwide obesity dynamics and their determinants. *Int J Obes Relat Metab Disord* 2004; **28**(Suppl. 3):S2–S9.

2 Working Group on Infant Growth: An evaluation of infant growth: the use and interpretation of anthropometry in infants. *WHO Bull World Health Organ* 1995; **73**(2): 165–174.

3 de Onis M, Garza C, Victora CG, Onyango AW, Frongillo EA, Martines J: The WHO Multicentre Growth Reference Study: planning, study design, and methodology. *Food Nutr Bull* 2004; **25**(1 Suppl.):S15–S26.

4 Kuczmarski RJ, Ogden CL, Grummer-Strawn LM et al: CDC growth charts: United States. *Adv Data* 2000; **8**(314):1–27.

5 Must A, Dallal GE, Dietz WH: Reference data for obesity: 85th and 95th percentiles of body mass index (wt/ht2) and triceps skinfold thickness. *Am J Clin Nutr* 1991; **53**(4): 839–846.

6 World Health Organization: The WHO Child Growth Standards; Available from: www.who.int/childgrowth/standards/en/ (accessed 5 October 2007).

7 Cole TJ, Bellizzi MC, Flegal KM, Dietz WH: Establishing a standard definition for child overweight and obesity worldwide: international survey. *BMJ* 2000; **320**(7244): 1240–1243.

8 Cole TJ, Flegal KM, Nicholls D, Jackson AA: Body mass index cut offs to define thinness in children and adolescents: international survey. *BMJ* 2007; **335**(7612):194–202.

9 Oken E, Gillman MW: Fetal origins of obesity. *Obes Res* 2003; **11**(4):496–506.

10 Rogers I: The influence of birthweight and intrauterine environment on adiposity and fat distribution in later life. *Int J Obes Relat Metab Disord* 2003; **27**(7):755–777.

11 Victora CG, Adair L, Fall C et al: Maternal and child undernutrition: consequences for adult health and human capital. *Lancet* 2008; **371**(9609):340–357.

12 Lobstein T, Baur L, Uauy R: Obesity in children and young people: a crisis in public health. *Obes Rev* 2004; **5**(Suppl. 1): 4–104.

13 Leguizamon G, von Stecher F: Third trimester glycemic profiles and fetal growth. *Curr Diab Rep* 2003; **3**(4):323–326.

14 Das UG, Sysyn GD: Abnormal fetal growth: intrauterine growth retardation, small for gestational age, large for gestational age. *Pediatr Clin North Am* 2004; **51**(3):639–654, viii.

15 Yu Z, Sun JQ, Haas JD, Gu Y, Li Z, Lin X: Macrosomia is associated with high weight-for-height in children aged 1–3 years in Shanghai, China. *Int J Obes (Lond)* 2008; **32**(1): 55–60.

16 Moschonis G, Grammatikaki E, Manios Y: Perinatal predictors of overweight at infancy and preschool childhood: the GENESIS study. *Int J Obes (Lond)* 2008; **32**(1):39–47.

17 Hediger ML, Overpeck MD, McGlynn A, Kuczmarski RJ, Maurer KR, Davis WW: Growth and fatness at three to six years of age of children born small- or large-for-gestational age. *Pediatrics* 1999; **104**(3):e33.

18 Lucas A, Fewtrell MS, Cole TJ: Fetal origins of adult disease-the hypothesis revisited. *BMJ* 1999; **319**(7204):245–249.

19 Gillman MW: The first months of life: a critical period for development of obesity. *Am J Clin Nutr* 2008; **87**(6): 1587–1589.

20 Monteiro PO, Victora CG: Rapid growth in infancy and childhood and obesity in later life—a systematic review. *Obes Rev* 2005; **6**(2):143–154.

21 Corvalan C, Gregory CO, Ramirez-Zea M, Martorell R, Stein AD: Size at birth, infant, early and later childhood growth and adult body composition: a prospective study in a stunted population. *Int J Epidemiol* 2007; **36**(3):550–557.

22 Karaolis-Danckert N, Buyken AE, Kulig M et al: How pre- and postnatal risk factors modify the effect of rapid weight gain in infancy and early childhood on subsequent fat mass development: results from the Multicenter Allergy Study 90. *Am J Clin Nutr* 2008; **87**(5):1356–1364.

23 Karaolis-Danckert N, Gunther AL, Kroke A, Hornberg C, Buyken AE: How early dietary factors modify the effect of rapid weight gain in infancy on subsequent body-composition development in term children whose birth

weight was appropriate for gestational age. *Am J Clin Nutr* 2007; **86**(6):1700–1708.

24 Dennison BA, Edmunds LS, Stratton HH, Pruzek RM: Rapid infant weight gain predicts childhood overweight. *Obesity* (Silver Spring) 2006; **14**(3):491–499.

25 Stettler N, Zemel BS, Kumanyika S, Stallings VA: Infant weight gain and childhood overweight status in a multi-center, cohort study. *Pediatrics* 2002; **109**(2):194–199.

26 Stettler N, Kumanyika SK, Katz SH, Zemel BS, Stallings VA: Rapid weight gain during infancy and obesity in young adulthood in a cohort of African Americans. *Am J Clin Nutr* 2003; **77**(6):1374–1378.

27 Rolland-Cachera MF, Deheeger M, Bellisle F, Sempe M, Guilloud-Bataille M, Patois E: Adiposity rebound in children: a simple indicator for predicting obesity. *Am J Clin Nutr* 1984; **39**(1):129–135.

28 Rolland-Cachera MF, Deheeger M, Maillot M, Bellisle F: Early adiposity rebound: causes and consequences for obesity in children and adults. *Int J Obes* 2006; **30**:S11–S17.

29 Whitaker RC, Pepe MS, Wright JA, Seidel KD, Dietz WH: Early adiposity rebound and the risk of adult obesity. *Pediatrics* 1998; **101**(3):E5.

30 Cole TJ: Children grow and horses race: is the adiposity rebound a critical period for later obesity? *BMC Pediatr* 2004; **4**:6.

31 Freedman DS, Kettel Khan L, Serdula MK, Srinivasan SR, Berenson GS: BMI rebound, childhood height and obesity among adults: the Bogalusa Heart Study. *Int J Obes Relat Metab Disord* 2001; **25**(4):543–549.

32 Food and Agricultural Organization: Human Energy Requirements Report of a Joint Expert Consultation, Rome, 2004.

33 Owen CG, Martin RM, Whincup PH, Smith GD, Cook DG: Effect of infant feeding on the risk of obesity across the life course: a quantitative review of published evidence. *Pediatrics* 2005; **115**(5):1367–1377.

34 Owen CG, Martin RM, Whincup PH, Davey-Smith G, Gillman MW, Cook DG: The effect of breastfeeding on mean body mass index throughout life: a quantitative review of published and unpublished observational evidence. *Am J Clin Nutr* 2005; **82**(6):1298–1307.

35 Harder T, Bergmann R, Kallischnigg G, Plagemann A: Duration of breastfeeding and risk of overweight: a meta-analysis. *Am J Epidemiol* 2005; **162**(5):397–403.

36 Toschke AM, Martin RM, von Kries R, Wells J, Smith GD, Ness AR: Infant feeding method and obesity: body mass index and dual-energy X-ray absorptiometry measurements at 9–10 y of age from the Avon Longitudinal Study of Parents and Children (ALSPAC). *Am J Clin Nutr* 2007; **85**(6): 1578–1585.

37 Stettler N: Nature and strength of epidemiological evidence for origins of childhood and adulthood obesity in the first year of life. *Int J Obes (Lond)* 2007; **31**(7):1035–1043.

38 Kramer MS, Matush L, Vanilovich I et al: Effects of prolonged and exclusive breastfeeding on child height, weight, adiposity, and blood pressure at age 6.5 y: evidence from a

large randomized trial. *Am J Clin Nutr* 2007; **86**(6): 1717–1721.

39 Parsons TJ, Power C, Logan S, Summerbell CD: Childhood predictors of adult obesity: a systematic review. *Int J Obes Relat Metab Disord* 1999; **23**(Suppl. 8):S1–S107.

40 Rees R, Kavanagh J, Harden J et al: Young people and physical activity: a systematic review matching their views to effective interventions. *Health Educ Res* 2006; **21**(6):806–825.

41 Moore LL, Nguyen US, Rothman KJ, Cupples LA, Ellison RC: Preschool physical activity level and change in body fatness in young children. The Framingham children's study. *Am J Epidemiol* 1995; **142**(9):982–988.

42 World Health Organization: A Guide for Population-Based Approaches to Increasing Levels of Physical Activity: Implementation of the WHO Global Strategy on Deit, Physical Activity and Health. Geneva: WHO, 2007.

43 Reilly JJ, Kelly L, Montgomery C et al: Physical activity to prevent obesity in young children: cluster randomised controlled trial. *BMJ* 2006; **333**(7577):1041.

44 Steinbeck K: Obesity in children: the importance of physical activity. *Aust J Nutr Diet* 2001; **58**(1):S28–S32.

45 Malina RM: Adherence to physical activity from childhood to adulthood: a perspective from tracking studies. *Quest* 2001; **53**(3):346–355.

46 Lobstein T, Baur L, Uauy R: Obesity in children and young people: a crisis in public health. *Obes Rev* 2004; **5**(Suppl. 1):4–104.

47 Magarey A, Daniels LA, Boulton TJ: Prevalence of overweight and obesity in Australian children and adolescents: reassessment of 1985 and 1995 data against new standard international definitions. *Med J Aust* 2001; **174**(11): 561–564.

48 Epstein LH, Goldfield GS: Physical activity in the treatment of childhood overweight and obesity: current evidence and research issues. *Med Sci Sports Exerc* 1999; **31**(11): S553–S559.

49 Sallis JF, Prochaska JJ, Taylor WC: A review of correlates of physical activity of children and adolescents. *Med Sci Sports Exerc* 2000; **32**(5):963–975.

50 Ziviani J, Macdonald D, Jenkins D, Rodger S, Batch J, Cerin E: Physical activity of young children. *Physical & Occup Therapy in Pediatrics* 2006; **26**(1):4–14.

51 Boreham C, Riddoch C: The physical activity, fitness and health of children. *J Sports Sci* 2001; **19**:915–929.

52 Cavill N: Health enhancing physical activity for young people: statement of the United Kingdom Expert Consensus Conference. *Pediatr Exerc Sci* 2001; **13**(1):12.

53 Steinbeck KS: The importance of physical activity in the prevention of overweight and obesity in childhood: a review and an opinion. *Obes Rev* 2001; **2**(2):117–130.

54 National Association for Sport & Physical Education: Active Start: A Statement of Physical Activity Guidelines for Children Birth to Five Years. Reston, Va: National Association for Sport & Physical Education, 2002.

55 Burdette HL, Whitaker RC: Resurrecting free play in young children: looking beyond fitness and fatness to attention, affiliation, and affect. *Arch Pediatr Adolesc Med* 2005; **159**(1):46–50.

56 Eastman W: Active living physical activities for infants, toddlers and preschoolers. *Early Child Educ J* 1997; **24**(3): 161–164.

57 Christiansen CH, Baum CM: Occupational Therapy Performance, Participation, and Well-being. Thorofare, NJ: SLACK Incorporated, 2005.

58 Cech D, Martin S: Functional Movement Development Across the Life Span, 2nd edn. Philadelphia, USA: W.B. Saunders Company, 2002.

59 Goran MI, Reynolds KD, Lindquist CH: Role of physical activity in the prevention of obesity in children. *Int J Obes Relat Metab Disord* 1999; **23**(Suppl. 3):S18–S33.

60 Dowda M, Pate RR, Trost SG, Almeida MJ, Sirard JR: Influences of preschool policies and practices on children's physical activity. *J Community Health* 2004; **29**(3): 183–196.

61 Andersen RE, Crespo C, Bartlett S, Cheskin L, Pratt M: Relationship of physical activity and television watching with body weight and level of fatness among children: results from the their National Health and Nutrition Examination Survey. *J Am Med Assoc* 1998; **279**(12):938–942.

62 Dixon HG, Scully ML, Wakefield MA, White VM, Crawford DA: The effects of television advertisements for junk food versus nutritious food on children's food attitudes and preferences. *Soc Sci Med* 2007; **65**(7):1311–1323.

63 Eisenmann JC, Bartee RT, Wang MQ: Physical activity, TV viewing, and weight in U.S. youth: 1999 Youth Risk Behavior Survey. *Obes Res* 2002; **10**(5):379–385.

64 Lowry R, Wechsler H, Galuska DA, Fulton JE, Kann L: Television viewing and its associations with overweight, sedentary lifestyle, and insufficient consumption of fruits and vegetables among US high school students: differences by race, ethnicity, and gender. *J Sch Health* 2002; **72**(10): 413–421.

65 Wake M, Hesketh K, Waters E: Television, computer use and body mass index in Australian primary school children. *J Paediatr Child Health* 2003; **39**(2):130–134.

66 Committee on Public Education: Children, adolescents, and television. *Pediatrics* 2001; **107**(2):423–426.

67 Zimmerman FJ, Christakis DA: Children's television viewing and cognitive outcomes: a longitudinal analysis of national data. *Pediatr Adolesc Med* 2005; **159**(7):619–625.

68 Tremblay MS, Willms JD: Is the Canadian childhood obesity epidemic related to physical inactivity? *Int J Obes Relat Metab Disord* 2003; **27**(9):1100–1105.

69 Bryant MJ, Lucove JC, Evenson KR, Marshall S: Measurement of television viewing in children and adolescents: a systematic review. *Obes Rev* 2007; **8**(3):197–209.

70 Vandewater EA, Rideout VJ, Wartella EA, Huang X, Lee JH, Shim MS: Digital childhood: electronic media and technology use among infants, toddlers, and preschoolers. *Pediatrics* 2007; **119**(5):e1006–e1015.

71 Story M, Kaphingst KM, Robinson-O'Brien R, Glanz K: Creating healthy food and eating environments: policy and

environmental approaches. *Annu Rev Public Health* 2008; **29**:253–272.

72 Cochran M: International Handbook of Child Care Policies and Programs, Greenwood Publishing Group, 1993.

73 Story M, Kaphingst KM, French S: The role of child care settings in obesity prevention. *Future Child* 2006; **16**(1): 143–168.

74 Capizzano J, Adams G: Hours that children under five spend in child care: variation across states. Washington: Urban Institute. Report No.: B-8, 2000.

75 Australian Bureau of Statistics: Australian Bureau of Statistics. Child Care Australia, 2005.

76 Anderson PM, Butcher KE: Childhood obesity: trends and potential causes. *Future Child* 2006; **16**(1):19–45.

77 Anderson PM, Butcher KF, Levine PB: Maternal employment and overweight children. *J Health Econ* 2003; **22**(3): 477–504.

78 Lumeng JC, Gannon K, Appugliese D, Cabral HJ, Zuckerman B: Preschool child care and risk of overweight in 6- to 12-year-old children. *Int J Obes (Lond)* 2005; **29**(1):60–66.

79 Gable S, Lutz S: Nutrition socialization experiences of children in the Head Start program. *J Am Diet Assoc* 2001; **101**(5):572–577.

80 Kranz S, Siega-Riz AM, Herring AH: Changes in diet quality of American preschoolers between 1977 and 1998. *Am J Public Health* 2004; **94**(9):1525–1530.

81 Fox MK, Pac S, Devaney B, Jankowski L: Feeding infants and toddlers study: what foods are infants and toddlers eating? *J Am Diet Assoc* 2004; **104**(1 Suppl. 1):s22–s30.

82 Hughes SO, Patrick H, Power TG, Fisher JO, Anderson CB, Nicklas TA: The impact of child care providers' feeding on children's food consumption. *J Dev Behav Pediatr* 2007; **28**(2):100–107.

83 Faith MS, Kerns J: Infant and child feeding practices and childhood overweight: the role of restriction. *Matern Child Nutr* 2005; **1**(3):164–168.

84 Kramer MS, Kakuma R: The optimal duration of exclusive breastfeeding: a systematic review. *Adv Exp Med Biol* 2004; **554**:63–77.

85 Klesges RC, Eck LH, Hanson CL, Haddock CK, Klesges LM: Effects of obesity, social interactions, and physical environment on physical activity in preschoolers. *Health Psychol* 1990; **9**(4):435–449.

86 Bellows L, Anderson J, Gould S, Auld G: Formative research and strategic development of a physical activity component to a social marketing campaign for obesity prevention in preschoolers. *J Community Health* 2008; **33**(3):169–178.

87 Brown WH, Pfeiffer KA, Mclver KL, Dowda M, Almeida MJCA, Pate RR: Assessing preschool children's physical activity: the Observational System for Recording Physical Activity in Children-Preschool Version. *Res Q Exerc Sport* 2006; **77**(2):167–176.

88 Bower J, Hales D, Tate D, Rubin D, Benjamin S, Ward D: The childcare environment and children's physical activity. *Am J Prev Med* 2008; **34**(1):23–29.

89 Benjamin SE, Ammerman A, Sommers J et al: Self-assessment for Child Care (NAP SACC): Results from a pilot intervention. *J Nutr Educ Behav* 2007; **39**(3):142–149.

CHAPTER 30

Working with schools

Goof Buijs[1] and *Sue Bowker*[2]
[1] Schools for Health in Europe Network, Netherlands Institute for Health Promotion, Woerden, The Netherlands
[2] Health Improvement Division, Department of Public Health and Health Professionals, Welsh Assembly Government, Cardiff, UK

Summary and recommendations for research and practice

- Dealing with obesity in schools includes promoting healthy eating, physical activity and mental health.
- School-based interventions have proven moderately effective in preventing obesity, with strong evidence where a whole school approach has been adopted.
- There is evidence to support the use of multi-faceted, school-based interventions to reduce obesity and overweight in schoolchildren, particularly girls.
- Interventions include nutrition education, physical activity promotion, reduction in sedentary behavior, behavioral therapy, teacher training, curricular material and modification of school meals and tuck shops.
- The health promoting school approach offers the most suitable framework for introducing and implementing obesity-prevention programs in schools.
- Action in schools on preventing obesity should be seen as part of a wider intervention framework in the school community and actively involving parents.
- School-based programs on preventing obesity that include active participation of students are promising.
- Better use should be made of countries' experiences on developing and implementing school-based programs on preventing overweight.

Preventing Childhood Obesity. Edited by
E. Waters, B.A. Swinburn, J.C. Seidell and R. Uauy.
© 2010 Blackwell Publishing.

Introduction

In Europe, close to one in four school children is overweight, with numbers rapidly increasing. Similar trends are observed worldwide. There is a growing concern about the rising prevalence rates of obesity among the general population, and specifically for our younger generation. The prevention of obesity is regarded as a major public health concern both at the international and at the national level; and an integrated approach is required to halt and reverse this trend. In most policy documents on obesity (such as the 2005 European Union Green Paper on the prevention of overweight[1] and the WHO paper on the challenge of obesity in the European region[2]) the focus is on children and young people. Schools are regarded as a key setting for health promoting interventions, and can contribute to the improvement of children's health by promoting healthy eating and physical activity, by providing a suitable environment which encourages their participation and by developing their skills.

This chapter describes the role schools can play in the prevention of obesity. Since the early 1990s, school health promotion has strongly evolved. Several reviews have demonstrated the effectiveness of this approach. It is now also clear that when dealing with the prevention of obesity in schools, it is not only the promotion of healthy eating and physical activity that should be included, but also aspects of mental health promotion (such as self-esteem, body image, dieting, eating disorders). But schools cannot, and do not have to, do it all on their own, since they are part of a broader community. The health-promoting school approach offers a rich body of evidence indicating that healthy students learn better and that improving knowledge, competencies and health status of children will improve learning outcomes.[3] Some successful and promising examples of dealing with obesity prevention via the school setting are described here.

So far, there is a lack of long-term evidence of effective and comprehensive approaches for the issue of obesity prevention in the school setting. A recent review on school-based obesity interventions by Shaya[4] concluded that no persistence of positive results in reducing obesity in school-age children has been observed. However, the review by Stewart-Brown[5] demonstrated that effective programs on school health promotion in general adopted whole-school approaches. It is clear that action against obesity should be part of overall strategies on promoting healthy lifestyles.

Dealing with healthy eating and physical activity in schools

The period that children spend in schools, usually from age 4 through to adolescence (16–18 years) is very important for their mental and physical development. The school historically and still today is seen by many as a site for health messages and activities.[3]

During the period of industrialization in the mid-nineteenth century, churches and charities in Europe started schools in order to support the social development of children and to care for them when both parents were working in cities. Rules for healthy living were taught at school, including proper hygiene measures, regular eating, enough physical activity and sufficient sleep. From the beginning of the twentieth century, health education in schools was introduced mainly by the medical profession because of the spread of infectious diseases and the role prevention could play. Medical care was provided through special school doctors and nurses, later also dental care, by specialized school dentists. Added to this was the introduction of school meals and physical education in schools, for example, in the UK, at the turn of the twentieth century.

During this time, in public health there was a shift from communicable to non-communicable diseases, and the recognition that good health is related to lifestyle. There has been a dramatic shift in morbidity and mortality, from infectious diseases to lifestyle-related causes such as cardiovascular diseases and cancers; and an increase in the prevalence of mental health problems. From the 1960s, this was recognized by a change in health education in schools, towards trying to influence health behaviors of children, mainly by providing information about risks related to specific diseases. However, it became clear that knowledge itself was insufficient to change an individual's lifestyle.

The last two decades have seen a shift towards the more holistic and ecological approach of health promotion. Based on the Ottawa charter,[6] it became clear that promoting health in a school setting should include teaching in the classroom (or "health education"), but also take the school environment and ethos into account, as well as considering links with the wider community. The charter states that health promotion is a process concerned with enabling people to gain more control over their own health and over their environment. This multi-faceted approach has strongly influenced the health-promoting schools concept, which has implied a shift in dominant paradigms over the years. This in turn had a great impact on the introduction of new health promotion programs and interventions for schools on healthy eating and physical activity (see Box 30.1).

Eating habits and diet have a significant influence on the health and well-being of children. More specifically, the overall health and nutrition of the child is recognized as one of the factors that influence academic performance, among other factors such as gender, ethnicity, quality of school and school experience, and socio-economic status.[4] Past studies have focused on the effects of a lack of nutrients or malnutrition on decreased school attendance and performance. A number of studies have demonstrated the positive effects of breakfast on school performance, but there are gaps in the literature about the long-term effects. A recent study in Canada[8] examined the impact of the quality of the whole diet, not just certain nutrients or meals on academic performance. Components of a high quality diet were defined as a high consumption of fruit and vegetables and a moderate fat intake. This was one of the first studies of this kind and it demonstrated that children with overall

Box 30.1 The Class Moves!

Many schools will support healthy eating messages by making fruit available at break times, by allowing pupils to have bottles of water on their desks, and by ensuring that any vending machines are filled with healthy options rather than drinks high in sugar and snacks high in saturated fat, salt and sugar.

Similarly, physical activity may be promoted in primary schools by encouraging activity with playground markings, and the inclusion of programs such as The Class Moves![7] It was developed in the Netherlands and has now been modified and translated for use in Wales and Scotland, The Class Moves! provides activities in the classroom for 4–12-year-olds, which can be undertaken at the desk as a short refreshing break from concentration.

between this connection; prospective studies suggested concentration increases for a brief time after physical activity or that there is an increased rate of learning per unit of school time, but that these effects are not sufficient to increase academic performance.[9]

Since obesity is now recognized as one of the major public health threats, increased attention has been given to developing integrated programs for schools. When dealing with the issue of obesity in a school setting the two issues of healthy eating and physical activity are usually addressed. The focus in these programs is on "energy balance". We now know that the most effective way is to integrate these issues into more coordinated programs that promote healthy lifestyles and that are incorporated into the health-promoting school approach.[5]

healthy diets performed better in school than children with unhealthy diets. Therefore, enhanced learning can be regarded as an additional benefit of a healthy diet in childhood. Key messages for school-based programs and policies are the importance of promoting dietary adequacy and variety, increased fruit and vegetable intake and a moderate consumption of dietary fat (see Box 30.1).[4]

Physical activity has a long tradition in schools, and the importance of having enough physical exercise and participating in sport has been acknowledged since the nineteenth century. Nowadays, physical education is included in the curriculum in primary and secondary schools, and attention is given throughout the school program for promoting physical activity and sports. The school offers a wide range of options for increasing physical activity for school-aged children, not only through the curriculum (physical education, integration with science and other subjects), but also by offering after-school programs and supporting initiatives for safe walking and cycling to school, as well as using the school as a community resource for physical activity. Schools often have a wide range of facilities available, including a gym and outside play area, which can also be used by the local community. Many studies have been carried out to demonstrate the link between physical activity and academic performance, although there is a shortage of prospective, controlled research in this connection. Retrospective studies found a weak or no relationship

Context of health promoting schools

The importance of education for health outcomes and of health for learning outcomes is well established.[10] When health education became a topic in schools in the Western world during the nineteenth century, the focus was narrow, relating to the individual, and covering moral and physical issues, including hygiene, the prevention of infectious diseases and incorporating strict warnings, for example, on the dangers of using alcohol. The methods used for health education were based on the transmission of knowledge.

The health promoting school approach incorporates the following principles:[3]

- Health has physical, mental, social and emotional dimensions.
- Providing information does not necessarily improve student's health outcomes.
- More active involvement of learners promotes behavioral change.
- Individual behavior is influenced by social factors such as peer pressure.
- Physical and socio-cultural environments, including the school environments, influence individual and community well-being.

In Europe, the health-promoting school approach was introduced in 1992 and has since developed, supported by the European Network for Health Promoting Schools (ENHPS) and now the Schools for Health in Europe network (SHE network).

Forty-three countries in the European region are now members of this network. The basic values underpinning the health promoting school approach are:

- equity
- active participation of students
- development of students' action competence
- importance of the social and physical environment of the school
- integration of health promotion policies as part of school development.

In 1997, the first European conference on school health promotion resulted in the identification of ten principles for school health promotion,[11] including democracy, equity, empowerment and partnership. In this network it was recognized that health and education are closely linked. Health status is related to access to schools as well as the ability to learn. There is a lot of evidence indicating that healthy students learn better and that improving the knowledge, competencies and health status of children will improve learning outcomes.[3] Also, schools that use the health promoting school approach improve at a faster rate than schools that do not use this approach. Effects have been demonstrated in improving learning environments, student concentration and performance, staff health and well-being, and better student achievements.[12]

Many studies have been carried out to investigate the effectiveness of the whole school approach. Overall, it can be concluded that the school health promotion programs that were effective in changing young people's health or health-related behavior were likely to be complex, multi-factorial and involve activity in more than one domain (curriculum, school environment and community). Also, programs that are intensive and implemented over a long period of time are more effective than programs of short duration and low intensity. Finally, school health promotion can be effective, particularly in improving mental health and in promoting healthy eating and physical activity.[5]

Recent evidence[3] makes clear that a whole school approach, which encourages and recognizes student participation and which addresses the building and maintenance of a caring school social environment, may be the most effective way to achieve both health and educational outcomes. Important influences that build health protective factors and reduce risk-taking behavior, are: the way a school is managed; how the school encourages student participation in shaping policies, practices and procedures; how teachers relate to and treat students; and how the school engages with its local community and parents in partnership work.

The supporting role of the school management is recognized as an important factor to start the process of introducing and implementing the health-promoting school approach.

Selection of good practice

Below is a selection of effective or promising initiatives to tackle obesity through the school setting based on the health-promoting school approach.

Food and fitness implementation plan (Wales)

The Food and Fitness Implementation Plan[13] in Wales was developed following the work of a Task Group and consultation with a wide audience including children and young people. Healthy schools were seen as a key component of work to improve nutrition and levels of physical activity. As part of their work, schools are required to consider these issues and to develop a whole school food and fitness policy. The plan looks specifically at the food and drink consumed throughout the whole school day, which has led to the development of a related strategy, called Appetite for Life.[14,15]

The importance of developing high quality physical education and practical cookery skills is also reinforced. Some examples of work here include the provision of a mobile cooking classroom—the Cooking Bus. The Cooking Bus visits primary schools in the most deprived areas of Wales and provides practical cooking lessons to pupils, as well as running a teacher training session and providing a session for parents of young children. This is supported by a change in the curriculum from September 2008, which makes it compulsory for pupils aged 7–13 to learn about food. They will have opportunities to practise, safely and hygienically, a broad range of practical food preparation and cooking tasks and to consider current healthy eating messages and nutritional needs. With regard to physical activity there is support via the Physical Education and School Sport program to develop the physical education curriculum, and this is complemented by out-of-school activities.[16] Food and fitness programs in the community, plus training of key workers and evaluation complete the plan.

Growing Through Adolescence (Scotland)

The WHO resource *Growing Through Adolescence*, developed by NHS Health Scotland,[17] combines nutrition and physical activity within the context of energy balance. This teacher training pack also makes the link with the issue of mental health. There is evidence that increasing numbers of young people are unhappy with their body size and shape and are more frequently becoming involved in dieting and unhealthy eating patterns. The resource explores the biological, social and emotional issues around health using a participative training approach and it aims to enable teachers to be confident with these issues in the classroom and in the health promoting school.

Planet Health (United States)

"Planet Health" is a school-based program on obesity prevention developed in the United States for middle school students (age group 11–14 years). Planet Health helps academic, physical education and health education teachers to guide middle school students in the following areas:

- learning about nutrition and physical activity while building skills in language arts, maths, science and social studies;
- understanding how health behaviors are interrelated;
- choosing healthy foods, increasing physical activity, and limiting TV and other screen time.

Gortmaker[18] demonstrated that Planet Health prevents obesity in girls, reduces television viewing in girls and boys, increases fruit and vegetable consumption in girls, and prevents disordered eating behaviors in girls. There is a similar program for upper elementary schools (ages 9–12 years) called "Eat well and keep moving".

Toolkit for overweight prevention in schools (the Netherlands)

In the Netherlands, a toolkit has been developed for schools on preventing overweight.[19] It provides an overview of available programs on healthy eating and physical activity for primary and secondary schools that have been developed at a national and regional level. It also describes strategies to deal with the issue as part of a health-promoting school approach. The toolkit has been developed for regional professionals as guidance for supporting their schools.

The nutrition-friendly school initiative (WHO)

In 2007, the WHO initiated the global nutrition-friendly school initiative, a school-based program to tackle undernutrition and overweight.[20] It is a standardized framework that serves as a tool for developing a school environment which promotes the nutritional well-being of school-aged children. The initiative is designed to be easily integrated into existing school programs or to be implemented on its own where there are no ongoing programs. The WHO initiative provides suggestions at both a national and a school level on how to implement the nutrition friendly school programs. At the school level, practical guidelines are given for developing a food and nutrition policy for schools, including: assembling a core action group; developing an action plan; evaluating the plan, and; incorporating changes into school policy. Box 30.2 shows the five elements of the nutrition friendly school initiative.

Conclusions

Since obesity is now recognized as one of the major public health threats, increased attention has been given to developing integrated programs for schools. We now know that the most effective way is to integrate these issues into more coordinated programs that promote healthy lifestyles, and that are incorporated into the health promoting school approach.

Although there has been a lack of effective and comprehensive school-wide approaches for obesity prevention in the school setting, some promising examples are now available. The review by Stewart-Brown[5] demonstrated that effective programs on obesity prevention adopted whole-school approaches.

Initiatives and new programs on preventing obesity in schools are currently developing in most countries throughout the world. But a more systematic approach on the international and national level is needed, making use of the knowledge that is already available within the health-promoting school approach. Exchange of experiences, research, evaluation and

Box 30.2 Elements of the WHO nutrition-friendly school initiative

1. Have a written school policy on nutrition.
   - Develop an action plan for implementing the initiative, including a monitoring and evaluation system.
2. Enhance awareness and capacity building of the school community.
   - includes parents, schools, community, local retailers and farmers
   - training for all school staff
   - media and publicity.
3. Develop a nutrition and health-promoting school curriculum.
   - life skills
   - education materials.
4. Create a supportive school environment.
   - school meals
   - breakfast clubs
   - vending machines policies
   - fruit, vegetable and milk subscriptions
   - access to water.
5. School nutrition and health services.
   - Inform parents about children's health and provide a referral health system for children needing attention.

implementation and sharing of good practice is needed.

The use of evidence of interventions on healthy eating and physical activity in the school setting and in the broader context of health promoting schools is much more developed compared to other settings. Experiences and lessons learned in the school setting can set an example for other settings, such as the local community and the workplace.

References

1 Commission of the European Communities: European Commission: Green Paper: Promoting healthy diets and physical activity: a European dimension for the prevention of overweight, obesity and chronic diseases, Brussels, 2005.
2 Branca F, Nikogosian H, Lobstein T: The Challenge of Obesity in the WHO European Region and the Strategies for Response. Summary. WHO Europe, 2007.
3 St. Leger L, Kolbe L, Lee A, McCall D, Young I: School health promotion: achievements, challenges and priorities. In: McQueen D, Jones C, eds. Global Perspectives on Health Promotion Effectiveness. Springer, 2007.
4 Shaya F, Flores D, Gbarayor C, Wang J: School-based obesity interventions: a literature review. *J Sch Health* 2008; **78**(4): 189–196.
5 Stewart-Brown S: What is the Evidence on School Health Promotion in Improving Health of Preventing Disease and Specifically, What is the Effectiveness of the Health Promoting School Approach? Copenhagen: WHO European Region, 2006.
6 WHO: The Ottawa charter for health promotion. *Health Promot Int* 1986; **1**(4):3–5.
7 Fysio Educatief, Welsh Assembly Government and Health Education Board for Scotland: The Class Moves! Cardiff: Welsh Assembly, 2002.
8 Florence MD, Asbridge M, Veugelers PJ: Diet quality and academic performance. *J Sch Health* 2008; **78**:209–215.
9 Rye J, O'Hara Tompkins N, Eck R: The role of schools in promoting physical activity and healthy weight in youth:a white paper from the policy research and engagement project, College of Human Resources and Education, West Virginia University, 2006.
10 Davis J, Cooke S: Educating for a healthy, sustainable world: an argument for integrating Health Promoting Schools and Sustainable Schools. *Health Promot Int.* 2007; **22**(4): 346–353.
11 WHO: The Health Promoting School—An Investment in Education, Health and Democracy. Copenhagen: World Health Organization, 1997.
12 National Foundation for Educational Research and Thomas Coram Research Unit: Evaluation of the impact of the National Healthy School Standard. London: Department of Health and Department for Education Skills, 2004.
13 Welsh Assembly Government: Food and Fitness—Promoting Healthy Eating and Physical Activity for children and Young people in Wales. 5 Year Implementation Plan, 2006.
14 Welsh Assembly Government: Appetite for Life. Welsh Assembly Government, 2006.
15 Welsh Assembly Government: Appetite for Life Action Plan. Welsh Assembly Government, 2007.
16 Active Young People in Wales: Sports Update, 58, Sports Council Wales, 2006
17 Young I: Growing Through Adolescence: A Training Pack Based on a Health Promoting School Approach to Healthy Eating. NHS Health Scotland, 2005.
18 Gortmaker SL, Peterson K, Wiecha J et al: Reducing obesity via a school-based interdisciplinary intervention among youth: Planet Health. *Arch Pediatr Adolesc Med* 1999; **153**(4):409–418.
19 Bessems K, Ruiter S, Buijs G: Toolkit Overgewicht: preventie van overgewicht binnen de setting school. [Toolkit for overweight prevention in schools]. Woerden: NIGZ, 2006.
20 World Health Organization: Nutrition-Friendly Schools Initiative, Part 1: NFSI Framework. Geneva: World Health Organization, 2007.

CHAPTER 31

Working in primary care

C. Raina Elley[1] and *Karen Hoare*[2]
[1]Department General Practice and Primary Care, School of Population Health, University of Auckland, Auckland, New Zealand
[2]School of Nursing and Goodfellow Unit, School of Population Health, University of Auckland, Auckland, New Zealand

Summary and recommendations for research and practice

- Primary care is an important setting to assess and reduce risk of childhood obesity during the antenatal, infancy, childhood and adolescent stages.
- Maternal nutritional advice, smoking cessation and early detection and management of gestational diabetes during the antenatal period, as well as infant nutritional advice and breastfeeding promotion, address risk factors of childhood and subsequent obesity.
- Trajectories of weight gain in infants, and body mass index (BMI) gain in children and adolescents, are the best available assessment tools to identify the risk of childhood obesity.
- There is little evidence of effective interventions in primary care to prevent or treat childhood obesity long term, but effective interventions to improve nutrition, increase physical activity and reduce sedentary behaviors in the short to medium term exist.
- Multi-component programs in health care settings with intensive and long-term follow-up and family involvement seem most promising, but more research is needed.
- Systematic screening and implementation of evidence-based management of children at risk of obesity are needed in primary care, which may

require changes at a policy, as well as practice, level.
- Primary care collaboration with community groups, schools, industry and local authorities may be effective in reducing the risk of childhood obesity at a community level.

Introduction

Childhood obesity is of central concern to primary care professionals, both for the immediate psychological and physical effects it may have for the child, but also for the increased likelihood of the child developing adult obesity and the increased risk of diseases such as Type 2 diabetes, cardiovascular disease and cancer. The risk of childhood obesity begins prior to the birth of the child, with genetics as well as the antenatal environment influencing risk of later obesity. Primary care has a potential role to play at this stage. During infancy and childhood, primary care professionals also have numerous opportunities to assess, manage and monitor potential overweight and obesity in children, from the times of postnatal care and breastfeeding to immunization visits, preschool checks and during visits for minor illnesses. This chapter addresses each stage, discussing assessment, and suggesting ways of translating evidence into primary care at a practice and policy level to reduce childhood obesity.

Antenatal and infancy

Assessment and monitoring

Maternal nutrition and well-being are areas where health professionals may influence subsequent

Preventing Childhood Obesity. Edited by
E. Waters, B.A. Swinburn, J.C. Seidell and R. Uauy.
© 2010 Blackwell Publishing.

childhood obesity rates and their consequences. Barker showed an association between low birth weight and weight at the age of 1 year in determining the risk of cardiovascular disease (CVD) in later life, especially in children who showed "catch-up" growth or became obese. Barker's research prompted international studies and public health recommendations to promote maternal nutrition and infant growth, largely through primary health care.[1] Fetal and early postnatal nutrition were thought to be the "common soil" that program the metabolic syndrome. This "common soil" hypothesis, postulated originally in 1984, suggested that early nutrition was a common link in the development of Type 2 diabetes and CVD, implying that CVD is not a complication but shares genetic and environmental antecedents with Type 2 diabetes.[2] Experimental rat studies have demonstrated that poor maternal nutrition is associated with increased insulin resistance and elevated blood pressure in the offspring.[3] Accelerated weight gain during infancy is also associated with increased insulin resistance as well as overweight and higher leptin and blood pressure levels in adolescence and adulthood.[3] Maternal over-nutrition is also of concern, as higher birth weights are associated with higher BMI during childhood and adulthood, as well as increased risk of obesity and diabetes.

Management

Therefore, the management of maternal nutrition is important in reducing obesity during childhood and later (and for many other reasons). Early detection and careful management of gestational diabetes in primary care is essential with not only the potential for congenital abnormalities and macrosomia if poorly controlled, but also increased adiposity and insulin levels even at the age of 5 years.[3] In the UK, the NICE guidance on maternal and child nutrition recommends the provision of information on the benefits of a healthy diet and practical and tailored advice on healthy eating throughout pregnancy.[4] Low birth weight is associated with subsequent obesity, so smoking cessation interventions in pregnancy are also important as they have been shown to reduce smoking rates and improve birth weight.[5]

As breastfeeding reduces risk for both CVD and Type 2 diabetes, and other benefits of breastfeeding are incontestable, breastfeeding promotion is of paramount importance in primary care and community health facilities. Philip and Radford argue that the risks of being formula fed are now well established.[6] A systematic review commissioned by the World Health Organization (WHO) and published in 2007 found that breastfed individuals were less likely to be considered as overweight/obese.[7] Scholten et al's more recent study examined longitudinal data from 2,347 children born in 1996/97 and found that children who were breastfed for more than 16 weeks had a lower BMI at 1 year than non-breastfed children. A high BMI at 1 year was strongly associated with a high BMI between the ages of 1 and 7 in the same model.[8]

In the UK it is a requirement that approved NICE guidance is implemented within the NHS, and for primary care this means through primary care trusts.[9] One example of this is the UNICEF Baby Friendly Initiative that promotes breastfeeding. The Baby Friendly Initiative is a worldwide program developed by the WHO and UNICEF and was launched in 1991.[10] Baby Friendly accreditation requires that community health care facilities implement seven points (Table 31.1). Achievement of the seven points is

Table 31.1 The seven-point plan for the protection, promotion and support of breastfeeding in community health care settings.

1	Have a written breastfeeding policy that is routinely communicated to all health care staff.
2	Train all staff involved in the care of mothers and babies in the skills necessary to implement the policy.
3	Inform all pregnant women about the benefits and management of breastfeeding.
4	Support mothers to initiate and maintain breastfeeding.
5	Encourage exclusive and continued breastfeeding, with appropriately-timed introduction of complementary foods.
6	Provide a welcoming atmosphere for breastfeeding families.
7	Promote cooperation between health care staff, breastfeeding support groups and the local community.

audited by UNICEF and once full accreditation is achieved, a health care facility is re-audited every two years.

Childhood

Assessment and monitoring

The US Preventive Services Task Force state that there is insufficient evidence to recommend for or against screening for overweight in children.[11] One of the WHO criteria for screening is the availability of effective treatment, which is largely lacking in this area. However, the American Academy of Pediatrics Committee already recommend that primary care pediatricians perform regular screening in children using body mass index (BMI = weight in kg/[height in m]^2).[12] The UK set targets in 2002 to "halt the year-on-year rise in obesity among children under 11 by 2010" recommending monitoring of child adiposity through a national scheme to measure all children (including BMI) upon entry to infant school and senior school through primary care trusts.[13]

The use of BMI to identify overweight children is widely recommended for children aged 2–18.[12,14] However, the use of BMI is controversial, as it may not distinguish between weight increases due to fat and those due to fat-free mass, which vary by individual and particularly by ethnic group.[11,15] Even so, BMI has reasonable correlation with adiposity. The Centers for Disease Control and Prevention BMI percentile charts or the use of locally recommended BMI charts where available, to assess age and gender-specific BMIs, are recommended.[14,15]

Overweight is defined by the US Centers for Disease Control and Prevention as being above the 95th percentile of BMI.[11] Other countries, such as Australia, have used the 85th percentile as the cut-off for "overweight" and 95th percentile for "obesity"[14] and the UK recommend tailored clinical intervention with a BMI at or above the 91st percentile.[15] However, choosing such cut-offs presents the problem that they are linked to the current range of BMI distribution in the reference population instead of being linked to morbidity or health outcomes. Waist circumference is not recommended for routine measurement in children at present, but it measures fat around the dangerous abdominal region, and therefore may be a better indicator of the risk of developing insulin resistance,

metabolic syndrome and long-term health problems and may have a place in routine clinical measurement in the future.[14,16]

It is important to recognize adverse weight trajectories in childhood both for treatment and prevention, as childhood overweight is predictive of adult overweight and obesity and eating patterns are often established early, so systematic screening may be worthwhile.[12] When overweight or obesity are identified, assessment of the nutritional and physical activity patterns of the child and their family should be undertaken; in particular, the nutritional quality of the food, portion size, snacking behaviors, meals eaten in front of the television, meals eaten with the family, and consumption of breakfast, fast foods and sugar-sweetened beverages. Participation in organized sport or activities, informal physical play, transport to school or other sources of physical activity can be assessed, as well as time spent in sedentary activities such as television watching and computer or other screen games.

The psycho-social setting within the family or school may be influencing these patterns. If a child is identified as being over the 95th percentile in BMI, assessment of obesity-related co-morbidities may be indicated, especially if there is also a family history of co-morbidity, such as Type 2 diabetes, early CVD or familial hyperlipidemia. Occasionally, a pathological cause can precipitate obesity in childhood and may also be associated with reduced height, such as a hypothalamic lesion, Cushing's syndrome, hypothyroidism or growth hormone deficiency, all of which require more detailed assessment and specialist referral.

It is important to communicate the results of screening to parents in a sensitive way, and to use effective approaches to address the issue, such as motivational interviewing.[12,17] Parent perceptions vary and the best way to discuss these issues with parents needs further research. Some parents report they are made to feel guilty while others are left feeling that the general practitioner (GP) has thought they are unnecessarily concerned about their child's weight.[18] Qualitative research has suggested that parents may also interpret growth charts and perceive "overweight" differently from health professionals.[19] In a study of maternal anxiety regarding overweight preschoolers, mothers were more likely to be concerned if a child became inactive or was teased by peers rather than worrying about their percentile on a growth chart.[19] An effective way to address the issue may be to establish shared goals and emphasize healthy diet and physical activity rather than focusing on the growth trajectory.

Management

There is currently sparse evidence for the effectiveness of treatment of childhood obesity in primary care.[14] There is some evidence to suggest that weight management programs for overweight or obese children involving weight maintenance rather than weight loss, behavioral strategies, family involvement (preferably motivated family), and an intensive and long-term approach may have some effectiveness, especially those combining dietary, physical activity and reduced sedentary behavior goals.[20] For example, physical activity and diet approaches combined are more effective than diet alone in specialist weight management programs.[15] There is some randomized controlled trial (RCT) evidence that interventions in health care settings can increase physical activity, reduce sedentary behavior and in those that are compliant with the program, weight increase can be slowed, with no adverse effects in terms of the child's growth or quality of life over 12 months, compared with usual dietetic advice.[20]

One barrier to delivering these interventions in primary care is the often brief nature of the primary care consultation (e.g. 10–15 minutes for GPs, although nurses may have longer). A few "brief" interventions based in primary care designed to improve physical activity patterns in school age children have had some early encouraging results. Interventions to lose weight have been less encouraging. For example a RCT showed that brief physical activity counseling was able to increase physical activity and reduce sedentary time in children over 12 months in the USA.[21] Although the counseling was delivered through primary care, computer-based diet and exercise assessment, goal setting and monthly mail and telephone counseling were also part of the intervention. In New Zealand, the Green prescription, an effective brief intervention delivered in primary care to increase physical activity among adults, has been adapted to improve physical activity in children (7–18 years) in a linked program called "Active Families". Although the

advice is initiated in primary care by the GP or practice nurse, the child and their family are referred to a community-based program over 12 months, aiming for 60 minutes of at least moderate intensity activity per day, as well as healthy eating. However, the effectiveness is not yet established.

Ford (US) (2000) tested a primary care intervention to reduce TV watching time over four weeks in a RCT.[22] Participants were 7–12-year-old African American children (not necessarily overweight) from 28 families. They compared 5–10 minute counseling with a longer intervention that also involved behavioral strategies, TV budgets and electronic TV time managers. Both groups decreased screen time by 14 hours per week but there was no difference between the groups. There was also a trend towards taking fewer meals in front of TV, and those with the TV electronic monitors did better than those without.

Further research is underway into primary care interventions such as the Live Eat and Play (LEAP) trial in Australia, and a subsequent Australian trial is planned of a multi-component intervention initiated in a hospital child obesity clinic but followed up three monthly in primary care, using computer assisted assessment and decision support.[23]

In general, principles of advice given by health professionals to parents or carers should encourage healthy eating, regular meals including breakfast, preferably with family and without distractions such as television, and reducing the consumption of sugar-sweetened beverages.[12,15] Physical activity of at least 60 minutes per day should be encouraged through play, recreational activities or with family, and through reduced sedentary behaviors involving, for example, television, computer or video games. These characteristics are all associated with reduced risk of overweight and obesity, although experimental evidence in primary care is scarce.[12] Training of primary care professionals in counseling techniques and lifestyle behavior change and the appropriate allocation of time and resources are needed.[15] Several countries have encouraged primary care organizations to collaborate or combine strategies with other community agencies or companies, such as supermarkets, schools, local exercise facilities, local authorities, planning agencies (e.g. of cycle tracks or walk ways) and industry.[15,24]

Adolescence

Assessment and monitoring

Assessment of the adolescent should include weight and height (BMI) and in those at risk such as those over the 95th percentile of BMI or with a family history of co-morbidity, waist circumference, blood pressure, serum fasting glucose, insulin and lipid levels, and liver function tests. Co-morbidities include psycho-social dysfunction or depression, bulimia or other eating disorder, obstructive sleep apnea, asthma, raised blood pressure, dyslipidemia, metabolic syndrome, insulin resistance or Type 2 diabetes, gall bladder disease, steatohepatitis, polycystic ovarian syndrome and orthopedic complications such as slipped capital femoral epiphyses.

Whether or not to involve the parents in consultations with older children about weight issues should be considered in light of the older child's maturity and competence to make decisions.[15] It is helpful to assess the adolescents' view about their weight, eating and physical activity patterns, as well as their social, cultural and ethnic context, previous attempts to change, readiness to change and confidence in their ability to make change.[15] There are also other issues of significance in this age group, such as peer pressures, issues of alcohol, drugs and sexuality. It is also a time of increased prevalence of eating disorders such as bulimia and anorexia. The HEEADSSS mnemonic (Table 31.2) may be useful to investigate the context of any potential weight issues. Questions to ask about eating could include: "What do you like or not like about your body?" and "Have there been any changes in your weight over the last year?"[25]

Management

The same principles of advice around diet, physical activity and sedentary behaviors would apply to this group but the issues and barriers are different from younger children and more research is needed which addresses this group.

Little evidence exists around primary care interventions for dietary change in overweight or obese adolescents. There has been some evidence of improvement in fruit and vegetable consumption over two years among adolescents using a primary care intervention in the US, but this involved a group of underweight adolescent girls who are likely to have very different population characteristics and responses.[26] Also, the intervention was intensive (bi-monthly meetings, self-monitoring and quarterly telephone calls).

There is a small amount of evidence for physical activity counseling in primary care among adolescents. In a Spanish trial, which assessed effectiveness of 5–10 minutes of physical activity counseling versus no counseling, significantly more adolescents were active in the intervention group compared with the control at 6 and 12 months.[27] The addition of more intensive follow-up did not improve increases in physical activity among adolescents in a US trial over 7 months.[28]

In the adolescent, there is some evidence for short- to medium-term effectiveness in weight loss for pharmaceutical treatments, such as phentermine, although this also causes severe insomnia.[14] Metformin may be useful in the obese adolescent with hyperinsulinemia.[14] A 6–12 month trial of orlistat or sibutramine, or bariatric surgery, such as lap banding, may be appropriate after specialist assessment, particularly in morbid obesity (e.g. BMI ≥ 40) or when co-morbidities exist, although evidence for long-term effectiveness in this age-group is lacking.[15,29] Management of co-morbidities identified is also required. Other minor medical sequelae of obesity may also require management such as musculoskeletal discomfort, heat intolerance or shortness of breath.[14]

Incorporating the evidence

Primary care initiatives need to work within the context of wider organizational and policy changes that support the advice given. At a practice level, the impact of simple advice should not be underestimated, even in light of limited evidence for specific primary care intervention. Partnership and goal-setting with parents, children and adolescents around

Table 31.2 The HEEADSS mnemonic.

H	Home environment
E	Education/employment
E	Eating
A	Peer-related Activities
D	Drugs
S	Sexuality
S	Suicide & depression
S	Safety from injury and violence

healthy diets and portion sizes, increasing physical activity and reducing sedentary activities may be effective in reinforcing healthy behaviors. In addition, approaches within everyday practice may need to change. For example, well child checks for the infant and preschool child should focus on "healthy" weights and not "gaining" weight.

At a policy level, health care practitioners often have a voice through overarching primary care organizations to influence the future shape of primary care in addressing issues such as childhood obesity in a systematic and population health focused way. The systematic implementation of evidence-based guidelines into usual primary care practice, such as the UNICEF Baby Friendly Initiative (community) would improve reach of our best evidence for preventing obesity. Electronic prompts and decision support within primary care practice management systems may be a way of prompting systematic screening and guidelines-based management for overweight and obesity in children.[30] Quality of care remains ad hoc where evidence-based guidelines are not systematically adopted at the primary care level.

Collaborations between primary care and community or school-based initiatives, facilitated at a policy level, may be needed to achieve a more effective approach to childhood obesity. This would also be in line with the Alma Ata declaration, which defines quality primary health care as integral to, and a central function of, the community and is based on practical, scientifically sound, culturally appropriate, and socially acceptable methods and technology, which is accessible to all age groups.[31] Furthermore, such an approach is consistent with Article 24 of the United Nations Convention on the Rights of the Child.[32]

References

1 Barker D, Gluckman P, Godfrey K, Harding J, Owen J, Robinson J: Fetal nutrition and cardiovascular disease in adult life. *Lancet* 1993; 341:938–941.

2 Singhal A, Lucas A: Early origins of cardiovascular disease: is there a unifying hypothesis? *Lancet* 2004; 363: 1642–1645.

3 Gillman MW, Barker D, Bier D et al: Meeting report on the 3rd International Congress on Developmental Origins of Health and Disease (DOHaD). *Pediatr Res* 2007; 61: 625–629.

4 National Institute for Health and Clinical Excellence (NICE): Maternal and child nutrition. 2008; Guidelines. Available from: www.nice.org.uk/guidance/index.jsp?action=byID&o =11943 (accessed April 2008).

5 Lumley J, Oliver SS, Chamberlain C, Oakley L: Interventions for promoting smoking cessation during pregnancy. *Cochrane Database Syst Rev* 2008; 2:13–14.

6 Phillip B, Radford A: Baby-friendly: snappy slogan or standard of care? *Arch Dis Child Fetal Neonatal Ed* 2006; 91: 145–149.

7 Horta B, Bahl R, Martines J, Victora C: Evidence on the long-term effects of breastfeeding. 2007; Available from: WHO http://whqlibdoc.who.int/publications/2007/ 9789241595230_eng.pdf (accessed 14 April 2008).

8 Scholtens S, Gehring U Brunekreef B et al: Breast feeding, weight gain in infancy and overweight at seven years of age. The prevention and incidence of asthma and mite allergy birth cohort study. *Am J Epidemiol* 2007; 165:919–926.

9 Whittaker S, Hill R: Policy on the Implementation of NICE Guidance. Central and North West Lond Mental Health NHS Trust, 2005.

10 UNICEF: About the Baby Friendly Initiative. 2006; Available from: www.babyfriendly.org.uk/page.asp?page=11 (accessed 14 April 2008).

11 US Preventive Services Task Force: Screening and interventions for overweight in children and adolescents: recommendation statement. *Pediatrics* 2005; 116:205–209.

12 Perrin EM, Finkle JP, Benjamin JT: Obesity prevention and the primary care pediatrician's office. *Curr Opin Pediatric* 2007; 19:354–361.

13 Patterson L, Jarvis P, Verma A, Harrison R, Buchan I: Measuring children and monitoring obesity: Surveys of English Primary Care Trusts 2004–2006. *J Public Health* 2006; 28:330–336.

14 National Health & Medical Research Council: Clinical Practice Guidelines for the Management of Overweight and Obesity in Children and Adolescents. 2003; Available from: www.obesityguidelines.gov.au (accessed 21 April 2008).

15 National Institute for Health and Clinical Excellence (NICE): Obesity: guidance on the prevention, identification, assessment and management of overweight and obesity in adults and children. 2006; Guidelines. Available from: www.nice. org.uk/guidance/index.jsp?action=download&o=30361 (accessed April 2008).

16 McCarthy HD: Body fat measurements in children as predictors for the metabolic syndrome: focus on waist circumference. *Proc Nutr Soc* 2006; 65:385–392.

17 Schwartz RP, Hamre R, Dietz WH: Office-based motivational interviewing to prevent childhood obesity: a feasibility study. *Arch Pediatr Adolesc Med* 2007; 161:495–501.

18 Edmunds LD: Parents' perceptions of health professionals' responses when seeking help for their overweight children. *Fam Pract* 2005; 22:287–292.

19 Jain A, Sherman S, Chamberlin L, Carter Y, Powers S, Whitaker R: Why don't low-income mothers worry about their preschoolers being overweight? *Pediatrics* 2001; 107:1138–1146.

20 Hughes AR, Stewart L, Chapple J et al: Randomized, controlled trial of a best-practice individualized behavioral program for treatment of childhood overweight: Scottish Childhood Overweight Treatment Trial (SCOTT). *Pediatrics* 2008; **121**:e539–e546.

21 Patrick K, Calfas KJ, Norman GJ et al: Randomized controlled trial of a primary care and home-based intervention for physical activity and nutrition behaviors: PACE+ for adolescents. *Arch Pediatr Adolesc Med* 2006; **160**:128–136.

22 Ford BS, McDonald TE, Owens AS, Robinson TN: Primary care interventions to reduce television viewing in African-American children. *Am J Prev Med* 2002; **22**:106–109.

23 Wake M: Better outcomes for obese children in general practice: randomized controlled trial of a new shared-care model vs usual care. 2008; Registered trial. Available from: www.anzctr.org.au/trial_view.aspx?ID=82549 (accessed 28 April 2008).

24 King A: The Primary Health Care Strategy. Wellington, New Zealand: Ministry of Health, 2001.

25 Goldenring J, Rosen D: Getting into adolescent heads: an essential update. *Contemp Pediatr* 2004; **21**:64–90.

26 DeBar LL, Ritenbaugh C, Aickin M et al: Youth: a health plan-based lifestyle intervention increases bone mineral density in adolescent girls. *Arch Pediatr Adolesc Med* 2006; **160**:1269–1276.

27 Ortega-Sanchez R, Jimenez-Mena C, Cordoba-Garcia R, Munoz-Lopez J, Garcia-Machado ML, Vilaseca-Canals J: The effect of office-based physician's advice on adolescent exercise behavior. *Prev Med* 2004; **38**:219–226.

28 Saelens BE, Sallis JF, Wilfley DE, Patrick K, Cella JA, Buchta R: Behavioral weight control for overweight adolescents initiated in primary care. *Obes Res* 2002; **10**:22–32.

29 Holterman A-X, Browne A, Dillard BE et al: Short-term outcome in the first 10 morbidly obese adolescent patients in the FDA-approved trial for laparoscopic adjustable gastric banding. *J Pediatr Gastroenterol Nutr* 2007; **45**:465–473.

30 Rogers L, Gerner B, Wake M, Gunn J: LEAP trial. *Aust Fam Phys* 2007; **36**:887–888.

31 World Health Organization: Report of the International Conference on Primary Health Care. Geneva, Switzerland: World Health Organization, 1978.

32 Office of the United Nations High Commissioner for Human Rights. Convention on the Rights of the Child. 1989; Available from: www2.ohchr.org/english/law/crc.htm (accessed 28 April 2008).

CHAPTER 32

Working with minority groups in developed countries

Lisa Gibbs,[1] *Mulugeta Abebe*[2] *and Elisha Riggs*[1]
[1] Jack Brockhoff Child Health and Wellbeing Program, McCaughey Centre, Melbourne School of Population Health, University of Melbourne, Melbourne, Australia
[2] Merri Community Health Services, Melbourne, Australia

Summary and recommendations for research and practice

- Ethnic diversity adds to the complexity of developing and implementing effective community-based obesity prevention research and programs.
- Models of cultural competence in public health research provide guidance in working with minority groups in developed countries.
- Working with minority groups requires researchers and practitioners to be reflective about their own cultural framework.
- Flexibility in communication styles, research processes, program strategies and methodologies increases the potential for meaningful involvement of minority groups.
- Respectful, participatory approaches allow for mutual knowledge exchange and support relevant research and program outcomes.
- Culturally competent community-based research and programs may help to address health inequities that operate in relation to ethnicity and overweight/obesity.

Introduction

Incorporating the evidence

The complexity of developing community-based obesity prevention interventions is well established. It

Preventing Childhood Obesity. Edited by
E. Waters, B.A. Swinburn, J.C. Seidell and R. Uauy.
© 2010 Blackwell Publishing.

arises from the range of socio-environmental influences on changes in weight status at a population level[1] and the subsequent need for multi-level, sustainable strategies in different settings and contexts.[2] The lack of uniformity in "real-world" settings is increasingly recognized as a challenge for study design, implementation and evaluation.[3] This is further complicated by the global increase in population diversity in developed countries.[4]

The evidence on health inequities for minority groups in developed countries is well established and highlights the need for consideration of diversity in obesity prevention efforts. It requires a flexible, culturally competent approach to the design and implementation of interventions (see Box 32.1). Culturally competent strategies for public health research and interventions have recently been developed to guide this process and are used as the basis for this chapter.[5,6] These strategies are designed to assist researchers to shift from an expert-driven to a participatory approach with increasing understanding and capacity for accommodating the added complexity inherent in cross-cultural exchanges. The intention is to encourage a culturally reflective process among researchers and health promotion practitioners who are working with minority groups in developed countries. This chapter is particularly relevant to those involved in public health and health promotion community-based research and interventions. The term "interventions" is a research term that potentially has negative connotations to lay readers. Therefore, for the remainder of the chapter the alternative terms, "programs", "initiatives" and "strategies" are used.

Box 32.1 Case study 1: a shift in the cultural framework for organized sport

The media release below describes a culturally appropriate community strategy to address increased energy levels late at night for young Muslim men. This was caused by a shift in eating patterns during the period of Ramadan. The issue first came to the attention of the organizers because of local residents' concerns about loud, impromptu soccer games occurring in local parks with open grassed areas in the middle of the night. Instead of trying to ban the informal games, the youths were supported through the provision of an indoor venue and an organized competition.

Kicking goals for youth during Ramadan
August 7, 2007
While most of us are sleeping, players in the annual Ramadan Soccer Program are just getting started for the night at the City of Melbourne's Carlton Baths Community Centre.

During Ramadan—for three weeks in late September to mid October, from 11pm to 3am—the centre is alive with young soccer lovers, most young Muslim men bursting with energy after their evening meal which has broken the daily fasting central to Islam's holiest time of the year.

The Carlton Parkville Youth Services YMCA in partnership with the Victoria Police, the City of Melbourne, the Carlton Baths Community Centre YMCA and St Jude's Church host the annual event which began in 1999. It kicked off in response to an acute need for recreational and support programs during Ramadan, for the young men residing in and around Office of Housing Estates within the City of Melbourne most who are recent immigrants from northern Africa.

The program aims to provide a safe and appropriate space for young men to gather and play sport during the month of fasting, and to help build relationships between the young men, the police and the local community.

This unique and responsive program has proved popular since its inception, and has become an established component of Ramadan activities in Carlton. It received Victorian Multicultural Commission recognition for "Service Delivery to the Multicultural Community—Youth Services".

In 2005, an average of 39 players a night took part—last year numbers rose to an average of 70 players nightly.

Reprinted with permission from YMCA

Chapter 17 highlights the socio-cultural influences on eating and physical activity and considers how this might affect community-based obesity prevention programs. In this chapter, we build on these considerations and focus on issues arising as a consequence of the circumstances of many minority groups. For the purposes of this chapter, the focus is on minority groups as defined by ethnicity. Ethnicity has been shown to be a predictor of overweight and obesity, even after taking into account socio-economic disadvantage.[7] There has been debate about the usefulness of the body mass index (BMI) as a measure of overweight and obesity across populations without consideration for different body types. A review of BMI for Asian populations determined that the World Health Organization BMI cut-off points for overweight and obesity should be retained as international classifications.[8] However, methods were proposed by which countries could make decisions about the definitions of increased risk for their population.

Various inconsistent terms and concepts are used in the health literature to describe a group or individual's ethnicity.[9] Terms include: ethnicity, race, culturally and linguistically diverse background, disadvantaged group or under-privileged group. These terms are influenced by biological origins and social groupings and can be misused. They can often be inappropriate, crude, confusing, limited, inaccurate, potentially stereotyping and can prevent generalizability of research. For the purposes of this chapter, ethnicity refers to an individual identifying as belonging to a particular social group with similar country of origin, spoken language, cultural practices and/or religious beliefs. It is acknowledged that 'minority' can be defined in many different ways and the particular needs of other minority groups such as people with disabilities also need to be addressed but they are not covered in this chapter. There is likely to be a general recognition by public health researchers and practitioners that diversity in ethnicity is often accompanied by diversity in values, beliefs, knowledge and attitudes regarding health.

There may be less awareness of other issues often associated with migration that can impact on health status and health behaviors. These include but are not limited to the following:
• **Migration circumstances** vary from skilled migration, family sponsored, humanitarian and refugee,

and reflect the circumstances of the individuals and families in their home country. The health status of a skilled migrant may be very different from a person who has fled a country affected by famine and/or war. Their visa status may also determine their level of access to employment and support services in their host country.

- Relocation to another country is often a period of disruption in terms of **housing, employment and secure income**. These issues are likely to take precedence over non-critical health considerations.
- Lack of **health education** in home countries and **limited family support and social connectedness** in the host country may reduce the capacity of families to engage in health promoting practices.
- **Acculturation** can increase awareness and knowledge of healthy lifestyle options in the host country. However, this takes time. In many cases it is the children who acquire this knowledge first, but without the benefit of an adult's maturity in decision making. Therefore, while they are in a position to inform the family choices, the transfer of knowledge may not take place. This is supported by recent research findings in Australia which show that use of the English language at home is a strong protective factor against overweight and obesity for boys.[10] This suggests that parents with greater proficiency in the main language of the host country may have greater access to nutritional information to support healthy dietary habits.

These are all likely to be issues affecting minority groups and their interaction with obesity prevention research and programs.

Who should represent the community?

Guidelines on culturally competent strategies in health research and programs consistently call for participatory approaches based on developed relationships and partnerships.[11,12] The challenge in implementing this approach is in knowing who the appropriate partner is, that is, who represents the community. This will vary considerably. For new and emerging communities it may be a gradual process of getting to know community members and networks and identifying individuals with capacity and influence in their community who are interested in supporting the research and program initiatives. Some minority groups will have established community organizations or community leaders who are expected to take that role. However, there may also be competing interests between different groups within a given cultural community. In these cases it is very important to allow an initial period of time to explore these different roles and to be transparent about who is being consulted. It is also important to determine if the community leaders are able to truly represent the interests of the target community members. For example, is the male religious leader of a community able to represent the daily experiences of a mother trying to provide healthy meals for her family? In these cases, it is clearly valuable to engage mothers but this should be negotiated through the community leader as a trusted and respected community representative. There are many cultural differences in accepted ways to communicate between genders and so the gender of the researcher and the setting of interactions with research or program participants need to be negotiated in advance.

As always, it is important to be aware of potential power differences in research and community program relationships. This is particularly important in interactions with minority groups if previous traumatic experiences or gendered roles have contributed to a feeling of vulnerability, suspicion of perceived authority figures, or lack of experience with research.

The benefits of this considered approach to identifying and engaging community representatives are self-evident. The time involved in building trusted relationships will save time and resources as the research and community program progresses.[13] However, can this culturally competent approach be supported in a community context with multiple minority groups? In these circumstances it is extremely valuable to conduct preliminary pilot work on the feasibility of the study design and the methodology to ensure appropriate time and resources have been allocated to meet the needs of culturally diverse communities.[11]

How can community involvement be supported?

Factors likely to impact on the way in which community groups are engaged in the research and

Box 32.2 Case study 2: different health beliefs

A wealthy man from a rural area of Africa was overweight and continually unwell. His wife who had learnt about healthy eating told him to eat less meat and fat. Instead, the man sought the advice of a local healer practised in traditional medicine. The healer diagnosed dirty blood and attached a device to the man's forehead to drain the "dirty" blood. When sufficient blood had poured from the wound, the healer declared him cured.

program processes are explored below, and highlight the need for reflection on which aspects of the study design and methodology are fixed and which can be customized to the group and setting.

A culturally competent approach to public health research and programs provides the framework for shared understanding and development of appropriate strategies through its underlying reliance on community-based participation (see Box 32.2).[14]

Different communication styles

In developed countries we have well-established ways of communicating and working which are so entrenched that it is easy to forget that they are a product of our own cultural framework. In order to work effectively in partnership with minority groups, it is necessary to reflect on those processes and the inherent power imbalance they support in our interactions with communities. In particular, reliance on print-based communication as well as emails and formal meetings for group decision-making is likely to undermine the potential for communities to make valuable contributions, and for those contributions to be valued. Instead, reliance on personal conversations held informally in normal daily settings can greatly enhance the process of developing common understandings and agreements for each stage of the research and community program.[4,15,16]

The use of alternative mediums such as story telling and art can also be an effective way of exploring issues in community programs. A traditional African story, *The Cat Olympics*, clearly conveys the concept of different body types:

A running race for cats was held and there were three cats, a US cat, a European cat and an Ethiopian cat. They started the race and the Ethiopian cat won very easily. When they asked the cat, "How did you manage to win by such a distance?" he replied, "Because I am a tiger, not a cat."

This is a story about comparing groups. Although the three cats were all the same size, the Western cats were overweight and the Ethiopian cat was lean and small as there is not much food to eat, so it looked the same size as the others, but was in fact a different type of cat altogether.

Understanding of historical context

Recognition of the diversity among and within minority groups is an important first step to developing an understanding of how to work together. An important component of this diversity is the historical context of the group and the circumstances of migration. Developing an understanding of the history of the group you are working with and sharing your own cultural history provides a cultural framework for a strong partnership. For example, in Australia, colonization, the stolen generation and cultural genocide are embedded as part of the historical context. Yet they have clearly been experienced quite differently by white Australians and indigenous Australians.

Engaging community members

Representation of minority groups in community-based obesity prevention programs requires a commitment to a range of strategies to overcome the potential for low literacy, limited health knowledge, limited understanding of the role of research, and mistrust of authority. Some of these strategies include overlapping strategies, support from trusted community leaders, oral communication/personal contact using interpreters, and recording of verbal rather than signed consent.[4,11,16,17]

Recruitment for research in Western countries focuses on individual participation. However, this may be inconsistent with the cultural framework of some minority groups that may function and prefer to respond to research as family groups, social groups or even as communities. This requires flexibility in the research and community program design, including flexibility in relation to the number of participants involved in interviews and focus groups and the inclusion and exclusion criteria for participation. For example, if the intention is to recruit people from specific countries such as Pakistan, Iraq and Lebanon and the community is being accessed through an Arabic cultural support organization, it is possible that people from other countries such as Saudi Arabia, Egypt, Syria, or from Palestinian territories may also be interested in participating, especially if they are part of a cultural social network that is participating as a group. It is important to be aware that if they have migrated, owing to persecution in their home country, excluding them from participation due to "research rigor" would be inappropriate and could create further feelings of exclusion.

Similarly, any research or community program targeting families needs to first understand the concept of family for the minority groups in question. In many cases, gender roles, intergenerational and community responsibilities in child rearing need to be understood with regard to their role in influencing eating and physical activity behaviors and choices. For example, decisions about food choices may be driven by the mother as the person responsible for preparing food, or grandparents who are responsible for child care, or fathers ensuring cultural practices are maintained. Cultural identification may also shift as a result of marriage. For example, a woman may describe herself as belonging to the cultural group of her husband rather than her own cultural background.

Appropriate community settings

When approaching minority groups it is most valuable to operate via the community settings they are currently utilizing, such as cultural or religious meeting places.[4,16,18,19] However, this is not always possible if minority groups are part of a wider community study. Schools are currently being widely used as a community-based setting for obesity prevention. The level of involvement family members of minority groups have with the school will obviously greatly impact on the effectiveness of school-community based initiatives. The level of interaction between families and schools varies considerably in migrant home countries. In many African countries, for example, the whole family visits the school only once a year for Parents' Day. Other than that, they would normally only attend if there for the recognition of a child's achievement or if the child were in trouble.

Engagement of families directly in community-based initiatives needs to accommodate not just cultural considerations in intergenerational and gender roles in decision making and child care. The impact of migration and differing levels of acculturation can also dramatically affect decision-making roles within the family. As the child is often the first member of the family to master the language of the host country and to gain some understanding of mainstream culture and systems, parents have to defer to their knowledge and in doing so can lose power in decision making. Children thereby become the power brokers in the family, driving food purchasing and activity decisions without the constraint of the disempowered adults. For example, children may perceive fast food and soft drinks as accepted diet in their host country and refuse to eat healthy traditional foods. The challenge in the development of obesity prevention programs is to engage parents and support their role as guardians of their children's health and/or to engage children as the drivers of changed behaviors.

What messages and strategies to use?

Effective health promotion/social marketing uses messages that have relevance and importance to the target community.[20] This is particularly relevant in obesity prevention because of the range of cultural values and beliefs in relation to food and physical activity, health and weight, as described in Chapter 17 and illustrated in Box 32.2.

In particular, the community program strategies need to accommodate different cultural frameworks which will impact directly on the relevance of the message. For example, for many families from developing countries obesity prevention messages will create confusion because:

- Overweight and obesity are perceived as a sign of health and wealth[21] (represented by the tie resting on the belly) in the home country and are seen as a sign of laziness and poor health in developed host countries.
- It is often difficult to maintain healthy traditional diets with unfamiliar food products in the host country.
- Foods high in fat that are seen as healthy and desirable in famine-affected countries are seen as

Box 32.3 Case study 3: food values—"I love you so much like I do for barbeque"

How do you know a person is healthy in Kenya?—if they eat meat, butter and milk. For many Kenyans, eating as much of these products as possible equates to being physically fit and strong. Low fat milk has no meaning, except perhaps to represent milk that is of poorer quality. Milk comes from a cow and is healthy.

The importance of meat, milk and butter is highlighted in the expression used to express deep love for someone—"Ninakupenda sana kama nyama choma!" This phrase translates literally to: "*I love you so much like I do for barbeque.*"

unhealthy in developed countries (see Box 32.3). Conversely, foods such as vegetables may be seen as part of a poverty diet in the home country but are seen as healthy and desirable in the host country.

- Physical activity is a product of poverty in the home country, for example, walking or riding long distances because of the cost of transport. Sport is only for the young. Family duties then take over unless sport represents a way of achieving wealth. In developed countries it is seen as a healthy and desirable activity for adults and families.

This contrast between life experiences in developing versus developed countries shows the importance of reframing obesity prevention health messages and community program strategies to address conflicting experiences. It also highlights the importance of including strategies which promote healthy environments and policies and thereby minimize reliance on conscious behavioral change.[22]

Responding to community needs

Shared recognition and prioritizing of health priorities should ideally determine the direction of community initiatives and the framing of health messages. This can operate in many different ways, for example, the community may identify the health issue and seek research or program support to address it. Alternatively, the health or academic sector may identify the health issue and seek community support to identify ways to address it. For example, obesity prevention programs targeting reduction of soft drink consumption could

use the most relevant health message/s from the following for the community group involved:

- promoting the health benefit of reducing soft drink consumption;
- promoting water as safe to drink—migrants who have come from countries with contaminated water supplies may not be aware of this;
- promoting oral health—this is particularly relevant in cultural groups such as some African communities where the "white" smile is highly valued;
- promoting a switch from soft drinks to water as a way of saving money.

Working closely with representatives of the community is the best way to determine the messages and strategies that are likely to be most relevant to the community members.

Conclusion

There are additional complexities involved in developing a community-based obesity prevention research and program with minority groups in developed countries. However, these additional considerations can be negotiated successfully provided culturally competent strategies are adopted, which rely on respectful partnerships at all stages of the research and intervention process and thus allow for mutual knowledge exchange. Reflection on the researcher/practitioner's cultural framework and allowance for diversity both within and across minority groups will also demonstrate the need for greater flexibility in strategies and processes. This will result in more meaningful and sustainable outcomes for the groups involved and increased capacity for researchers and practitioners to work effectively in culturally diverse settings. At a broader level, culturally competent community outcomes will potentially address the established health inequities operating in relation to ethnicity and overweight/obesity.

References

1 Swinburn B, Egger GJ, Raza F: Dissecting obesogenic environments: the development and application of a framework for identifying and prioritising environmental interventions for obesity. *Prev Med* 1999; **29**:563–570.
2 Summerbell C, Waters E, Edmunds L, Kelly S, Brown T, Campbell K: Interventions for preventing obesity in children. *CochraneDatabase Syst Rev* 2005; **3**:CD 001871.

3 Mercer SL, Vinney JD, Fine LJ, Green L, Dougherty D: Study designs for effectiveness and translation research. Identifying trade-offs. *Am J Prev Med* 2007; **33**(2):139–154.

4 Daunt D: Ethnicity and recruitment rates in clinical research studies. *Appl Nurs Res* 2003;**16**(3):189–195.

5 Waters E, Gibbs L, Renzaho A, Riggs E, Kulkens M, Priest N: Increasing Cultural competence in public health and health promotion. In: Heggenhougen K, ed. *Encyclopedia of Public Health*. Oxford, UK: Elsevier Inc., 2008:38–44.

6 Gibbs L, Waters E, Renzaho A, Kulkens M: Moving towards increased cultural competency in public health research. In: Williamson A, DeSouza R, eds. Researching with Communities: Grounded Perspectives on Engaging Communities in Research. London: Muddy Creek Press, 2007:339–355.

7 Waters E, Ashbolt R, Gibbs L et al: Double disadvantage: the influence of ethnicity over socioeconomic position on childhood overweight and obesity: findings from an inner urban population of primary school children. *Int J Obes.* 2008;**3**(4): 196–204.

8 WHO Expert Consultation: Appropriate body mass index for Asian populations and its implications for policy and intervention strategies. *Lancet* 2004; **363**(9403):157–163.

9 Bhopal R: Glossary of terms relating to ethnicity and race: for reflection and debate. *J Epidemiol Community Health* 2004; **58**(6):441–445.

10 Renzaho A, Oldroyd J, Burns C, Waters E, Riggs E, Renzaho C: Over and undernutrition in the children of Australian immigrants: assessing the influence of birthplace of primary carer and English language use at home on the nutritional status of 4 to 5 year olds. *Int J Paediatr Obes.* 2009;**4**(2): 73–80.

11 National Health and Medical Research Council. Cultural Competence in Health: A Guide for Policy, Partnerships and Participation. Commonwealth of Australia, 2006.

12 Pacific Health Research Committee. Guidelines on Pacific Health Research. Auckland: Health Research Council, 2004.

13 Gibbs L, Gold L, Kulkens M, Riggs E, Gemert CV, Waters E: Are the benefits of a community-based participatory approach to public health research worth the costs? *Just Policy* 2008; **47**:52–59.

14 Israel B, Schulz A, Parker E, Becker A: Review of community-based research: assessing partnership approaches to improve public health. *Annu Rev Public Health* 1998; **19**: 173–202.

15 Lipson JG, Meleis AI: Research with immigrants and refugees. In: Hinshaw AS, Feetham SL, Shaver JLF, eds. Handbook of Clinical Nursing. London: Sage, 1999: 87–106.

16 Brown B, Long H, Gould H, Weitz T, Milliken N: A conceptual model for the recruitment of diverse women into research studies. *J Womens Health Gend Based Med* 2000; **9**(6):625–632.

17 Keyzer J, Melnikow J, Kupperman M et al: Recruitment strategies for minority participation: challenges and cost lessons from the power interview. *Ethn Dis* 2005; **15**: 395–406.

18 Green J, Waters E, Haikerwal A et al: Social, cultural and environmental influences on child activity and eating in Australian migrant communities. *Child Care Health Dev* 2003; **29**(6):441–448.

19 Lindenberg C, Solorzano R, Vilaro F, Westbrook L: Challenges and strategies for conducting intervention research with culturally diverse populations. *J Transcult Nurs* 2001; **12**(2):132–139.

20 Blair JE: Social marketing: consumer focused health promotion. *AAOHN J* 1995; **43**(10):527–531.

21 Renzaho A: Fat, rich and beautiful: changing socio-cultural paradigms associated with obesity risk, nutritional status and refugee children from sub-Saharan Africa. *Health Place* 2004; **10**(1):105–113.

22 World Health Organization. Ottawa Charter for Health Promotion. Ottawa: Department of Health and Welfare, World Health Organization; 1986.

CHAPTER 33

Developing country perspectives on obesity prevention policies and practices

Juliana Kain,[1] *Camila Corvalán*[2] and *Ricardo Uauy*[1,3]

[1] Institute of Nutrition and Food Technology, University of Chile, Santiago, Chile
[2] School of Public Health, Faculty of Medicine, University of Chile, Santiago, Chile
[3] Nutrition and Public Health Intervention Research Unit, London School of Hygiene and Tropical Medicine, London, UK

Summary and recommendations for research and practice

- Developing countries are faced with the double burden of malnutrition. However, as income rises, the problem of obesity becomes progressively more important.
- In most developing countries there is no net food energy shortage, but limited access to healthier foods, which are more expensive, and this defines consumption patterns.
- Poverty is often associated with obesity; increased consumption of low-cost energy-dense foods and decreased physical activity are the main causes.
- In transitional societies, foods provided by government feeding programs to stunted children may contribute to rising obesity rates.
- Micronutrient-rich foods with no excess of energy should be provided to stunted children early on, to promote linear growth, lean body mass gain and prevent later obesity.

Introduction

The double burden of malnutrition

Undernutrition is no longer the dominant form of human malnutrition from the standpoint of popula-

tion public health relevance. The coexistence of the dual expressions of under- and overnutrition are now apparent globally: in 2001, the estimated number of people worldwide suffering from overweight equaled those with undernutrition. Close to a billion people were estimated to be overweight or obese and an equal number who were underweight, with the former being predominantly adults in developed countries and the latter being predominantly children in developing countries.[1-6] Figure 33.1 shows how overweight and obesity coexist with underweight; the global geographic distribution maps show the proportion of healthy life years lost from conditions related to excess and insufficient energy intake relative to expenditure.

There is clearly a need for a common agenda to address the double burden as in some regions, such as Northern Africa and the Middle East, most of South, Southeast and East Asia, there is an appreciable loss of disability-adjusted life years (DALYs) from both conditions. In Europe and most of the Americas the problem is largely related to obesity. The double burden existing within the same nation is the next level of aggregation in a descending hierarchy. De Onis[4,7,8] has provided a perspective on how under- and overnutrition operate within the same countries, specifically with reference to children. The percentages of children in different Latin American nations who are underweight and overweight relative to the international reference median are shown in Figure 33.2. However, this graph needs to be interpreted in the light of the cut-off standards used. At each end of a

Preventing Childhood Obesity. Edited by
E. Waters, B.A. Swinburn, J.C. Seidell and R. Uauy.
© 2010 Blackwell Publishing.

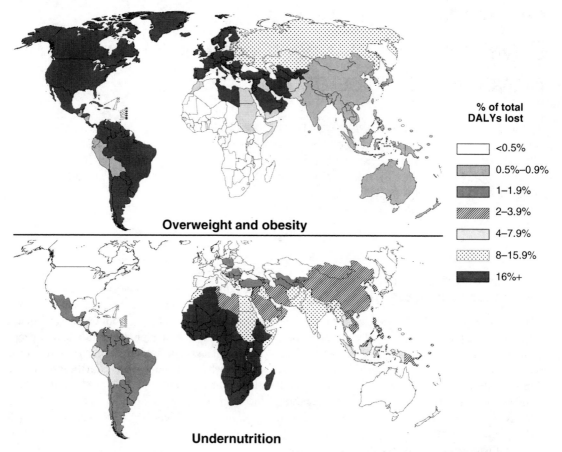

% of total DALYs lost

☐	<0.5%
▨	0.5%–0.9%
▨	1–1.9%
▧	2–3.9%
☐	4–7.9%
⠿	8–15.9%
■	16%+

Overweight and obesity

Undernutrition

Figure 33.1 Global geographic distribution maps of the proportion of Disability-Adjusted Life Years (DALYs) burden from conditions related to excess energy (overweight and obesity) in the upper panel and DALYs burden related to undernutrition (underweight) in the lower panel. (Adapted from R Uauy, The role of the international community forging a common agenda in tackling the double burden of malnutrition. SCN News #32, 2006).

Gaussian distribution, 2.5% of any reference population would, itself, have values beyond 2 standard deviations. In this respect, the burden is only dual on a population basis where the prevalence in both directions exceeds >2.5% on the horizontal axis. Guyana and Haiti are the countries with a single burden of undernutrition. For most of the other nations a greater burden is caused by energy excess, indicating that overweight has emerged as the dominant malnutrition problem even in this young age group.[9,10]

De Onis and Blossner[4] conclude that, "attention should be paid to monitoring levels and trends of overweight in children. This, however, should not be done at the expense of decreasing international commitments to alleviating undernutrition." Within the same community or even within a given household, the presence of both over- and undernutrition takes on some interesting dimensions. Caballero[11] has scrutinized the phenomenon of persons with high and low body weights living in the same household; the findings are summarized in Figure 33.3. On a continuum of gross national product, only the poorest countries have a low rate of the intra-household dual burdens; this is partly explained by the low prevalence of obesity limiting the opportunity for association. However, as incomes rise, one can observe the curious occurrence of a mixture of the extremes of body composition status existing within the same family unit.

Under and Overweight in Latin American Children

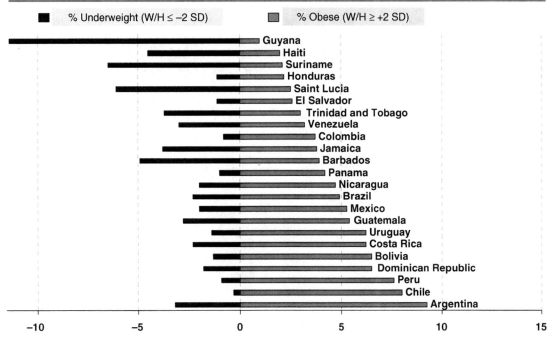

Legend: ■ % Underweight (W/H ≤ −2 SD)   ▨ % Obese (W/H ≥ +2 SD)

Countries (top to bottom): Guyana, Haiti, Suriname, Honduras, Saint Lucia, El Salvador, Trinidad and Tobago, Venezuela, Colombia, Jamaica, Barbados, Panama, Nicaragua, Brazil, Mexico, Guatemala, Uruguay, Costa Rica, Bolivia, Dominican Republic, Peru, Chile, Argentina

Axis: −10, −5, 0, 5, 10, 15

Figure 33.2 The percentage of children in Latin American nations with weight-for-height Z-scores either below (underweight) or above (obese) 2 standard deviations of the international reference WHO standard. The obesity figures are likely underestimates considering the present WHO 2006 reference in terms of obesity. (Adapted from De Onis[8]).

Households having both under and overweight members data from selected countries

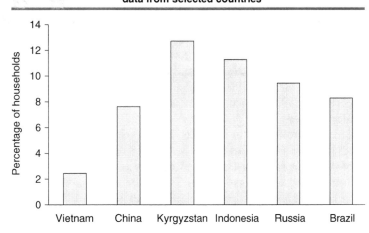

Figure 33.3 Percent of households having individuals with high- and low-body weights in the same household. As gross national product increases the intra-household dual burdens also increases. (Adapted from Caballero[11]).

Finally, within a given individual, namely a malnourished young child, there can be a quick transition, over a few years or even months, from being wasted (underweight for height) to being overweight or even obese (excess weight for height). Moreover, in many cases, these children remain stunted (low height for age), making them more vulnerable in an urban setting to obesity and diabetes, both of which are linked to excess body fat resulting from sedentary lifestyles and consumption of high-energy density diets. In fact, the model of the malnourished child during recovery serves to illustrate many of the features of the nutrition transition mirroring the rapid shift in diet from low- to high-energy density food, as well as a progressively sedentary life style, that moves stunted populations from underweight to overweight and obesity.[12]

More recently, the influence of postnatal growth on later development of obesity and nutrition-related chronic disease has been documented. Postnatal growth is clearly related to prenatal growth with some of the metabolic changes associated with prenatal nutritional sufficiency affecting postnatal physiology and behavior which, in turn, affect growth.[13–15] In 2005, Stein et al reviewed the evidence linking child growth and chronic diseases in five cohorts from transitional countries (China, India, Guatemala, Brazil and the Philippines) concluding that growth failure in early childhood and increased weight gain in later childhood were associated with increased prevalence of risk factors for cardiovascular disease (i.e. body composition, blood pressure, glucose metabolism).[16] These results correspond to studies from cohorts that originated in the 1970s and early 1980s. The clear progression of the obesogenic environment in most countries around the world suggests that the present impact of these early life factors in determining the rise in adult chronic diseases is likely to be underestimated.

Postnatal growth, on the other hand, is also associated with later adult disease independent of prenatal growth. Studies from developed countries show a consistent positive association between infant size and later body size but inconsistent associations with later disease.[17] In transitional countries, it is important to clarify the relative importance of growth in different postnatal periods in order to implement interventions. In Brazil, India and Guatemala, growth in

infancy (0–1 years) and late childhood (over 2 years) were described as critical periods predicting adult body composition. Weight gain in infancy was related to higher fat-free mass in adulthood, while rapid weight gain in late childhood was associated with a higher acquisition of fat mass. In India, greater increases in body mass index (BMI) between 2 and 12 years were strongly associated with glucose intolerance and Type 2 diabetes in adulthood.[15]

Access to food, poverty and childhood obesity

Income level is the main determinant of access to food. The proportion of family income that is spent on food serves to define the population income categories in most developing countries. If family income is less than the cost of one basic food basket the family is defined as indigent; those with income below the cost of two food baskets are classified as poor, in this case they actually spend more than 50% of their income on basic foods.[18]

Food security depends on the households' access to food rather than overall availability of food. In rural areas, household food security depends mainly on access to land and other agricultural resources which facilitate domestic production. In urban areas, however, food is mainly purchased in the market. A variety of foods, therefore, needs to be available and affordable in urban markets for adequate food security. In most developing regions there is plenty of food in the stores, yet families living under poverty conditions are unable to buy food of sufficient quantity and/ or quality and thus will be food insecure.[19,20]

Poverty and food insecurity go hand in hand. Food security in poor households often fluctuates dramatically, depending on changes in agricultural production in response to seasonal and environmental conditions. Fluctuating market prices affect poor producers as well as the urban or rural poor. In an open market economy, farmers and their families are also affected by falling global market prices for food commodities. In most cases, they depend on products they place in the market and this means that their income will vary with commodity prices which are beyond their control. In the urban setting, the poor rely on food purchases that are commonly affected by rampant inflation. This income instability means that families may be able to cope with their food bills for one week, but are unsure of what will happen the following week as they are not able to build up food reserves. In practice, the lesson is that they eat as much as they can since they do not know when they will fall below the food sufficiency line.[20,21]

Household food insecurity is defined as limited or uncertain availability of nutritionally adequate and safe foods, and limited or uncertain ability to acquire acceptable foods in socially acceptable ways.[18,22] The possible paradoxical association of hunger and food insecurity with childhood obesity was first raised in a case report in 1995.[23] The author speculated that this association may be because of "an adaptive process to food shortages whereby increasing the consumption of inexpensive energy dense foods results in increasing body mass". Plausible mechanisms that may explain this association include cheaper cost and over-consumption of energy-dense foods, overeating when foods become available, metabolic changes that may permit more efficient use of energy, fear of food restriction, and higher susceptibility to hunger, disinhibition and environmental cues.[24,25]

Socio-economic disadvantage in childhood is positively associated with an increased risk of obesity in adulthood. Lissau and Sorensen[26] showed that 9–10-year-old children in Copenhagen rated as dirty and neglected by school personnel were 9.8 times more likely to be obese 10 years later. Olson et al in 2007[27] attempted to explain why food insecurity as it is experienced in rich countries such as the USA results in adult obesity. After following 30 rural women with at least one child, their most important conclusion was that growing up in a poor household appeared to "super-motivate some women to actively avoid food insecurity in adulthood by using food to meet emotional needs after deprivation". As the authors point out, this behaviour towards food may be a possible mechanism for explaining the association between childhood poverty and adult obesity.

Drewnowski, in 2007,[28] demonstrated that much of the past epidemiologic research is consistent with a single parsimonious explanation: obesity has been linked repeatedly to consumption of low-cost foods. Refined grains, added sugars, and added fats are inexpensive, tasty and convenient. The fact that energy-dense foods cost less per megajoule than nutrient-dense foods, means that energy-dense diets provide not only cheaper energy, but may be preferentially selected by the lower-income consumer. In other words, the low cost of dietary energy (dollars/megajoule), rather than specific food, beverage, or macronutrient choices, may be an important predictor of weight gain amongst poorer populations.

In examining the childhood obesity epidemic from the perspective of economics, Cawley[29] reports that the market has contributed to the recent increase in childhood overweight in three main ways. First, the real price of food fell, particularly energy-dense foods; second, rising wages increased the "opportunity costs" of food preparation for people in the workforce, encouraging them to spend less time preparing meals; and third, technological changes created incentives to use prepackaged food rather than to prepare foods.

Several economic rationales justify government intervention in markets to address these problems. First, because free markets generally under-provide information, governments may intervene to provide consumers with nutrition information they need. Second, because society bears the soaring costs of obesity, the government may intervene to lower the costs to taxpayers. Third, because children are not what economists call "rational consumers"—they cannot evaluate information critically and weigh the future consequences of their actions—the government may step in to help them make better choices. The government could disseminate information to consumers directly, it could protect children from the marketing of unhealthy foods and could also apply taxes and subsidies that discourage the consumption of these or encourage physical activity. It could also require schools to remove vending machines for soft drinks and candy. From the economic perspective, policy-makers should evaluate these options on the basis of cost–effectiveness studies.

Until recently, it was commonly thought that nutrition-related chronic diseases were associated with wealthy societies, but it has been shown in almost all categories of developing countries that nutrition imbalances are most frequent among the poor.[30] This is especially evident in migrant populations; for example, in northern Mexico, there has been a dramatic increase in obesity and diabetes among indigenous populations who have become progressively urbanized and have abandoned their traditional diets in favor of a Western pattern of consumption and decreased physical activity with serious consequences for health.[31] The availability of foods, income and advertising are the main determinants of the demand for certain foods among the poor, particularly sugary drinks and high fat salty and sweet snacks.[28]

Table 33.1 illustrates policy instruments and activities that can be applied at different stages of the food supply chain to reduce obesity, as well as the feasibility of implementing them. As this table demonstrates, most policy instruments are feasible to implement if the different actors involved (government, food companies, marketers, consumers, the public, scientific community, etc.) place the health of the population as a high priority. These policy options are pertinent to countries in the epidemiological transition as well as to industrialized countries. As shown in the table, we considered that price control and export quotas may be more likely applicable in developing countries since governments play a stronger role in trade policies.

Rising food prices and poverty

The sharp increase in food prices over recent years will affect poor people in both developed and developing countries. The main causes for this sharp increase are: the high price of energy with oil prices at an all-time high; farmers growing crops, especially maize, to produce biofuel (ethanol) rather than food; growing demand for food, especially from China; shifting from traditional staples toward higher-value foods like meat and milk, which in turn needs grains to feed livestock.[32]

The nutrition of the poor will certainly be affected by high food prices if governments do not take steps to address this issue. Von Braun[33] recommends policy actions in three areas, one of which is to expand comprehensive social protection to meet the needs of the poor, such as food or income transfers and nutrition programs focused on early childhood. In this situation, nutrition programs are very praiseworthy, but as shown in the next section, it is important to consider the nutritional status of the children and the quality of the diet, in order to prevent future obesity.

Including obesity prevention considerations in nutrition programs in developing and transitional societies

In areas of the world such as Latin America, South and East Asia where populations are progressively becoming urban and sedentary and energy availability is not a limiting factor, poverty is related to adequate or even excess energy relative to physical activity levels, but diets are of poor quality in terms of factors that protect from positive energy balance. Thus, there is a need to incorporate improving the quality of diets as a complement to food security: that is, progressive increases in fruits and vegetables and low-fat milk to the specifications of feeding programs for young children and women of reproductive age. The combined objectives of promoting healthy growth while preventing obesity are often not recognized as intertwined components of good nutrition; rather they are often considered as opposite poles of the malnutrition spectrum. Providing complementary foods to young children with the worthy objective of preventing malnutrition without considering the need to avoid obesity in stunted children may in fact do potential harm. Nutrition programs that aim to prevent malnutrition may have built-in mechanisms that can easily promote positive energy balance and thus increase risk for obesity.

This is particularly relevant when feeding underweight, stunted children who may be of normal or even excessive weight for stature. Thus, it is of utmost importance to define what is normal weight and height and to apply normative standards to assess growth and to establish energy intake recommendations that are consistent with good nutrition and health during childhood and beyond. A critical issue in defining the nature of this problem is recognizing that underweight children are usually stunted, thus most malnourished children will be of low weight and length for age, but will have a near normal weight for length/height. They are underweight and stunted, but not wasted. Since recovery in length for age is incomplete if nutrition improvement occurs after 24–36 months of age, these children when given additional food will gain significantly more weight for age, than length for age. In older children, little or no gain in length for age is observed.[34] The recommendations for

Table 33.1 Potential supply-side and demand-side interventions in the food supply chain to modify food consumption, for example, in this case to reduce obesity.

Link in the food supply chain	Food policy instruments with nutritional impact	Examples of impact on food consumption affecting obesity	Feasibility of implementation
Food production	• Subsidies or price supports[a] (fruits-vegetables/lean meats and low-fat dairy)	• Subsidies for production of low-fat options • Price guarantees for fruits and vegetables	Very difficult
	• Import and export quotas[a]	• Export incentives for staple foods and oil seeds. • Restrictions and/or tariffs on high fat/high sugar foods	Uncertain
Food processing	• Quality grading	• Definition of the level of quality (changes in the criteria for selecting quality, e.g., lean versus fatty meats, high versus low-fat dairy products)	Difficult
	• "Identity standards"	• "Identity standards"—switch to low-fat milk and yoghurt, "lean meats"	Possible
	• Nutrition labeling	• Descriptors in nutrition labelling (e.g., low-fat milk, lean animal products, low-fat dairy, foods with added sugar, low glycemic index)	Very likely
Distribution, marketing, and advertising of food	• Advertising campaigns for lower energy-density products	• Changes in the demand of government programs for milk products (e.g. low-fat to replace full-fat milk)	Difficult
	• Nutrition labeling	• Use % fat or % lean in the labeling of ground meat	Very likely
	• Portion size	• Use % fat in labeling dairy foods	Likely
	• Marketing standards	• Labeling in restaurant menus (total energy, quantity and quality of fat, low in trans or saturated fat and low in sugar) according to portion size • Standardization of the various sector descriptors: agricultural, health, marketing, trade • Reduce marketing of unhealthy foods to children	Very likely
Food choices and consumption	• Public information campaigns to promote good nutrition	• Nutrient profiles for consumer orientation (sugar/salt/saturated fat)	Very likely
	• Promotion of specific products	• Icon to orient food choices (e.g. ticks)	Likely

[a]The likelihood of applying these policy instruments is greater in developing countries.

Box 33.1 Recommendations for reducing the risk of promoting unhealthy weight gain in child nutrition programs

1. Promote and support exclusive breastfeeding for six months, with the introduction of complementary foods and continued breastfeeding thereafter—up to 2 years of age or longer as mutually desired by the mother and infant.
2. Promote the appropriate introduction of safe, nutritionally adequate, and developmentally appropriate complementary foods. This is critical after 6 months and must continue until 3 years of age in order to support optimal linear growth. Stunting is difficult to modify after the age of 3.
3. Ensure that the needs of nutritionally-at-risk infants and children are met, giving special attention to linear growth of preterm and/or low birth weight infants. Prevent excess weight gain in order to decrease risk of obesity in later life.
4. Monitor growth and avoid rapid weight gain at all stages of life, especially in infancy. Children should keep a healthy weight from early on. Create an environment that supports healthy food choices and promote physical activity patterns concordant with a healthy lifestyle.
5. Identify children at schools and health centers, with individual and or social risks for overweight and obesity early, establishing dietary and physical activity measures to prevent unhealthy weight gain.
6. Implement programs for treatment of childhood obesity early to prevent present and future adverse consequences.
7. Monitor growth using appropriate standards, take necessary actions to prevent stunting in all children and avoid unhealthy weight gain in all children.[35]

preventing obesity among participants of nutrition programs are shown in Box 33.1.

Conclusions

Developing countries are faced with the double burden of malnutrition, but as income rises (household and national), obesity becomes progressively more important. In most developing countries there is no net food energy shortage. However, there is limited access to healthier foods, which are more expensive, and this plays an important role in determining consumption patterns. Poverty is associated with obesity, with increased consumption of low-cost energy-rich foods and decreased physical activity being the likely causes. In transitional societies, foods provided by government feeding programs to stunted children may contribute to rising obesity rates. Finally, micronutrient rich foods with no excess of energy, should be provided to stunted children early on, to promote linear growth, lean body mass gain and prevent later obesity.

References

1 Zhai F, Wang H, Du S et al: Lifespan nutrition and changing socio-economic conditions in China. *Asia Pac J Clin Nutr* 2007; **16**(Suppl. 1):374–382.
2 Popkin B: The nutrition transition in low-income countries: an emerging crisis. *Nutr Rev* 1994; **52**:285–298.
3 Adair L, Popkin B: Are child eating patterns being transformed globally? *Obes Res* 2005; **13**:1281–1299.
4 de Onis M, Blossner M: Prevalence and trends of overweight among preschool children in developing countries. *Am J Clin Nutr* 2000; **72**:1032–1039.
5 Mendez M, Monteiro C, Popkin B: Overweight exceeds underweight among women in most developing countries. *Am J Clin Nutr* 2005; **81**:714–721.
6 Amuna P, Zotor F: Epidemiological and nutrition transition in developing countries: impact on human health and development. *Proc Nutr Soc* 2008; **67**:82–90.
7 de Onis M, Garza C, Victoria C, Onyango A, Frongillo EA, Martines J: The WHO multicentre growth reference study: planning, study design, and methodology. *Food Nutr Bull* 2004; **25**:S1–S86.
8 de Onis M: The use of anthropometry in the prevention of childhood overweight and obesity. *IJO* 2004; **28**:S81–S85.
9 Uauy R, Albala C, Kain J: Obesity trends in Latin America: transiting from under- to overweight. *J Nutr* 2001; **131**: 893S–899S.
10 Uauy R, Monteiro C: The challenge of improving food and nutrition in Latin America. *Food Nutr Bull* 2004; **25**: 175–182.
11 Caballero B: A nutrition paradox—underweight and obesity in developing countries. *NEJM* 2005; **352**:1514–1516.
12 Uauy R, Alvear J: Effects of Protein Energy Interactions on Growth in Protein Energy Interactions, Scrimshaw NS and Beat S, eds. Lausanne Switzerland: IDECG, 1992:151–182.
13 Adair L: Filipino children exhibit catch-up growth from age 2 to 12 year. *J Nutr* 1999; **129**:1140–1148.
14 Cameron N, Preece M, Cole T: Catch-up growth or regression to the mean? Recovery from stunting revisited. *Am J Hum Biol* 2005; **17**:412–417.
15 Sachdev H, Fall C, Osmond C et al: Anthropometric indicators of body composition in young adults: relation to size at

birth and serial measurements of body mass index in childhood in the New Delhi birth cohort. *Am J Clin Nutr* 2005; **82**:456–466.

16 Stein A, Thompson A, Waters A: Childhood growth and chronic disease: evidence from countries undergoing the nutrition transition. *Matern Child Nutr* 2005; **1**:177–184.

17 Popkin B: Global nutrition dynamics: the world is shifting rapidly toward a diet linked with non-communicable diseases. *Am J Clin Nutr* 2006; **84**:289–298.

18 Keenan D, Olson C, Hersey J, Parmer S: Measures of food insecurity/security. *J Nutr Educ* 2001; **33**:S49–S58.

19 Coates J, Frongillo E, Rogers B, Webb P, Wilde P, Houser R: Commonalities in the experience of household food insecurity across cultures: what measures are missing? *J Nutr* 2006; **136**:1438S–1448S.

20 Habicht J-P, Pelto G, Frongillo E, Rose D: Conceptualization and instrumentation of food insecurity. Paper presented at the Workshop on the Measurement of Food Insecurity and Hunger, 15 July 2004. Panel to Review the US Department of Agriculture's Measurement of Food Insecurity and Hunger. 2004: at www7.nationalacademies.org/cnstat/Habicht_etal_paper.pdf. (accessed 20 April 2008).

21 Tanumihardjo SA, Anderson C, Kaufer-Horwitz M et al: Poverty, obesity, and malnutrition: an international perspective recognizing the paradox. *J Am Diet Assoc* 2007; **11**:1966–1972.

22 Bickel G, Nord M: Measuring Food Security in the United States: Guide to Measuring Household Food Security. Rev 2000. Alexandria, VA: US Department of Agriculture/Food and Nutrition Services/office of Analysis, Nutrition, and Evaluation, 2000.

23 Dietz W: Does hunger cause obesity? *Pediatrics* 1995; **95**:766–767.

24 Casey P, Simpson P, Gossett J et al: The association of child and household food insecurity with childhood overweight status. *Pediatrics* 2006; **118**:e1406–e1413.

25 Provencher V, Drapeau V, Tremblay A, Despres JP, Lemieux S: Eating behaviours and indices of body composition in men and women from the Quebec Family Study. *Obes Res* 2003; **11**:783–792.

26 Lissau I, Sorensen T: Parental neglect during childhood and increased risk of obesity in young adulthood. *Lancet* 1994; **343**:324–327.

27 Olson C, Bove C, Miller E: Growing up poor: long-term implications for eating patterns and body weight. *Appetite* 2007; **49**:198–207.

28 Drewnowski A: The real contribution of added sugars and fats to obesity. *Epidemiol Rev* 2007; **29**:160–171.

29 Cawley J: Markets and childhood obesity policy. *Future Child* 2006; **16**:69–88.

30 Popkin B: The shift in stages of the nutrition transition in the developing world differs from past experiences! *Public Health Nutr* 2002; **5**:205–214.

31 Neufeld LM, Hernández-Cordero S, Fernald LC, Ramakrishnan U: Overweight and obesity doubled over a 6-year period in young women living in poverty in Mexico. *Obesity* 2008; **16**:714–717.

32 Kharas H: Global Food Prices: A Global Crisis: at www.brookings.edu/interviews/2008/0423_food_prices_kharas.aspx (accessed 2 May 2008).

33 von Braun J: Rising food prices. What should be done? at www.ifpri.org/themes/food prices/food prices.asp (accessed 27 April 2008).

34 Uauy R, Rojas J, Corvalan C, Lera L, Kain J: Prevention and control of obesity in preschool children: importance of normative standards. *J Pediatr Gastroenterol* 2006; **43**:1–12.

35 Uauy R, Kain J: The epidemiological transition: need to incorporate obesity prevention into nutrition programmes. *Public Health Nutr* 2002; **5**:1–8.

36 Uauy R: The role of the international community forging a common agenda in tackling the double burden of malnutrition. SCN News # 32, 2006.

CHAPTER 34

Preventing childhood obesity: looking forward

William H. Dietz
Division of Nutrition, Physical Activity, and Obesity, National Center for Chronic Disease Prevention and Health Promotion, Centers for Disease Control and Prevention, Atlanta, GA, USA

Introduction

As the foregoing chapters indicate, obesity has become a prevalent disease among children and adolescents worldwide and in most countries, the prevalence continues to increase. The causes of childhood and adolescent obesity are multiple and are still being elucidated but, as indicated, the rises in prevalence have been accompanied by marked changes in the food supply, opportunities for physical activity and media use. These shifts in the food and physical environments have changed in developed and developing countries. For example, in the United States, fast food restaurants have become ubiquitous, family meals have declined, soft drink consumption, television viewing and other screen time have increased dramatically, and the likelihood that children or adolescents walk to school or participate in physical education programs in school has declined. While these changes have accompanied the rise in the prevalence of obesity, and most of these changes have been associated with obesity in cross-sectional or longitudinal studies, few studies have shown that interventions directed at these targets successfully reduce the prevalence of obesity. It seems likely that no single change in the food, physical activity or media environment can account for the current epidemic. Because it also seems unlikely that any single change in any of the aforementioned behaviors will be powerful enough to reduce the prevalence of obesity, efforts to address multiple factors within the food, physical activity and media environments simultaneously would seem the most appropriate strategy to address the epidemic. To change these environments will probably require major shifts in social norms which will not be likely without a social movement of the breadth and scale of other social movements,[1] such as that which reduced tobacco consumption.

In this chapter, I use lessons learned from the efforts to control tobacco consumption as a potential model for obesity prevention and control. I compare and contrast the current status of efforts to prevent and control obesity to outline the needs and options for the way forward. Although this analysis focuses on the United States, parallels to experiences elsewhere may inform the way forward.

Recognition of the health effects

One of the first lessons from tobacco control was that as the prevalence of the adverse consequences of cigarette consumption were increasingly well-documented, efforts to increase public awareness of the health effects also grew, and generated an increased awareness of the adverse effects of smoking on health.[2] The rise and fall of cigarette consumption is shown in

Preventing Childhood Obesity. Edited by
E. Waters, B.A. Swinburn, J.C. Seidell and R. Uauy.
© 2010 Blackwell Publishing.

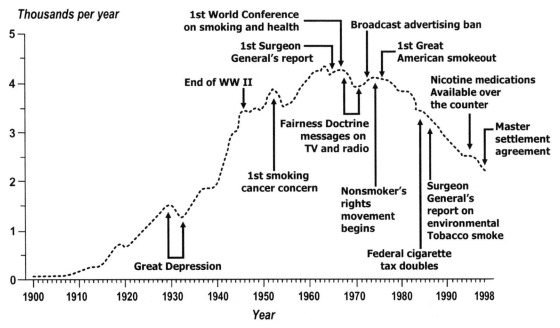

Figure 34.1 Annual adult per capita cigarette consumption and major smoking and health events–United States, 1900–1998.

Figure 34.1.[3] As is apparent, the rise in per capita cigarette consumption began in the 1900s and continued to rise in an almost linear fashion until the 1950s when the first reports linking tobacco to adverse health outcomes began to appear. Thereafter, as more data linking smoking and disease appeared, and as restrictions began to be instituted on advertising for cigarettes, per capita cigarette consumption began to plateau. The association of the increased awareness of the adverse health effects of tobacco with the plateau in cigarette consumption suggests that these two phenomena may be causally related.

With respect to obesity in the United States, the publication of annual state-based maps (www.cdc. gov/nccdphp/dnpa/obesity/trend/index.htm) derived from the Centers for Disease Control and Prevention's Behavioral Risk Factor Surveillance System that showed state-by-state changes in the prevalence of obesity prompted an increased awareness of the rapid changes in prevalence in the US population. These data were buttressed by National Health and Nutrition Examination Survey data that demonstrated that the prevalence of obesity in US children and adolescents was relatively stable until 1980, and then began to

increase steadily.[4,5] Although the adverse health effects of obesity were known to physicians and public health practitioners, the public may not have been aware of these effects.

In the United States, the rapid rise in prevalence was accompanied by stories in the media about obesity and its health consequences. For example, from 1999 to 2004, articles in the print media and newswires related to obesity increased from approximately 8,000 articles in 1999 to over 28,000 articles in 2004.[6] Perhaps in response to the intensive attention to the prevalence and consequences of obesity, its prevalence in children and adolescents of both genders, in black, white and Mexican American youth,[7] and adult females[8] in the United States appears to have begun to plateau. Furthermore, plateau or decreases in the prevalence of childhood obesity have also been reported in Arkansas[9] and Texas (D. Hoelscher, personal communication). Although there is no assurance that increased attention to the prevalence, health effects and causes of obesity contributed to the plateau in prevalence, it is possible that this plateau mirrors the experience with tobacco, where awareness of the adverse health effects of tobacco use was associated with a plateau in cigarette consumption, but not a decline. With respect to obesity, the stabilization of prevalence suggests we may be at or approaching a similar turning point.

The role of policy and environmental change

Although initiatives in the United States to change tobacco policy began at the state or local level, a number of federal reports helped provide the impetus for change.[10] For example, the 1964 Surgeon General's report on smoking and health compiled the evidence on the adverse consequences of smoking. Subsequent efforts by Surgeons General to focus on the health impact of tobacco use provided the scientific rationale for local efforts at control. Likewise, the Federal Trade Commission (FTC) ruled in 1964 that warning labels were required on cigarette packs, and that tobacco advertising should be strictly regulated. Although Congressional legislation temporarily pre-empted the FTC's authority to regulate tobacco advertising, the battle around advertising had begun. Eventually, a ruling mandating counter-advertising on television and, subsequently, a ban on tobacco advertising on television, was a very visible indication to the public that the adverse effects of tobacco were being addressed at the federal level.

However, the successful reduction in per capita cigarette consumption resulted from the implementation of a variety of policy initiatives in multiple settings.[3] These included the restriction of smoking in public buildings, evidence-based school curricula, counter-marketing, increased taxes on cigarettes, enforcement of laws that prohibited sales of cigarettes to minors, and smoking cessation programs. Almost all of these initiatives resulted from local or state-based efforts. For example, Arizona passed the first statewide ban on smoking in public places in 1973, and by 1975 similar legislation had been passed in 10 states.[10]

With respect to obesity, although a number of behaviors have been targeted for change, such as sugar-sweetened beverage intake, fruit and vegetable intake, television time, intakes of high-energy density foods, breastfeeding and physical activity, the portfolio of successful policy and environmental strategies to address these behaviors is limited. However, a number of communities in the United States and elsewhere have initiated efforts to begin to prevent and control obesity, and surveys like the School Health Policies and Programs Survey in the USA suggest that changes at multiple levels have begun in US schools.[11] Like the early efforts at tobacco control, these activities are local, but it is not yet clear how consistently these behaviors are being targeted, what policy initiatives are being employed, what critical mass of policy change is necessary to change the prevalence of obesity, and whether these topics are consistently the focus of evaluation.

Perception of a common threat

Another characteristic of social movements is the perception of a common threat. In 1967, as described above, application of the Fairness Doctrine to tobacco advertising led to radio and television counter-advertising of cigarettes.[12,13] The advertisements about the adverse health effects of cigarettes produced a decrease in cigarette consumption,[10] which led the tobacco industry to negotiate the elimination of radio and television advertising for cigarettes. Somewhat later, the public became aware of the efforts of the tobacco industry to conceal their knowledge of the health effects of tobacco and to market their products to adolescents.[14] These actions on the part of industry contributed to the recognition of cigarette smoking as a threat to youth, and passive smoke exposure as a threat to the health of non-smokers.[2] The efforts of the cigarette companies to persuade adolescents to smoke, to obscure the health effects of tobacco, and to resist efforts to control tobacco use quickly made them a common enemy.

Although survey data confirm that a 40% of Americans consider childhood obesity a serious problem,[15] and 27% of adults consider obesity the most important health issue for children,[16] many parents of obese children do not recognize that their child is obese.[17–19] These observations indicate that a disjunction exists between the public's concern about childhood obesity and the recognition that their child shares the problem. Use of the term "obesity" may contribute to the perception that obesity is not an immediate threat, because the term has a pejorative connotation, and in common use generally refers to individuals with severe obesity. The pejorative connotation of the term obesity may also explain why obesity is not an acceptable term for providers to use to discuss excess weight in adolescent[20] or adult patients.[21] Therefore, one of the earliest challenges in the evolution of a movement to address obesity is the need to identify a common frame that mobilizes support for policy initiatives or promotes behavior change. Because obesity is perceived as a social concern but not necessarily a personal threat, and because the term obesity is not a term that can be used to personalize the threat, further emphasis on the obesity epidemic or the health effects of obesity may not generate the commitment necessary to mobilize the public around environmental change.

A second issue with respect to the threat posed by obesity is the lack of a single readily identifiable widely accepted cause. Tobacco in any quantity is harmful, whereas the same cannot be said about food. Furthermore, efforts in the United States to identify fast food, sugar-sweetened beverages, television time, or television advertising as the factor(s) responsible for the epidemic of childhood obesity have not generated the political will necessary to change them, suggesting that they are not widely perceived as a significant threat.

A common frame

Consistent themes that led to efforts to control tobacco were the public's health, especially the need to protect youth, and the health of non-smokers.[2] With tobacco, the tobacco companies and their products quickly became the targets of efforts to reduce smoking. Limiting their ability to advertise and using economic strategies such as tobacco taxes to reduce purchases were readily accepted strategies. In contrast, it follows from the lack of perception of obesity as a common or immediate threat that other reasons to change the nutrition and physical activity environments may provide more persuasive incentives for a broad population approach to obesity. For example, many of the strategies to improve the diet and physical activity are shared with efforts to reduce global warming. Farm-to-market strategies may provide fruits and vegetables at lower cost without incurring the costs of fuel and the production of carbon dioxide that result from the transportation of fruits and vegetables across the country. Likewise, use of public transportation[22] or

walk-to-school programs[23] reduce car use and increase physical activity. Both of these examples engage groups that may not see these strategies as obesity prevention and control strategies, but might embrace them because of their impact on global warming.

Another alternative may be to frame the nutrition and physical activity strategies to address obesity in terms of social justice. In the United States, significant ethnic disparities exist with respect to access to parks and recreation facilities,[24] or supermarkets that provide healthy choices of fruits, vegetables, or other lower calorie food choices.[25] Access and the promotion of parks and recreation facilities is a recommended strategy to increase physical activity,[26] and access to supermarkets may improve food choices in neighborhoods where the population relies on corner shops for much of their food supply.[27] Characterization of access to healthy food choices and physical activity facilities as a reflection of social inequity may provide a more compelling rationale to generate change than the potential contribution of these inequities to obesity.

Although wellness is a more elusive concept than obesity, good nutrition and physical activity are generally recognized as important components of wellness. In the United States, the economic costs associated with chronic diseases have led to a growing interest in wellness as a way to contain those costs. A recent estimate suggested that 12% of the rise in medical costs between 1987 and 2000 were attributable to obesity related illnesses.[28] The observation that one third of children born in the year 2000 in the United States will develop Type 2 diabetes mellitus at some time during their lifetime[29] and the costs associated with this disease are likely to overwhelm an already burdened medical care system.

In 2005, US medical costs were approximately 15% of the gross domestic product (GDP), and by 2015, were expected to rise to 20% of the GDP.[30] The CEO of General Motors recently stated that medical costs paid by his company added to the costs of GM cars and, therefore, impaired GM's international competitiveness.[31] Furthermore, the rise in medical costs has increasingly led employers to begin shifting the payment of insurance plans to their workforce,[32] but also to the exploration and investment in worksite wellness programs. However, whether efforts in the business sector are sufficient to mobilize broader segments of the population remains uncertain. Furthermore, efforts to contain medical costs, as well as the increase in medical costs borne by consumers may drive changes in behavior and create a demand for environmental change.

Grass-roots mobilization

The history of social movements is characterized by grass-roots groups that mobilize in response to a common threat and are committed to change.[1] An important element of tobacco control was the development of a variety of groups with shared or overlapping agendas, which worked separately on some issues but together on others to limit tobacco use at the local and state level.[2] These efforts often began locally, but as a result of the communication that developed between the groups and the networks, these strategies spread to other venues. For example, regulations to require smoking and non-smoking areas in public buildings were implemented in Minnesota in 1975[2] and spread from there to other locales and states.

Although obesity has been recognized as a significant problem by a variety of elites, such as medical providers, public health authorities, philanthropies, and some business and government leaders, the public has not mobilized broadly around common strategies to improve nutrition and physical activity in children and adolescents. One potential explanation is that obesity is still widely perceived as an issue of personal or parental responsibility rather than one for which broad changes in policy are required. Nonetheless, as indicated above, a number of schools and communities have committed to change. Because many of these efforts have been supported by local organizations including philanthropic trusts, it remains uncertain whether these efforts are imposed on the community with only limited community mobilization, or are community based or community driven. Only the latter two scenarios are likely to mobilize substantial numbers of individuals with a sustained commitment to change. Furthermore, the efforts in communities to control obesity are not yet connected or coordinated. An important challenge is how to connect these local efforts to broaden the base of support necessary for the prevention and control of obesity.

Conclusion

Tobacco control has progressed because of a successful social movement that has been coupled with policy and environmental change. Surveillance led to an awareness of the adverse health effects of tobacco use and a broad appreciation of the human costs associated with tobacco use. Reports from the federal government regarding the hazards of tobacco use reinforced local initiatives. Cigarettes and the companies that produce them became a common enemy, galvanizing local communities and states to act to control access to tobacco and sales to minors. Successful control occurred because of the implementation of policy and environmental initiatives in a variety of venues, which were made possible because of shifts in social norms related to smoking.

If we are to successfully control obesity, it may be useful to conceptualize our approach to obesity prevention and control as a social movement. Although some data would suggest that we have successfully established obesity as a medical and public health concern, a number of key elements that characterize social movements are not yet in place. Obesity is not perceived as a common threat, and it is not clear that obesity is the appropriate frame to mobilize broad segments of the population. A variety of other frames may engage a broader segment of the population, and may improve nutrition and physical activity without specifically targeting obesity. To build the social movement necessary to address obesity, our efforts should be channeled to identifying strategies that resonate with a broad group of supporters, to remain flexible with respect to they way we promote and frame our objectives, and to link efforts in diverse settings to form a more comprehensive approach across settings and constituencies.

References

1 Davis GF, McAdam D, Scott WR, Zald MN eds: Social Movements and Organization Theory. Cambridge: Cambridge University Press, 2005.
2 Wolfson M: The Fight Against Big Tobacco. Hawthorne NY: Aldine de Gruyter, 2001.
3 Morbidity and Mortality Weekly Report. Tobacco use—United States, 1900–1999. 1999; **48**:986–993. www.cdc.gov/mmwr/preview/mmwrhtml/mm4843a2.htm (accessed 15 May 2008).

4 Troiano RP, Flegal KM: Overweight children and adolescents: description, epidemiology, and demographics. *Pediatrics* 1998; **101**:497–504.

5 Ogden CL, Carroll MD, Curtin LR, McDowell MA, Tabak CJ, Flegal KM: Prevalence of overweight and obesity in the United States, 1999–2004. *JAMA* 2006; **295**:1549–1555.

6 International Food Information Council Foundation: Figures retrieved from Lexis-Nexis searches on "obesity" or "obese" in U.S. and international newspapers and newswires. April 2008.

7 Ogden CL, Carroll MD, Flegal KM: Overweight and high body mass index (BMI)-for age among U.S. children and adolescents, 2003–2006. *JAMA* 2008; **299**:2401–2405.

8 Ogden CL, Carroll MD, McDowell MA, Flegal KM: Obesity among adults in the United States—no statistically significant change since 2003–2004. NCHS Data Brief, November 2007. www.cdc.gov/nchs/data/databriefs/db01.pdf (accessed 11 May 2008).

9 Arkansas Center for Health Improvement: Assessment of childhood and adolescent obesity in Arkansas. Year four (Fall 2006–Spring 2007). www.achi.net/publications (accessed 11 May 2008).

10 Department of Health and Human Services: Smoking and Tobacco Use: 2000 Surgeon General's Report—Reducing Tobacco Use. Washington DC, US Public Health Service, 2000. Available at www.cdc.gov/tobacco/data_statistics/sgr/sgr_2000 (accessed 10 May 2009).

11 Kann L, Brener ND, Wechsler H: Overview and summary: school health policies and programs study 2006. *J Sch Health* 2007; **77**:385–397.

12 Ibrahim JK, Glantz SA: The rise and fall of tobacco control media campaigns, 1967–2006. *Am J Public Health* 2007; **97**:1383–1396.

13 Bero L: Implications of the tobacco industry documents for public health and policy. *Annu Rev Public Health* 2003; **24**:267–288.

14 Ericksen M: Lessons learned from public health efforts and their relevance to preventing childhood obesity. In: Koplan JP, Liverman CT, Kraak VI, eds. Preventing Childhood Obesity; Health in the Balance. Washington DC: National Academies Press, 2005:343–375.

15 Evans WD, Finkelstein EA, Kamerow DB, Renaud JM: Public perceptions of childhood obesity. *Am J Prev Med* 2005; **28**:26–32.

16 Charleton Research Company for Research! America Endocrine poll 2006. www.endo-society.org/media.press/2006/OBESITYCITEDNUMBERONEKINDSHEALTHISSUE.cfm (accessed 10 May 2005).

17 Mamun AA, McDermott BM, O'Callaghan MJ, Najman JM, Williams GM: Predictors of maternal misclassifications of their offspring's weight status: a longitudinal study. *Int J Obes* 2008; **32**:48–54.

18 Baughcum AE, Chamberlin LA, Deeks CM, Powers SW, Whitaker RC: Maternal perceptions of overweight preschool children. *Pediatrics* 2000; **106**:1380–1386.

19 Maynard LM, Galuska DA, Blanck HM, Serdula MK: Maternal perceptions of weight status of children. *Pediatrics* 2003; **111**:1226–1231.

20 Cohen ML, Tanofsky-Kraff M, Young-Hyman D, Yanovski JA: Weight and its relationship to adolescent perceptions of their providers (WRAP): a qualitative and quantitative assessment of teen weight-related preferences and concerns. *J Adolesc Health* 2005; **37**:163e9–163e16.

21 Wadden TA, Didie E: What's in a name? Patients' preferred terms for describing obesity. *Obes Res* 2003; **11**:1140–1146.

22 Frank LD, Engelke PO, Schmid TL: Health and Community Design. Washington DC: Island Press, 2003.

23 Staunton CE, Hubsmith D, Kallins W: Promoting safe walking and biking to school: the Marin County success story. *Am J Public Health* 2003; **93**:1431–1434.

24 Cradock AL, Kawachi I, Colditz GA et al: Playground safety and access in Boston neighborhoods. *Am J Prev Med* 2005; **28**:357–363.

25 Karpyn A, Axler F: Food geography: how food access affects diet and health. www.thefoodtrust.org/pdf/Food%20Geography%20Final.pdf (accessed 11 May 2008).

26 Task Force on Community Preventive Services: Recommendations to increase physical activity in communities. *Am J Prev Med* 2002; **22**(4S):67–102.

27 Moore LV, Diez Roux AV, Nettleton JA, Jacobs DR Jr: Associations of the local food environment with diet quality——a comparison of assessments based on surveys and geographic information systems. *Am J Epidemiol* 2008; **167**:917–924.

28 Thorpe KE, Florence CS, Howard DH, Joski P: The impact of obesity on the rise in medical spending. Health Affairs 2004; Web Exclusive. *Health Aff* 2004 (20 October); 10.137/hlthaff..w4-480.

29 Narayan KMV, Boyle JP, Thompson TJ et al: Lifetime risk for diabetes mellitus in the United States. *JAMA* 2003; **290**:1884–1890.

30 Appleby J: Health care tab ready to explode. *United States of America and Today* 2005 (24 February); p. 1A.

31 Connolly C: U.S. firms losing health care battle, GM chairman says. *Washington Post* 2005 (11 February); Financial; p. E01.

32 Pear R: Nation's health spending slows but it still hits a record. *New York Times* 2005 (11 January); p. A15.

Index